get ready to get pregnant

get ready to get

pregnant

YOUR COMPLETE PREPREGNANCY
GUIDE TO MAKING A SMART
AND HEALTHY BABY

Michael C. Lu, MD, MPH

HARPER

NEW YORK · LONDON · TORONTO · SYDNEY

HarperCollins books may be purchased for educational, business, or sales promotional use. For information, please write: Special Markets Department, HarperCollins Publishers, 10 East 53rd Street, New York, NY 10022.

FIRST EDITION

Designed by Jennifer Daddio / Bookmark Design & Media Inc.

Library of Congress Cataloging-in-Publication Data

Lu, Michael C.
   Get ready to get pregnant : your complete prepregnancy guide to making a smart and healthy baby / Michael C. Lu.—1st ed.
      p. cm.
   Includes index.
   ISBN 978-0-06-174030-5
   1. Pregnancy—Nutritional aspects.   2. Mothers—Nutrition.   3. Prenatal care.
I. Title.

   RG559.L8 2009
   618.2'4—dc22

                                                                        2008044092

09 10 11 12 13   WBC/RRD   10 9 8 7 6 5 4 3 2 1

To the loves of my life:

My mom, Ming-Yueh,

My wife, Jessie, and

My daughters, Sasha and Avery.

ACKNOWLEDGMENTS

At the top of my list of people to thank are my parents, Ming-Yueh and Kun-Tsai Lu. My parents will probably never write a book because they never went to college or, in my mom's case, high school or even junior high. You see, my mom was only 11 when her father died, and as the oldest daughter she had to drop out of fifth grade to go work in a factory. She and my dad worked hard all their lives to put food on the table and still managed to put their four children through college. My parents may have never gone to college, but they taught me everything I ever needed to know about family, hard work, and sacrifice by the simple eloquence of their examples.

Right up there alongside my parents on the list is my wife, Jessie. This book would not have been possible without her untiring support and encouragement. For two years she patiently watched and waited as I spent vacations, weekends, and nights working on this book. She helped me with the research, offered me her wisdom and insight as a woman and a mother of two, and proofread countless drafts, all while she was going through medical school and residency training in psychiatry and raising two young children. When you get to the parts in Chapter 4 where I talk about balance, resilience, emotional intelligence, and positive mental health, believe me I know what I'm talking about because I'm married to a great role model.

My family has always been there for me, and so I want to take this opportunity to thank my sister Felicia, her husband, Joseph, and their children Jeff and Keson Lai; my brother Sam, his wife, Cheryl, and their children Kevin and Darren Lu; my brother William, his wife, Leslie, and their children Christine and Emily Lu; and, most important, my cousin Dennis Kao for believing in this book from the very beginning and helping to see it through.

When I count my blessings there are several people I have to count twice because they've been such amazing teachers and mentors to me: Gautam Chaudhuri, Alan DeCherney, Bill Dignam, Christine Dunkel Schetter, Thomas Garite, David Grimes, Neal Halfon, Gail Harrison, Calvin Hobel, Loretta Jones, Kirk Keegan, Milton Kotelchuck, Anne Pebley, and Bill Trueblood. They are great teachers in the way William Wordsworth talks about teaching: "What we have loved, others will love, and we will teach them how." Thanks for teaching me how.

I owe a debt of gratitude to the following experts who have generously answered questions, reviewed chapters, and offered me guidance and encouragement: Barbara Abrams, David Barker, Jennifer Culhane, Fran Curtis, Karla Damus, Christine Dunkel Schetter, Robert Goldenberg, Michael Gravitz, Gail Harrison, Dena Herman, Neal Halfon, Calvin Hobel, Brian Jack, Lorraine Klerman, Charles Lockwood, James McGregor, Merry-K Moos, Peter Nathanielsz, Jorn Olsen, Cheri Pies, Beate Ritz, Teresa Seeman, Mark Schuster, Madeleine Shalowitz, and Michelle Wilhelm. To paraphrase Isaac Newton, if I have seen farther it is by standing on the shoulders of these giants.

This book would not exist without the hard work and insight of a few key publishing professionals. Special thanks to my agents at Vigliano Associates, Dan Ambrosio and Kirsten Neuhau, for believing in this book and guiding me through every step of the way, and my editor at Collins, Caroline Sutton, for embracing this book with such enthusiasm and for helping to make this book as useful as possible for prospective parents through her queries, edits, and wisdom.

Most important, this book is dedicated to my two wonderful daughters, Sasha and Avery, who remind me everyday what my life's work is all about. And if my two little girls, the granddaughters of a girl who had to drop out of fifth grade to work in a factory, can now grow up to be anything they want to be, there is still hope yet for our future.

CONTENTS

Introduction		*1*
1	Get Ready	*11*
2	Nutritional Preparedness	*29*
3	Brain Foods and Toxic Foods	*75*
4	Stress Resilience	*105*
5	Immune Tune-Up	*141*
6	Healthy Environment	*171*
7	Preconception Care	*217*
8	From Here to Paternity	*255*
Epilogue		*285*
Appendices		*291*
Index		*323*

Angie and her husband came to see me last year for a prepregnancy consultation.

"We want to have another baby."

Planning a baby is an exciting time, but for Angie and her husband their excitement was tempered by some trepidation. Their two previous pregnancies were ended three months early by severe preeclampsia, a condition in which mom's blood pressure goes up so high that it can jeopardize the health and even the lives of mother and baby. Angie and her husband were afraid (for good reason) that she might get preeclampsia again in her next pregnancy. They wanted to know what they could do to prevent a repeat.

These days my appointment book is filled with patients who want me to help them get ready to get pregnant. Some are high-powered professionals who've deferred childbearing until their careers are established, and now want to make sure that they are doing everything right before they conceive. Others are infertile couples who want to make sure all systems are checked out and ready to go before they undergo fertility treatment. Still others are patients with chronic medical conditions like epilepsy or rheumatoid arthritis who want to make sure that the medications they are taking are safe for pregnancy. But many are simply healthy women who want a head start on making a smart and healthy baby.

And then there are patients like Angie who've had a problem pregnancy in the past—who have dealt with problems such as preeclampsia, preterm birth, stillbirth, and birth defects—and are at risk for recurrence of the same problem in their next pregnancy. Given Angie's history, there was a good chance that she would get preeclampsia again in her next pregnancy.

To prevent this from happening, I had to find and treat the underlying problem before she got pregnant again. This required some detective work. I reviewed her old records, performed a thorough history and physical exam, and ordered a bunch of laboratory tests including genetic analyses, searching for clues as to what might have happened in Angie's two previous pregnancies. But, alas, nothing turned up as suspect.

Then I did an endometrial biopsy to examine the linings inside the uterus. I did this based on my knowledge of the pathogenesis of preeclampsia. Preeclampsia is a disease of the placenta. One of the most consistent pathological features of preeclampsia is poor, shallow implantation; something went awry in early pregnancy so that the placenta was never able to implant properly inside the uterus. This poor, shallow implantation sets up the pathogenic processes that eventually lead to preeclampsia later in pregnancy. By looking at the linings inside the uterus, I was hoping to find anything that might interfere with proper implantation.

The endometrial biopsy came back with evidence of chronic inflammation. Eureka! This was the clue I was looking for! As one could imagine, had Angie gotten pregnant again the placenta would've had to implant into a womb that was chronically inflamed. Chronic inflammation could have interfered with proper implantation, and Angie might have ended up with severe preeclampsia a third time.

So I had to put out the fire inside Angie's womb before she got pregnant again. First I looked for any chronic infection that, if left untreated, could become a source for chronic inflammation. I found none. Then I put Angie on a special "anti-inflammatory diet" rich in omega–3 fatty acids and antioxidants, and got rid of a lot of "pro-inflammatory foods" from her diet. Knowing that chronic stress can cause chronic inflammation, I also put Angie on a stress-reduction plan, which included daily exercise and meditation. I showed Angie how to detoxify her home room by room, and get rid of any potential triggers of chronic inflammation, including some personal care and household products that she was using. Lastly, I put Angie on baby aspirin, which has anti-inflammatory properties, once a day for three months. I gave Angie an early draft of this book, which she and her husband read cover to cover and followed as their Bible.

Angie came back to see me three months later, and I repeated the endometrial biopsy. The biopsy came back negative; the chronic inflammation was gone! I gave her the green light to get pregnant, which she did within the next month.

I watched Angie's pregnancy with great care, closely monitoring her blood pressure and placental functions. Twenty-eight weeks (which was when Angie's previous pregnancies had ended in severe preeclampsia) came and went, and there were still no signs of preeclampsia.

Angie went on to deliver a normal, healthy baby at full term. Today her third baby is completely healthy, all because she did her homework *before* pregnancy.

Angie's story reveals two secrets I've learned over the years about making a smart and healthy baby. The first is **timing is everything.** Had Angie waited to see me until after she got pregnant, it would've been too late. This is because implantation begins very early in pregnancy, at seven days after conception. Seven days is before any home pregnancy test would turn positive, and long before most women start prenatal care. So had Angie shown up for early prenatal care, it still would've been too late for me to turn back the clock on implantation and stop the inexorable march toward preeclampsia.

The second secret of success that I've learned over the years is **preparation is key.** Angie had a healthy baby because she did her homework before pregnancy. When it comes to making a smart and healthy baby, getting ready *before* pregnancy is the first and perhaps most important step. But the question is *how?* This is why I wrote this book—to show prospective parents how to get ready for a pregnancy. This book is filled with information that prospective parents need to know before making a baby, such as how to get themselves nutritionally prepared for pregnancy, or, as Angie did, how to give their immune system a good tune-up before pregnancy.

why you should read this book *before* you get pregnant

If you are curious enough to open up this book, chances are the thought of having a baby has crossed your mind at least once or twice already. You might be actively trying to get pregnant. Or you might be waiting a year or two. Whatever you are thinking, I would like to invite you to read this book, cover to cover, BEFORE you get pregnant.

Even if you are planning to wait before having a baby.

This is because what you do or don't do right now can have consequences (good or bad) for your future pregnancy, even a year or two from now. Let me give you an example.

Ever heard of something called *dioxins?*

If you haven't, you should. Dioxins are toxic chemicals that pollute our environment. They may be harmful to the fetal brain. They can also disrupt normal development of the fetal endocrine and immune systems, similar to other so-called endocrine disruptors like diethylstilbestrol (DES) or polychlorinated biphenyls (PCB). But unlike DES and PCB, which are banned in the United States, dioxins are produced in large quantities in paper mills, pesticide manufacturers, incinerators, and other sources of combustion all across the United States. They pollute our environment and contaminate our food supply; more than 90 percent of human exposure to dioxins currently is through the food supply. Dioxins are very lipophilic, which means they like fat—they are stored in animal fat. We accumulate dioxins in our body by consuming animal fat. The more animal fat we eat, the more dioxins we accumulate. And the prevailing practice of feeding animal fat to animals to fatten them up further raises the dioxin content of the meat and dairy we consume.

There are two more things you should know about dioxins. First, they stay in your body for a very long time. Dioxins are stored in your body fat, with a half-life of up to seven years (that is, it will take up to seven years to get rid of half the amount of dioxins that are stored in your body today). Second, dioxins cross the placenta easily, which means your baby will get a hefty dose of what you've stored in your body fat. So even if you become a vegan once you get pregnant, it may be a little too late to avoid exposing your baby to all the dioxins that are already stored in your body fat.

This is why an Institute of Medicine expert panel recommended in 2003 that girls and young women drink low-fat or skim milk instead of whole milk and eat foods lower in animal fat *years before they become pregnant* in order to avoid accumulation of dioxins in their body.

If you wait until pregnancy, it's too late.

This is why you and your husband (or partner) should read this book BEFORE you get pregnant. *That's right. He, too, needs to read this book BEFORE you conceive.* This is because the DNA carried in his sperm can get damaged in a lot of different ways before conception takes place. Such DNA damage can get passed on to the next generation, which can result in birth defects and even childhood cancers.

The good news is that the average life cycle of sperm is only 42 to 76 days, which means that if your husband (or partner) follows my program for at least three months before conception, he can replace most of the damaged sperm with good sperm.

But if he waits until pregnancy, it's too late.

Over his lifetime, he will make trillions of sperm (as many as 12 trillion by some accounts). For most men, only one or two sperm will ever get chosen to pass on their genetic legacy. That's less than one in a trillion chance of being the chosen one. So tell him to make it a good one. Don't pass on damaged goods. He can start by reading this book.

what is unique about this book

This book is unique in three ways. First, this book is written to help prospective parents prepare for pregnancy. While there are plenty of good *pregnancy* books that teach prospective parents what to do once they are pregnant, there are very few *prepregnancy* books that teach them how to get ready for a pregnancy. As I mentioned before, if you wait until pregnancy, it may be too late. Increasingly doctors and researchers are learning that by the time a woman gets pregnant, she may have already missed a critical window of opportunity to bring forth her baby's fullest potential. The critical period for children's lifelong health and development does not begin with zero to five, or even pregnancy. It begins before conception. This book is full of information that both you and your husband (or partner) need to know before making a baby.

Second, this book is based on good science, which is more than I can say about many prepregnancy and pregnancy books out in the market today. Most haven't kept up with the latest advances in science and medicine. This book brings together in one place state-of-the-art knowledge about how to make a smart and healthy baby, based on over 1,000 scientific studies as well as my own research over the past decade. As a research scientist and a professor at UCLA, I can honestly say that this book summarizes the best of what we know today about preparing for pregnancy.

Third, this book gives the readers an action plan to get themselves ready for pregnancy. Each chapter in the book comes with ten concrete, specific action steps to take before getting pregnant, such as:

- Ten steps to get yourself nutritionally ready
- Ten "brain foods" you should eat more of, and ten "toxic foods" to avoid
- Ten steps to strengthen your stress resilience
- Ten steps to give your immune system a good tune-up

- Ten steps to detoxify your environment
- Ten things to talk to your doctor about during the prepregnancy check-up
- Ten steps to get your man ready for fatherhood

Each step is based on the best available scientific evidence as well as the most up-to-date clinical guidelines and public health recommendations. I believe I've put together in this book a state-of-the-art pregnancy preparedness program for the readers.

an overview of this book

This book has eight main chapters.

Each chapter is divided into two parts. The first part explains *why* it is important for you to work on certain things, be it nutritional preparedness or stress resilience, before pregnancy. Studies have shown that people are a lot more likely to change their health behaviors if they are given an explanation *why* they need to change.

The second part of each chapter explains *how*—*how* to put out the fire of chronic inflammation inside your body. *How* to detoxify your home before pregnancy. *How* to protect the sperm from DNA damage before conception. Studies have shown that people are a lot more likely to change their health behaviors if they know *how* to change *and* believe that they can make the change. Thus each chapter comes with an action plan, complete with ten simple, achievable action steps that you can follow to get yourself ready for pregnancy.

In Chapter 1, I introduce three of the most important scientific discoveries in recent years—fetal programming, epigenetics, and allostasis, and discuss how these three discoveries have revolutionized the science of making a smart and healthy baby.

In Chapter 2, I explain the importance of nutritional preparedness before pregnancy, and recommend a ten-step program to help you get yourself nutritionally ready for pregnancy. You are not only what you eat; you are what your mother ate. And you are not only what she ate during pregnancy; you are what she ate *before* pregnancy.

I get asked all the time by my patients about "brain foods"—what can they eat to help their babies grow a smart brain. They also want to know what foods they should avoid. In Chapter 3, I give you my top-ten list of "brain foods" of which you should eat plenty, along with my top-ten list of "toxic foods" that you should avoid before and during pregnancy.

In Chapter 4, I examine the difference between feeling "stressed" and "stressed out," and explain why feeling "stressed out" *before* and during pregnancy may be harmful to your unborn child. I prescribe a ten-step program to help you reduce your stress level and build up your stress resilience before pregnancy.

In Chapter 5, I explain why infection and inflammation pose perhaps the biggest threats to healthy pregnancy and fetal programming. The best way to avoid infection and inflammation during pregnancy is by giving your immune system a good tune-up before pregnancy. I recommend a ten-step program to remove any on-going sources of infection and inflammation that can cause further wear and tear on your immune system, and make lifestyle changes to improve your immune fitness before pregnancy.

In Chapter 6, I call attention to a silent pandemic of developmental neurotoxicity that is sweeping our nation today, and to all the reproductive and developmental toxicants in our air, water, food supplies, and consumer products that may be robbing our children of their fullest potential before they are born, or even conceived. The chapter then takes you through a ten-step program to build a cleaner, greener, and healthier nest for your baby, including steps you can take to detoxify your home, before pregnancy.

In Chapter 7, I discuss the importance of preconception care, and identify ten of the most important topics you should discuss with your doctor during the prepregnancy check-up.

Chapter 8 is written for dads-to-be. I tell them that their greatest contributions to making a smart and healthy baby come down to two things: making good sperm and giving good support. I prescribe a ten-step program to help dads-to-be get ready for pregnancy, including ways to protect their sperm from DNA damage before conception.

The book finishes with an epilogue and an appendix. The appendix contains "Are You Ready?," a Pregnancy Readiness Quotient (PRQ) self-test that you can take to assess how ready you are for pregnancy, as well as a compilation of articles, books, and websites that you can go to for more information.

As a father of two very smart and healthy girls, there is nothing in life that gives me greater joy than to watch them learn and grow every day. I couldn't ask for more. I'd like to share what I know with you.

And please share your stories with me. Let me know what you think—what worked and what didn't—so I can make this book more helpful for other moms- and dads-to-be in the future. You can send me your comments on my YouTube (www.youtube.com/getready2getpregnant) or Facebook page (keyword *get ready 2 get pregnant*).

Michael C. Lu, MD, MPH
September 2008

get ready

the greatest gift of all

My patient Paula taught me what heroism is all about.

One Sunday afternoon when I was away, I got a call from Paula.

"Michael, you've got to help me," she said, sounding distressed.

"What's going on?" I asked.

I've known Paula for a long time. She is a dear colleague and friend of mine. I had delivered her son J.J. three years before.

"I'm in the hospital," she said. "I have severe preeclampsia and they want to do a c-section right away."

At the time Paula was only 27 weeks pregnant with her second child. A baby born this premature can have a lot of long-term health problems and disabilities, including cerebral palsy and mental retardation. There was even a chance that a baby born this early might not survive.

"I don't want a c-section right now," Paula pleaded. "The baby is too premature."

I called the perinatologist on-call. Paula's preeclampsia was indeed very severe. Preeclampsia is a disease of pregnancy in which blood pressure goes up so high that it begins to cause damage to the body's vital organs. The diagnosis is made with a blood pressure above 140 (systolic) over 90 (diastolic). Paula came in with a blood pressure of 180 over 110. Of course, all the talk about an immediate c-section didn't help the matter. She freaked out and her blood pressure shot up to 210 over 140. The perinatologist on-call wanted to do a c-section right away, but Paula refused. The perinatologist pleaded with me to talk some sense into Paula so she would accept a c-section.

I called Paula back. "Paula, we've got a problem." I explained to her what could happen with a blood pressure this high. At 210/140, her brain could bleed and herniate. Her liver could rupture. Her kidneys could go into failure. Preeclampsia is an awful disease to get; it is a ticking time bomb. Preeclampsia is a leading cause of maternal death in the United States and around the world. It accounts for nearly 20 percent of all maternal deaths in the United States. I've seen four maternal deaths in my career; one of them was due to preeclampsia.

But I didn't have to tell Paula all this. She was a doctor and knew preeclampsia only too well. She knew that her health, and possibly her life, was in jeopardy, but Paula wasn't thinking about her own life. She was thinking about her baby—about the baby's survival, and the possibility of a lifetime of health problems and disabilities from being born so premature.

Since I was coming back later that day, Paula and the perinatologist agreed to hold off the c-section until I returned. As soon as I got back to L.A., I went into the hospital to talk to Paula. After reviewing her vital signs and lab results, I walked into her room.

"I am so glad to see you," Paula greeted me, a bit groggy from the magnesium infusion she was getting to prevent an eclamptic seizure.

I gave Paula a hug, sat down, and we talked for the next hour.

Walking into the room, I had already made up my mind what I was going to do. I was going to try to talk Paula into agreeing to an immediate c-section because the cure for preeclampsia is delivery of the baby and the placenta. Preeclampsia is a disease of the placenta. The placenta sends chemical messengers into the bloodstream (that's why the disease used to be called "toxemia"—toxins in the blood) that initiate a cascade of biochemical reactions that can constrict and damage blood vessels, thereby causing high blood pressure. Impaired blood flow causes damage to the body's vital organs, which can become permanent and irreversible if delivery is delayed for too long. Once the placenta is delivered, the disease process quickly reverses itself and the patient is cured. I was anxious to do the c-section because I took care of a patient who later died from severe preeclampsia during my residency training, and I didn't want that to happen to my dear colleague and friend. Not under my watch.

By the time I walked out of Paula's room, however, I had changed my mind. Instead of talking Paula into an immediate c-section, she talked me into waiting.

What changed my mind?

Paula and I talked about a lot of things that day, but one thing she said really stood out in my mind.

"You would jump in front of an on-coming train to save Sasha if you had to, wouldn't you?" Paula asked me.

Sasha is my daughter. She and her younger sister Avery and my wife Jessie are the loves of my life. "Of course I would," I answered.

"Preeclampsia is that on-coming train," Paula said. "And I'm jumping in front of that train to save my baby."

I will never forget that moment. There was an eerie calmness in Paula's voice, the same kind of calmness that I've heard from patients with terminal cancer who've come to accept their imminent death. The magnesium hadn't clouded her head; Paula knew exactly what she was doing. She knew she could go into kidney failure, her liver could rupture and her brain could herniate; there was even a chance she could die. But Paula was going to stare down the on-coming train for as long as she could. At 27 weeks, every day gained for the baby was a victory.

It became clear to me what I had to do. As Paula's obstetrician my job was to push her out of the way of the on-coming train right before the train was about to hit her. Paula's blood pressure had come down to 160 over 100 with blood pressure medications, which was still high, but in a range where I felt it was safe to wait. So I called off the c-section that day.

Paula's pregnancy lasted another 21 days. She stayed in the hospital the entire three weeks. I monitored her vital signs and labs closely. We waited nervously for the on-coming train. We went from day to day, celebrating each day gained as a victory for the baby.

At 30 weeks, I heard bells and whistles coming loud and clear around the corner. Paula's preeclampsia was worsening. Her kidneys started failing, and her blood pressure was getting out of control despite being maxed out on multiple blood pressure medications. So we went ahead with the c-section.

Paula delivered a baby girl weighing 2 ½ pounds. Her blood pressure returned to normal within a few weeks of delivery, and her beautiful baby girl did remarkably well in the NICU and is completely healthy today, thanks in large part to those three extra weeks her mommy bartered with her own life and health.

"*Giving birth is definitely a heroic deed,*" Joseph Campbell wrote in the *Power of Myth*, "*in that it is the giving over of oneself to the life of another.*" What Paula did was nothing short of heroic; it was an extraordinary act of self-sacrifice. As a doctor, Paula knew very well what she was doing. She chose to risk her own life for the health of her baby. But for Paula, this was no heroism. This was something that *any* mother would have done for her baby.

For the dads-to-be who are reading this book, some of you might have seen the movie *John Q* that came out in 2002. It was a cheesy movie, but it struck a chord deep within me as a dad. The story line is about a down-on-his-luck father (played by Denzel Washington) whose HMO insurance won't cover his son's heart transplant. He takes the hospital's emergency room hostage until the doctors agree to perform the operation. What about the heart? Where was he going to get a donor heart? It turned out that he was a match for his son, and so he was going to take his own life so that his son could have his heart. This is the stuff that makes great Hollywood melodrama, but there was something very real about it. This was something that *any* father would have done for his child. I'd gladly give my heart to Sasha or Avery if it means saving her life.

Most of us would jump in front of a train to save our kids. And most of us would readily give our hearts to our children so they could live. We'd give anything for their health. The good news is, as parents, you *can* give them good health. Not all of you can give your children a trust fund or down payment on their first house or a car for their sixteenth birthday, but all of you can give them the gift of health, which is worth more than any of these other gifts combined. Next to life, health is the greatest gift you can give your children.

fetal programming

Some of you might have seen reruns of the *Six Million Dollar Man*, a TV series in the 1970s about an astronaut (Steve Austin, played by Lee Majors) who was severely injured in a crash and was "rebuilt" with bionic parts that gave him strength, speed, and vision far above human norms. In the opening sequence, a team of scientists stand around the badly injured astronaut as the chief scientist announces, "*Steve Austin: astronaut. A man barely alive. We can rebuild him. We have the technology. We can make him better than he was. Better . . . stronger . . . faster.*"

Fast forward 30 years, and science is catching up with science fiction. Only this time we are not talking about repairing a broken man with bionic parts; we are talking about building a healthy baby from inside the womb. If we were to remake the *Six Million Dollar Man* today, the opening lines might go something like this: "*Steve Austin: future astronaut. A man barely conceived. We can build him. We have the technology. We can make him better . . . healthier . . . smarter.*"

Today we are close to being able to say that. We can build babies smarter and healthier, thanks to important scientific discoveries in recent years. We've cracked the human genome. We are beginning to learn how genes can get switched on or off during fetal development, making a life-long impact on health and function (this is called epigenetics, which I will talk about later in the chapter). Perhaps one of the most important scientific discoveries in recent years is fetal programming.

Fetal programming refers to the process whereby a stimulus or insult, at a sensitive or critical period of fetal development, induces permanent alterations in the structure and functions of the baby's vital organs, with lasting or lifelong consequences for health and disease. The idea of fetal programming was first introduced by Dr. David Barker and his colleagues at the University of Southampton in England. They made the link between poor fetal growth inside the womb (which resulted in low birth weight) and coronary heart disease, high blood pressure, diabetes, high choles-terol, metabolic syndrome, and a whole host of chronic adult diseases in later life.

Now when we think of risk factors for heart disease, most of us think of smoking, high blood pressure, high cholesterol, obesity, etc. But *low birth weight*? What does *low birth weight* have to do with heart disease 40 or 50 years later?

Barker and his colleagues hypothesized that, much like program-ming a computer, a baby's heart and other vital organs are "programmed" inside the womb. If something goes wrong during pregnancy, then these vital organs may not get "programmed" properly and may never function optimally over a lifetime. For example, if you were undernourished inside the womb, particularly in the second trimester when your pancreas was rapidly growing, you probably have a smaller pancreas than the average adult. A poorly developed pancreas may put you at greater risk for diabe-tes over your lifetime.

The so-called "Barker hypothesis" was met initially with a great deal of skepticism in the scientific community, but over the past decade a growing body of scientific evidence from animal, clinical, and epidemio-logical studies now supports this idea of fetal programming. Box 1.1 pro-vides a few examples of how the seeds of many childhood or adult diseases may be planted inside the womb, and how your baby's future health and disease susceptibility may originate in fetal life.

box 1.1: fetal origins of childhood obesity, adhd, autism, and schizophrenia

Here are three important examples of fetal programming:

1. *Maternal nutrition linked to childhood obesity.* Nutrition plays a major role in fetal programming. Animal studies have shown that poor fetal nutrition inside the womb results in permanent alterations in the structure and function of several vital organs including the pancreas, kidneys, and blood vessels, which can lead to diabetes, hypertension, and heart disease in later life. Poor fetal nutrition also turns on the baby's "thrifty genes," which help the body use and store energy more efficiently. This might be adaptive if the child were born into a world of famine and starvation. But if the child was instead born into a fast-food nation that supersizes everything, then these "thrifty genes" that got turned on prenatally will hang on to every last calorie of carbs and fats that the child eats, predisposing her to a lifelong struggle with obesity.

2. *Maternal stress linked to ADHD.* When mom is stressed out during pregnancy, her baby is immersed in a stress hormone called cortisol. Animal studies have shown that fetal overexposure to cortisol results in permanent alterations in the structure and function of the fetal brain. A growing body of research in humans now links maternal anxiety or stress during pregnancy to neurological disorders in children, including attention deficit hyperactivity disorder (ADHD). Magnetic resonance imaging (MRI) studies of the brain of individuals with ADHD reveal structural abnormalities in areas of the brain (hippocampus, amygdala, prefrontal cortex) that are particularly vulnerable to the neurotoxic effects of cortisol.

(continued)

3. *Maternal flu linked to autism and schizophrenia in child.* Maternal infections during pregnancy are linked to a number of psychopathologies in her offspring, including autism and schizophrenia. One recent study showed that if you get the flu in the first half of pregnancy, your baby has a three-fold increased risk of developing schizophrenia as an adult. It is hypothesized that the inflammation caused by an infection could interfere with hardwiring of the developing fetal brain, resulting in greater vulnerability to psychopathologies such as autism or schizophrenia in the offspring.

There is still much that we don't know about fetal programming, but already it is being hailed as a "paradigm shift" in science, with profound implications for what we do in clinical medicine and public health. For example, if we want to prevent heart disease, we have to start not by screening for blood pressure and cholesterol in adults, but by optimizing fetal programming of the heart and other vital organs inside the womb. After all, it is a lot easier to build a healthy baby than to repair a broken man. Of course this information doesn't do you much good if you are already 50 with hypertension and hypercholesterolemia (except giving you one more reason to blame your mother for all your troubles). But if you are a mom-to-be who'd give anything for your baby's health, doing all you can to optimize fetal programming is one of the most precious gifts you can ever give your child, and it's a gift that keeps on giving over your child's lifetime. To make a smart and healthy baby, fetal programming is key.

epigenetics: how genes get turned on and off

How does fetal programming work? How do the seeds of future health and diseases get planted inside the womb? Until recently, this was a big mystery. Epigenetics may be the key to unlocking this mystery.

Epigenetics is the study of how genes get turned on or off. Genes contain the instructions for how the body should work, and epigenetics are the on/off switches. There are several ways by which genes can get switched on or off; the most common way is by putting a small chemical molecule called methyl (which is made up of one carbon and three hydrogen atoms) directly in front of a gene, which permanently blocks the gene from ever being expressed. Conversely, if the methyl molecule is removed, then the gene is allowed to freely express itself. Generally speaking, methylation turns off or silences a gene, whereas de-methylation turns on a gene.

Fetal programming probably works by turning on or off genes. In a classic study, researchers were able to turn off a gene that can cause obesity in rat pups simply by feeding their mothers a diet rich in folic acid during pregnancy. *How does folic acid turn off a gene?* It turns out that folic acid is a rich methyl donor (it contains lots of methyl molecules), and mothers who ate a diet rich in folic acid methylated (and thereby turned off) their pups' obesity gene inside the womb. This study demonstrated how maternal nutrition in pregnancy can influence fetal DNA methylation, and that such epigenetic changes can have a lifelong and even intergenerational impact on health and function. So you are not only what you eat, but you are also what your mother ate during pregnancy.

It is probably too early to infer dietary advice from a study on mice, but its implications are quite profound. Imagine someday being able to switch on the genes that will confer upon your baby good health, intelligence, and longevity, and switch off those genes that will put your baby at risk for obesity, diabetes, and cancer before your baby is ever born. Over the next decade this may no longer be stuff only for science fiction. Already cancer researchers are looking for drugs that can switch on tumor suppressor genes, and switch off tumor promoter genes.

We shouldn't get too far ahead of ourselves though, because there is still much we don't know about the epigenetic basis of fetal programming. Much of what we've learned about fetal programming comes from animal studies, and we have to be careful about extrapolating too much from animals to humans because not all humans are rats. And by and large we still don't know how to switch on and off genes, and I'd be worried about the unseen dangers of such epigenetic manipulations. Still epigenetics reminds us just how critical those nine months of pregnancy are; your child's lifelong health and development may well depend on what he or she is exposed to inside the womb (e.g., nutrition, stress, infections, toxins). These stimuli or insults, at critical periods of fetal development, can switch on/off a gene, which may result in permanent alterations in the structure and functions of the baby's brain and other vital organs.

Epigenetics transcends the classic debate about nature versus nurture. How smart and healthy your future baby will be has to do with not only his or her genetic endowment; it also has to do with his or her environment, including those conditions inside the womb, which can reprogram gene functions without rewriting the genetic code. So if you want a smart and healthy baby, you'd better give your baby more than just good genes; you've got to prepare the womb environment for optimal fetal programming.

how to make a smart and healthy baby

"Everyone is a hero at birth," Joseph Campbell wrote in the *Power of Myth*, *"where he or she undergoes a tremendous transformation, from the condition of a little water creature living in a realm of amniotic fluid into an air-breathing mammal which ultimately will be standing."*

I love this imagery of the baby as a hero who personifies limitless human potentialities, an idea that Joseph Campbell borrowed from Otto Rank. But the truth is that the tremendous transformation begins long before birth, and that transformation inside the womb, from a single-cell organism into a little water creature, resulting in an air-breathing mammal, is what brings into being the full range of human potentialities.

This book is about how to make a smart and healthy baby. While a lot of things need to go just right, the five most important steps are:

Step 1: Get ready for pregnancy
Step 2: Grow a good placenta
Step 3: Use the right building blocks
Step 4: Send the right cues
Step 5: Keep out of harm's way

A key message is that these are all steps you can take—they are not complicated or hard to apply. Here I will briefly describe each step and discuss why the first step is the most important one.

STEP 1: GET READY FOR PREGNANCY

This is probably the most important step, and this is why I am devoting this entire book to helping you and your husband (or partner) get ready for pregnancy. A central message of this book is that what you do *before* pregnancy is just as important (if not more important) to making a smart and healthy baby as what happens *during* pregnancy. All of you know the importance of prenatal care. But as I will explain later, by the time you start prenatal care, you may have already missed a critical window of opportunity to bring forth your baby's fullest lifelong potentials. So if you want a smart and healthy baby in the future, you've got to start taking care of yourself now. In this book I will show you how to get ready to get pregnant.

STEP 2: GROW A GOOD PLACENTA

One of the earliest and most critical steps to making a smart and healthy baby is to grow a good placenta. Indeed, scientists have now traced the origins of several major pregnancy complications that manifest later in pregnancy, such as preeclampsia or preterm birth, to poor placental development in early pregnancy. The placenta plays a critical role in fetal programming. The placenta is the only pipeline to your baby for nine months; as such it plays a major role in nutritional programming. The placenta also controls how much cortisol crosses into fetal circulation; as such it plays a major role in stress programming of the fetal brain and other vital organs.

The placenta begins to grow very early in pregnancy, beginning with implantation at about seven days after conception. This is another good reason to get ready before pregnancy—at seven days post-conception most women aren't even aware that they are pregnant (this is three days before most home pregnancy tests turn positive, and about a week before most women miss their period), and yet the seeds of your baby's lifelong health and disease are already being planted. To grow a good placenta in early pregnancy, you've got to prepare your womb before pregnancy.

STEP 3: USE THE RIGHT BUILDING BLOCKS

To make a smart and healthy baby, you need to use the right building blocks—starting with a good egg and a good sperm. The egg carries your genetic materials, and the sperm those of your baby's father. The egg and sperm can get damaged in a lot of different ways. For example, tobacco, alcohol, drugs (e.g., steroids), poor diet, certain medical conditions such as diabetes and varicoceles (varicose veins around the testes), radiation and chemotherapy, sexually transmitted infections, and even testicular hyperthermia (e.g., overheating from hot tub), and an increasing number of environmental pollutants (e.g., phthalates, acrylamide, pesticides, and dioxins) can cause sperm DNA damage. Such DNA damage can get passed on to the next generation, which can result in birth defects and even some childhood cancers. In this book you will learn how to protect your eggs, and in Chapter 8 I will teach your baby's father how to protect his sperm so your future baby can be made with the best building blocks.

Once the egg and sperm become 1, 1 then becomes 2, and then 4, and then 8, and then 16, and the fertilized egg will continue to divide and grow until it becomes an air-breathing mammal with billions of living cells (the newborn brain alone has over 100 billion neurons). Where do all these cells come from? On the day you were born, every single cell, organ, or system inside your body came mostly from the foods your mother ate during those nine months of pregnancy. The foods she ate became the building blocks for your bones, muscles, heart, brain, and other vital organs. And as I will explain in Chapter 2, nutrition determines not only form but also function. You are what your mother ate, and your baby will be what you eat during pregnancy. Because it is hard to change your eating habits overnight, and some foods you eat are stored in your body for a long time, you should get into a habit of choosing the right building blocks for your baby now, before you get pregnant.

STEP 4: SEND THE RIGHT CUES

Your unborn baby takes cues from you about what the outside world is like. If you are anxious or stressed out all the time, the cue you send your baby, via stress hormones, is that the outside world is stressful and hostile. The baby responds by turning on her stress genes and turning up her stress response, in preparation for fight or flight. This heightened stress response can cause significant health and developmental problems in the long run. Indeed, a growing body of evidence now links maternal anxiety and stress during pregnancy to a whole host of health and developmental problems, including ADHD, in her offspring. So if you want a smart and healthy baby, you need to send more positive vibes during pregnancy (I will say more about fetal programming of the baby's stress response in Chapter 4).

How do you send positive vibes to your baby? I'm not suggesting that you sing Hosannah or play Mozart to your baby everyday, but I think keeping your stress level low and your stress resilience high is important. You want to tell your unborn baby that the world is safe and nurturing (much as you'd do after the baby is born), but it is a lot harder to do so when you are stressed out, anxious, or depressed. In Chapter 4, I will give you some practical advice on how to build up your stress resilience and develop positive mental health before pregnancy. Since your man can be an important source of either stress or support, in Chapter 8 I will teach him how to give good support (in addition to good sperm) starting before pregnancy.

STEP 5: KEEP OUT OF HARM'S WAY

The journey of life is full of danger, even inside the womb. Earlier I gave examples of a possible link between maternal flu during pregnancy and autism/schizophrenia in her offspring, as well as between maternal stress and anxiety during pregnancy and ADHD in childhood. There are many more dangers, often in places you wouldn't even expect, such as lead and trihalomethanes in your tap water, phthalates and bisphenol-A in your bottled water, perchloroethylene from dry-cleaning, and pesticides in parks, playgrounds, and golf courses. In Chapter 6 I will teach you how to keep out of harm's way (without becoming paranoid about everything around you).

even early prenatal care is too late

Most of you know the importance of prenatal care. But over the past decade, there has been a growing recognition among doctors and researchers that by the time most women start prenatal care, it may be too late. Early prenatal care is often too late to prevent some birth defects. For example, the neural tube is completely formed by day 28 post-conception. Many of you are aware of the benefit of folic acid supplementation for preventing neural tube defects (e.g., spina bifida or anencephaly). It turns out that if you start taking folic acid after the first 28 days of pregnancy, it does nothing to prevent neural tube defects, probably because neural tube formation is already complete by then.

Similarly, women with pre-gestational diabetes are at greater risk for having a baby with a congenital heart or neural tube defect, especially if the mother's blood sugars were out of control in early pregnancy. The heart begins to beat at 22 days post-conception. The neural tube is completely formed by 28 days post-conception. So by the time these women come into my office for prenatal care (usually after the first 22 to 28 days post-conception), there is little I can do to prevent fetal heart or neural tube defects, even if I could get their blood sugars under perfect control for the rest of pregnancy.

But the heart and neural tube aren't even the first vital organs to form in early pregnancy. As I mentioned earlier, the placenta begins to form very early in pregnancy, starting with implantation at seven days post-conception. This is important because we now know that many pregnancy complications that manifest later in pregnancy, such as preeclampsia or preterm birth, can trace their origins to aberrant placental development early in pregnancy.

Take preeclampsia, for example. As I mentioned earlier, preeclampsia is a disease of the placenta. One of the most consistent pathological findings of preeclampsia is poor, shallow implantation; something went awry in early pregnancy so that the placenta was never able to lay down good roots inside the uterus. This poor implantation sets up the pathogenic processes that eventually lead to preeclampsia months later. By the time most women start prenatal care, it may be too late to prevent the implantation problems that can cause major complications such as preeclampsia or preterm birth later in pregnancy.

Remember my patient Paula? Paula started prenatal care with me very early in pregnancy, at about five weeks' post-conception. But by the time she started prenatal care, it was too late for me to turn back the clock on implantation. Implantation was already well underway, and the inexorable march toward preeclampsia had already begun. I told her that for her next pregnancy, I'd like to see her *before* she gets pregnant. I will help you prepare for your preconception visit with your doctor in Chapter 7.

allostasis: how your body maintains balance

Perhaps the most important reason why early prenatal care may be too late has to do with allostasis and allostatic overload.

Allostasis describes the body's ability to maintain balance through change. A good example of allostasis is found in your body's stress response. When you are under stress, your body activates a stress response. Your sympathetic system kicks in and your adrenalin flows to make your heart pump faster and harder (with the end result of delivering more blood and oxygen to your vital organs, including the brain). Your hypothalamic-pituitary-adrenal (HPA) axis also kicks in to produce more cortisol, which has many actions to prepare you for fight or flight.

But as soon as the fight or flight is over, the body turns off the stress response. Your sympathetic response is counteracted by a parasympathetic response, which fires a signal via the vagal nerve to slow down your heart so you don't overwork your heart muscles. And your HPA axis is shut off by cortisol via a negative feedback loop. Negative feedback loops are common to many biological systems and work very much like a thermostat. When the room temperature falls below a preset point, the thermostat turns on the heat. Once the preset temperature is reached, the heat turns off the thermostat. Stress turns on your HPA axis to produce cortisol. Cortisol, in turn, turns off the HPA axis to keep your stress response in check. Your body has these exquisite built-in mechanisms for checks and balances to help maintain allostasis, or balance through change.

This stress response works well under acute stress; it tends to break down under chronic stress. It works well for stress you can fight off or run from, but it doesn't work as well for stress from which there is no escape. In the face of chronic and repeated stress, your stress response is always turned on. It is not allowed to shut down and recover. Over time your stress response gets worn out. This is when you go from being "stressed" to being "stressed out." And your body goes from allostasis to "allostatic overload," which describes the cumulative toll of all the wear and tear on your body from chronic stress.

Bruce McEwen at the Rockefeller University illustrates the concept of allostasis as two kids balancing on a seesaw—maintaining balance through change. But what would happen if instead of two 25-lb kids, it's

Kern County Library
Southwest Branch Library
RENEW BY:
Phone: 661-664-7716
Telecirc 24/7: 866-290-8681
Online: kernlibrary.org
email: info@kernlibrary.org
Mobile App: SJVLS ValleyCat
(Apple ,Android)

****

Read the Book. Attend Events.
Join the Discussion.
Learn more about the
One Book Project at KCLonebook.org

Checked Out Items 10/16/2019 15:24
ALMARAZ, WENDY CONSUELO

Item Title	Due Date
* Making a baby : everything you need to know to get pregnant	11/6/2019
* The sinus cure : seven simple steps to relieve sinusitis and other ear, nose and throat conditions	11/6/2019
* Get ready to get pregnant : your complete prepregnancy guide to making a smart and healthy baby	11/6/2019

* Indicates items checked out today

Items are due on the date listed and must be returned or renewed on or before that date to avoid fees.

Please keep this slip for your records.

two 500-lb sumo wrestlers riding on the seesaw? Sooner or later that see-saw would break from all that extra load (allostatic overload).

You might be healthy now. But if you keep putting your body under chronic stress, and I am talking about both biological and psychological stress, sooner or later your body's allostatic systems are going to get worn out. Your stress response, immune system, and metabolic functions be-come imbalanced, and as a result your body produces too much cortisol, too much inflammation, and too much insulin, which could lead to a whole host of chronic diseases over time.

This is why even early prenatal care is often too late. If you enter pregnancy carrying two 500-lb sumo wrestlers on your back, there may be little that your body or your doctor can do. If you want a smart and healthy baby, you cannot keep on abusing your body and then expect to restore allostasis overnight when you get pregnant. You've got to start taking care of yourself now, long before you get pregnant.

what is your pregnancy readiness quotient (prq)?

To sum up the three key points I made in this chapter:

First, to make a smart and healthy baby, you need to optimize fetal programming. Fetal programming is just what it sounds like—much like "programming" a computer, a baby's brain and other vital organs are be-ing "programmed" inside the womb. If something goes wrong during pregnancy, then these organs may not get programmed properly and may never function optimally over a lifetime. The difference may be whether your baby gets an Apple II with 4K or a Mac Pro with 16 gigabytes of memory for a brain.

Second, to optimize fetal programming, you need to optimize your own health *before* pregnancy. An important concept I introduced in this chapter is allostasis, which describes the body's ability to maintain bal-ance through change. But if you enter pregnancy carrying two 500-lb sumo wrestlers on your back, your body isn't going to be able to maintain that balance very well, and your baby isn't going to get good fetal programming.

Third, if you want a smart and healthy baby, don't wait until you are pregnant to get ready because even early prenatal care may be too late. Early prenatal care is too late to prevent some birth defects and implantation errors. Most important, early prenatal care is too late to restore your body's allostasis quickly enough to optimize fetal programming.

So do you think you are ready to make a smart and healthy baby? Take the Pregnancy Readiness Quotient (PRQ) self-test in Appendix A and see just how ready you are. You can use this self-test to help you identify areas that you need to work on before you get pregnant.

nutritional preparedness

Most of you have heard the expression "you are what you eat." But did you know that you are also what your mother ate? The day you were born, every cell, organ, and system inside your body came primarily from the foods your mother ate during those nine months of pregnancy. Your mother's nutrition provided the building blocks from which you were made. Not only that, the way your body functions also has a lot to do with what your mother ate. As I mentioned in the first chapter, if you were undernourished inside the womb during the second trimester, when your pancreas was rapidly developing, you probably have a smaller pancreas than the average adult. A poorly developed pancreas might not work as well over the long haul, putting you at greater risk for developing diabetes as an adult.

Indeed, a growing body of research now suggests that high blood pressure, diabetes, heart disease, obesity, metabolic syndrome, and a whole host of chronic adult diseases may have their origins inside the womb, and poor maternal nutrition appears to play a major role. In this chapter I will talk about how to get yourself nutritionally ready for pregnancy in order to optimize fetal programming.

you are what your mother ate . . .
before pregnancy?

It is perhaps not too hard to see that you are what your mother ate during pregnancy. But *before pregnancy*? What does what she ate *before pregnancy* have to do with how smart or healthy you are? And what does what you eat now, perhaps months before you conceive, have to do with how smart or healthy your future baby is going to be? Because this is the basis for the rest of the chapter, I will first make the case why you should start eating healthily now, before you get pregnant.

1. GIVE YOUR BODY A GOOD
NUTRITIONAL TUNE-UP

Remember the idea of allostatic overload that I talked about in Chapter 1? It refers to the toll on your body from chronic stress. While the idea is best understood in the context of chronic *psychological* stress, it is pertinent to chronic *nutritional* stress as well. For example, every time you eat, your blood sugar goes up. This triggers an insulin response, which shuttles blood glucose into the cells and restores normal blood sugar level. This is called allostasis, which describes the body's ability to maintain balance through change. Normally your body can handle this type of challenge with relative ease. But if you keep stressing your body with a diet high in added sugars and refined carbohydrates, sooner or later your insulin response is going to get worn out (sooner if you are overweight). Your body becomes somewhat insensitive or resistant to the actions of insulin, so it no longer shuttles blood glucose into the cells and restores normal blood sugar level efficiently.

When you become pregnant, you will bring to bear on your pregnancy this state of insulin insensitivity and resistance. Pregnancy itself is an insulin-resistant state, and so your blood sugar is going to get even higher. Because blood sugar crosses the placenta easily, if your blood sugar is high your baby's blood sugar is going to be high as well. As I'll explain later in the chapter, all this excess blood sugar during critical periods of fetal development could permanently alter the forms and functions of the fetal pancreas, fat cells, and other vital organs and systems, leading to greater susceptibility for diabetes, obesity, and other metabolic diseases over a lifetime.

Even if you try to eat better during pregnancy, it may be too late. You won't be able to undo overnight all the wear and tear on your body's insulin response and other metabolic functions from all your overindulgences over the years. And you won't be able to restore allostasis quickly enough to optimize fetal programming. So how do you get your pancreas, fat cells, and insulin receptors to work the way they are supposed to during pregnancy? You need to make some changes now before you get pregnant—switch to a diet high in complex carbohydrates with a low glycemic load, eat more fiber and less fat, and exercise regularly, as I will explain later in this chapter.

2. START A NUTRITIONAL SAVINGS ACCOUNT FOR YOUR FUTURE BABY

Eating healthily before pregnancy is like depositing money in a bank. You are creating a nutritional savings account now from which your future baby can withdraw funds. Studies have shown that women who are underweight before pregnancy are at greater risk for having a low birth weight baby, perhaps caused by a lower nutritional reserve from which the baby can draw sustenance. Similarly, short birth spacing is associated with greater risk for low birth weight and other pregnancy complications in the subsequent pregnancy, which is often attributed to maternal nutritional depletion. Pregnancy takes a lot out of women (nutritionally and otherwise); it takes time to replete what nutritional stores were depleted during a prior pregnancy—time that is not allowed by short birth spacing. So give yourself enough time to build up your nutritional reserves before pregnancy, and make sure you are making good deposits into the baby's nutritional savings account.

3. GET RID OF JUNK FROM YOUR BODY'S NUTRITIONAL STORES

Nutritional stores work both ways. Just as good nutrients get stored in the body, bad stuff can also get stored, sometimes for a very long time. I gave the example of dioxins in the Introduction. Remember, dioxins are stored in your body fat, and the half-life of some dioxins can be as long as seven years. Say you're 25: Even if you are eating healthily now, those bacon cheeseburgers and all the bad saturated fats you took into your body with impunity when you were in college come back to bite you. If you lose some weight, you can get rid of some dioxins from your body's fat stores. Other substances like methylmercury can also stay in the body for a long time by binding to a protein and getting concentrated in an organ such as the brain, kidneys, and liver. So don't wait until you are pregnant to "clean house"; start getting rid of junk from your body's stores.

4. BREAKING UP IS HARD TO DO

Foods provide us not only sustenance but also comfort. Think about some of your favorite foods. They are loaded with not only good taste but also good feelings. That's why they are so hard to give up, even though you know they aren't all that good for your baby. While pregnancy is a time when women are more motivated to change behaviors (including eating habits) than just about any other time in their lives, it is also a time of new stress and uncertainties, during which women are more in need of their "comfort foods." There is now growing evidence from animal studies that abdominal fat stores, together with fats and carbs, actually send a signal to the brain to blunt our stress response. That is why they are called "comfort foods"; they actually make us feel better. It takes time to change your eating habits, to give up bad ones and to pick up good ones. Give yourself plenty of time before pregnancy to fine-tune your eating habits so that you don't have to feel guilty about what you eat during pregnancy.

5. TIMING IS EVERYTHING

There is a lot going on in early pregnancy. As I mentioned before, your baby's heart begins to beat at 22 days after conception. Her neural tube is formed by 28 days after conception. That is about three to four weeks into the pregnancy, and only a week or two after your missed period (if you have a 28-day cycle). Most women will not have started prenatal care by then. Many women may not even be aware that they are pregnant.

And yet some of the baby's most vital organs are already formed or forming. For example, most of you are well aware of the benefit of folic acid supplementation for preventing neural tube defects. But as you might expect, folate supplementation that begins more than four weeks after conception has shown no benefit, probably because the neural tube is already completely formed. Timing *is* everything.

There are many more reasons why you should begin to eat healthily before pregnancy, but I hope I have made a sufficiently strong case to convince you that if you want a smart and healthy baby, you need to get yourself nutritionally ready *before* pregnancy.

ten steps to nutritional preparedness

Many of you are familiar with the idea of "emergency preparedness"; most of us living in California have (or know we should have) an "earthquake preparedness" plan, complete with a checklist of items we should have on hand and a plan for survival in case of an earthquake. What I am trying to do in this chapter is to get you to begin to think about a "nutritional preparedness" plan for pregnancy, complete with a checklist of steps you can take to get yourself nutritionally ready for pregnancy:

Step 1: Achieve a healthy weight
Step 2: Eat a balanced diet every day
Step 3: Make every calorie count
Step 4: Go low on glycemic load
Step 5: Load up on smart fats
Step 6: Dump the dumb fats
Step 7: Eat high-quality proteins

(continued)

> **Step 8:** Eat a rainbow of fruits and vegetables
> **Step 9:** Take a daily multivitamin containing folic acid
> **Step 10:** Eat more brain foods and less toxic foods

The goal of nutritional preparedness is to optimize your nutritional status before you get pregnant. Let's turn our attention now to each of the ten steps.

1. ACHIEVE A HEALTHY WEIGHT

Step one is to achieve a healthy weight before pregnancy. Being overweight puts you at risk for a number of pregnancy complications, including gestational diabetes, preeclampsia, and cesarean delivery. Being severely overweight also puts your baby at risk for birth defects like spina bifida, delivery complications, and even fetal death. Being underweight puts your baby at risk for preterm birth and growth retardation.

What is an ideal weight for you? It depends on your height. The National Institutes of Health recommends an ideal prepregnancy weight-for-height, or body-mass-index (BMI), of 18.5 to 24.9. If your prepregnancy BMI is under 18.5, you are considered *underweight*. If your BMI is 25 to 29.9, you are considered *overweight*; and if your BMI is 30 or greater, you are considered *obese*. You can look up your BMI in Table 2.1, or log onto the website for the National Heart, Lung, and Blood Institute at www. nhlbi.nih.gov and use their BMI calculator to calculate your BMI.

To use the table, find your height in the left-hand column labeled Height. Move across to your weight (in pounds). The number at the top of the column is your BMI. For example, if you are 5'5" and weigh 168 lbs, your BMI is 28. To get your BMI to under 25, you need to lose at least 18 lbs.

How do you shed those 18 lbs? Here are five things you can do:

- **Set realistic goals and timelines for weight loss.** It's hard to lose weight. If you can't lose 18 lbs, try losing 10. Any weight

table 2.1: body mass index

Body Mass Index (BMI) Table

BMI	19	20	21	22	23	24	25	26	27	28	29	30	31	32	33	34	35
Height										**Weight (in pounds)**							
4'10" (58")	91	96	100	105	110	115	119	124	129	134	138	143	148	153	158	162	167
4'11" (59")	94	99	104	109	114	119	124	128	133	138	143	148	153	158	163	168	173
5' (60")	97	102	107	112	118	123	128	133	138	143	148	153	158	163	168	174	179
5'1" (61")	100	106	111	116	122	127	132	137	143	148	153	158	164	169	174	180	185
5'2" (62")	104	109	115	120	126	131	136	142	147	153	158	164	169	175	180	186	191
5'3" (63")	107	113	118	124	130	135	141	146	152	158	163	169	175	180	186	191	197
5'4" (64")	110	116	122	128	134	140	145	151	157	163	169	174	180	186	192	197	204
5'5" (65")	114	120	126	132	138	144	150	156	162	168	174	180	186	192	198	204	210
5'6" (66")	118	124	130	136	142	148	155	161	167	173	179	186	192	198	204	210	216
5'7" (67")	121	127	134	140	146	153	159	166	172	178	185	191	198	204	211	217	223
5'8" (68")	125	131	138	144	151	158	164	171	177	184	190	197	203	210	216	223	230
5'9" (69")	128	135	142	149	155	162	169	176	182	189	196	203	209	216	223	230	236
5'10" (70")	132	139	146	153	160	167	174	181	188	195	202	209	216	222	229	236	243
5'11" (71")	136	143	150	157	165	172	179	186	193	200	208	215	222	229	236	243	250
6' (72")	140	147	154	162	169	177	184	191	199	206	213	221	228	235	242	250	258
6'1" (73")	144	151	159	166	174	182	189	197	204	212	219	227	235	242	250	257	265
6'2" (74")	148	155	163	171	179	186	194	202	210	218	225	233	241	249	256	264	272
6'3" (75")	152	160	168	176	184	192	200	208	216	224	232	240	248	256	264	272	279

Source: Evidence Report of Clinical Guidelines on the Identification, Evaluation, and Treatment of Overweight and Obesity in Adults, 1998. NIH/National Heart, Lung, and Blood Institute (NHLBI)

loss will help. It will make your body more metabolically efficient and less insulin resistant, even if you don't achieve your ideal body weight. Be patient. Give yourself enough time to achieve a healthy weight before pregnancy.

- **Decrease caloric intake.** There is one simple formula to weight loss:

weight change = calories in minus calories out

A key component to successful weight loss is to reduce your caloric intake. Since 1993, the National Weight Control Registry has maintained a registry of people who have lost more than 30 lbs and kept them off for over a year. Over 3,000 women and men have now joined this registry. What was their secret of success? First and foremost, *they all ate fewer calories.* On average they ate 1,400 calories a day. They also switched to a lower fat diet, cut back on sugars and sweets, and ate more fruits and vegetables. Sample menus with reduced calories (1,200 to 1,600 calories) can be found at the National Heart, Lung, and Blood Institute website.

- **Exercise (increase calories out).** The other secret of success was that they all exercised regularly. They burned, on average, 400 calories a day, which translates to about an hour of brisk walking or half an hour of vigorous activity a day.

- **Keep track of your weight and nutrition.** The men and women who made the registry also weighed themselves frequently; nearly half did so daily. It's easy to eat more than you should; keeping a food diary can make you more aware of how much you are eating. Maintaining balanced, healthy nutrition is still important while you are trying to lose weight; beware of those fad diets and crazy weight-loss programs that deprive your body of the essential nutrients it needs before and during pregnancy. Make sure you are getting enough calcium, B-vitamins, and zinc; nutrients that are commonly lacking in weight-loss diets.

- **Get help.** You don't have to do this all on your own. There are successful weight-loss programs that have been proven to work, such as Weight Watchers (for more information go to www.WeightWatchers.com). If you need to lose a lot of weight,

I'd recommend working with a registered dietician, especially someone who specializes in working with pregnant women and can continue to help you through your pregnancy. Talk to your doctor about the appropriateness of weight-loss medications and surgery for you.

- **Maintain a healthy weight.** It's hard to lose weight, but it is even harder to keep the weight off. This is especially true in pregnancy. All too often women who lose a lot of weight right before they get pregnant gain it all back, plus some more, as soon as they get pregnant. It's as if the body is fighting for all the weight it lost, and you end up gaining 70-plus pounds during pregnancy. This defeats the purpose of weight loss and isn't healthy for the pregnancy. I'd recommend that you work with a registered dietician to help you keep the weight off before and during pregnancy. Once you've achieved a healthy weight, you should try to maintain a stable weight for at least **three to six months** to allow the body to adjust to the new, healthier weight, before attempting to conceive.

If you are underweight, here are several things you can do to achieve optimal weight before pregnancy:

- **Set a realistic goal for weight gain.** You are aiming for a BMI between 18.5 to 24.9. Remember this weight gain needs to be healthy weight; if you gain 20 pounds on chocolate cake and doughnuts the weight gain probably won't help your pregnancy much.
- **Increase caloric intake.** To gain 1 to 1 ½ pounds a week, you will need to eat an additional 500 to 750 calories daily.
- **Use nutritional supplements.** To help you gain weight, you can use specially formulated nutritional supplements that are nutritionally balanced, calorically concentrated, and easily

absorbed. Regular supplements such as Ensure, Instant
Breakfast, Sweet Success, Boost, Sustacal, ReSource, Deliver
2.0, and TwoCal HN provide one-third to two-thirds more
calories, 50 percent more protein, and three times the amount
of carbohydrates per serving compared to a glass of milk.
Avoid unbalanced dietary supplements, including high-protein
supplements.

- **Get help.** Given our society's fixation on thinness, gaining
weight may be a hard thing to do for some of you. If you feel
conflicted about your body image, talk to your doctor about it,
or ask your doctor to refer you for counseling.

2. EAT A BALANCED DIET EVERYDAY

Healthy eating takes planning. It's all too easy, when you are late for
work, to just grab coffee and a bagel on the go or skip breakfast altogether. And it's all too easy, at the end of the day, to pick up some fast-
food on the way home if you are too tired to cook and there is nothing in
the refrigerator. We all know better, but we don't always make the best
spur-of-the-moment choices about what we eat, especially when we are
stressed out, tired, or hungry.

You need to plan ahead. You should eat a balanced, healthy diet everyday, which should include the following:

- **Whole grain foods:** such as oatmeal, whole-wheat bread, and
brown rice. You should eat 5 to 7 servings of whole grain foods
a day. A serving of whole grain equals
½ cup of cooked brown rice or whole grain pasta;
1 slice of whole grain bread;
½ regular whole grain muffin; or
1 cup of whole grain cereal.
For example, to get 5 servings of whole grain foods a day, you
could eat a cup of whole grain cereal (1 serving) for breakfast,
a sandwich with 2 slices of whole-wheat bread (2 servings)

for lunch, and 1 cup of brown rice or whole grain pasta
(2 servings) for dinner.

- **Plant oils:** such as olive, canola, and flaxseed oil. You can use up to 6 teaspoons of plant oils a day.
- **Vegetables and fruits:** vegetables and fruits are a great source of vitamins, minerals, and phytochemicals with antioxidant properties. They can help reduce oxidative stress and inflammation during pregnancy. The Centers for Disease Control and Prevention and a number of organizations including the National Cancer Institute recommend that all Americans consume at least 5 servings of vegetables and fruits (preferably 3 servings of vegetables and 2 servings of fruits) a day. Here are a few examples of what constitutes a serving:

  1 medium-size fruit;

  ½ cup fresh, frozen, or canned fruit (in 100 percent juice) or vegetables;

  ¾ cup (6 oz) of 100 percent fruit or vegetable juice;

  ¼ cup dried fruit; or

  1 cup of raw leafy greens

- **Nuts and legumes:** nuts and legumes (beans, peas, lentils) are excellent sources of protein, fiber, vitamins, and minerals. I recommend eating ½ to 1 cup of legumes, and a small handful of raw, natural, unsalted or lightly salted nuts or seeds a day.
- **Fish, poultry, and eggs:** fish, poultry, and eggs are excellent sources of animal proteins. Fish and some eggs also contain high levels of omega–3 polyunsaturated fatty acids. Growing concerns about methylmercury levels in fish, however, has led to public health warnings about consumption of fish and other seafood by pregnant women, or women who are planning to get pregnant (see EPA/FDA Advisory on Fish and Shellfish in Box 2.2). I recommend eating

  4 to 6 oz of wild coldwater fish twice a week;

> 4 to 6 oz of drug- and hormone-free, de-skinned free-range chicken or turkey 2 to 3 times a week, and
>
> 1 DHA-fortified egg, from drug- and hormone-free, free-range chicken 2 to 3 times a week.

- **Dairy or calcium supplement:** Dairy products are an excellent source of calcium. The United States Department of Agriculture (USDA) recommends that you drink 3 cups of milk a day; I'd add that you should drink non-fat or low-fat milk and eat dairy products made from skim milk. You can also take a calcium supplement; each 500 milligram tablet of calcium carbonate (e.g., TUMS) contains about the same amount of calcium as drinking one 8 oz glass of milk. Other excellent sources of calcium include green, leafy vegetables, tofu and other fortified soy products, fortified orange juice, and almonds.

- **Multivitamin:** The U.S. Public Health Service recommends that all women of childbearing ages take a daily multivitamin containing at least 400 micrograms of folic acid to prevent two common and serious birth defects: spina bifida and anencephaly. The CDC estimates that 50–70 percent of these birth defects could be prevented if this recommendation were followed before and during early pregnancy.

You should minimize consumption of red meat and butter, which contain high amounts of saturated fats. You should also reduce your intake of refined carbohydrates such as white rice, white bread, potatoes, and pasta, along with sweets, which can spike up your blood sugar and insulin. If you are actively trying to get pregnant, you should avoid alcohol altogether. You can get more information on how to eat a balanced meal from the USDA's Dietary Guidelines for Americans at www.mypyramid.gov, or the Healthy Eating Pyramid developed by Walter Willett and colleagues from Harvard School of Public Health at http://www.hsph.harvard.edu/nutritionsource/what-should-you-eat/pyramid/.

Now you know what to eat, let's talk about how you can eat healthier.

- **Use a menu planner,** such as the USDA's MyPyramid Menu Planner at www.mypyramid.gov. There you can create your own personalized menus. You can also get reports on how your food choices measure up to your goals, how much each food contributes to recommended goals and limits, and what steps you can take to improve your diet.
- **Shop from a list.** Make a shopping list based on the menus you've created for the week. It's all too easy to forget what you need, so shop from a list.
- **Eat three meals and two snacks a day.** The Institute of Medicine recommends that pregnant women eat three meals plus at least two snacks a day (in mid-morning and mid-afternoon; some experts suggest adding a snack before bedtime), which is probably a good habit for you to get into now.
- **Don't skip meals.** Skipping meals when you are pregnant causes a placental stress hormone called corticotropin-releasing hormone (CRH) to go up, and may increase the risk of preterm delivery. Skipping meals may also cause you to binge later—especially on foods high in fats and refined carbo-hydrates—as a physiological response to starvation. This creates lows and highs in blood sugar and sends your insulin and other endocrine responses on a roller-coaster ride.

  Breakfast is the meal that many people skip, but it's the one meal you really shouldn't skip. If you skip breakfast, you might go 12 hours or more without nourishment. You wouldn't go 12 or more hours without feeding a newborn baby; why would you do that to your unborn child during pregnancy? Always start the day off with a good breakfast, and get into the habit of not skipping meals (especially breakfast) and eating snacks between your meals now, before you get pregnant.

- **Consult a registered dietician** if you have any special dietary requirements (e.g., hypertension, diabetes, gastric bypass, celiac disease, phenylketonuria, veganism). Try to find a dietician who specializes in preconception and pregnancy nutrition counseling so she can continue to provide guidance to you throughout your pregnancy.

3. MAKE EVERY CALORIE COUNT

A calorie is a unit of energy. Your body needs energy to function, and during pregnancy your baby needs energy to grow. But eating too many calories can make you fat, especially if you're eating "empty calories" high in energy but low in nutritional values. Here are my recommendations to help you get the most out of every calorie:

- **Determine how many calories your body needs a day.** Your energy requirement depends on a number of factors including your age, BMI, level of physical activity, and health status. For example, if you are a healthy 25-year-old, 5'4", 125 lbs, and you workout 30–60 minutes a day, your body requires 2,200 calories a day. But if you are 35, 5'4", 150 lbs, and sedentary, you will need to reduce your total daily caloric intake to less than 1,800 calories in order to start moving toward a healthier weight. You can look up your energy requirements at www.mypyramid.gov.

  Contrary to popular belief, you don't have to "eat for two" during pregnancy, at least as far as energy requirements are concerned. Your energy requirement is the same in the first trimester as before pregnancy, and goes up by only 350 calories a day in the second trimester and 500 calories a day in the third trimester. So for the most part you can stick to the balanced, healthy diet you started before pregnancy, with some minor adjustments in the second and third trimesters.

- **Count your calories.** Once you determine how many calories your body needs, you can adjust your daily caloric intake accordingly. A Burger King Whopper plus fries easily exceed 1,000 calories (which is more than half the daily energy requirements for most American women); counting (or at least watching) your calories helps make every calorie count. This has been made simple by web-based menu planners such as the one at www.mypyramid.gov. Just enter the foods you eat, and the planner will automatically add up your total calories. You can also find the caloric content of most common foods by going to the USDA National Nutrient Database website at www.ars.usda.gov., or by reading food labels for caloric content.

- **Avoid empty calories.** "Empty calories" describes foods that are high in calories but low in nutritional values. Examples of foods containing mostly empty calories include candies, sodas, crackers, cookies, chips, French fries, butter, dressings, and most processed foods made with lots of added sugars, *trans* fats, or partially hydrogenated oils, beer, wine, and any alcoholic beverages. You should keep your empty calories to no more than 265 calories a day; you can keep track of your empty calories (so-called "extra calories") using MyPyramid Menu Planner at www.mypyramid.gov.

- **Make food substitutions.** Substitute baked skinless chicken breast for fried chicken. Replace French fries with baked yams. Use low-fat or non-fat salad dressings instead of creamy dressings. Add lettuce, tomato, and onions to sandwiches and burgers instead of cheese, mayo, or bacon. Snack on fruits instead of chips and crackers. Most important, substitute whole, natural foods for processed foods. Play around with the menu planner on MyPyramid and see how your choices of foods and add-ons affect the calorie count (e.g., one sweet baked potato with no add-ons gives you 101 calories, but one medium fries with ketchup gives you 478 calories with 238 empty calories).

- **Realize that size matters.** Watch your portion size, and avoid the temptations to supersize.

- **Bring snacks to work.** Get into the habit of bringing healthy snacks to work. This way you will have control over what you eat at work, rather than relying on what is available through the vending machines. Unsalted or lightly salted nuts, trail mix with raisins, almonds, walnuts, and pumpkin seeds, celery and carrots, and other fruits and vegetables make great snacks and offer healthy substitutes to candies, potato chips, and other junk foods.

- **Avoid fast-foods.** Avoid the temptations of eating fast-foods as much as you can. Most fast-foods are high in calories, total fat, saturated fat, cholesterol, salt, and added sugar (mostly from carbonated soft drinks), and are low in dietary fiber, calcium, vitamins A and C, folate, fruits, and vegetables. Try to limit your fast-food consumption to no more than once or twice a month, if at all. Should you end up at McDonald's or other fast-food restaurants, try to make healthy choices such as salad with low-calorie dressing or a chicken breast sandwich and tell 'em to "hold the mayo and fries."

- **Avoid stress eating.** Some people tend to overeat when they are under stress. Moreover, they tend to reach for "comfort foods" that are high in fats and added sugar. If you are one of them, try to recognize when you are stress eating and develop other strategies for coping with your stress (see Chapter 4).

Let's now turn to the specific contents of nutrition. Nutrients are categorized as macronutrients and micronutrients. Macronutrients consist of carbohydrates, proteins, and fats, whereas micronutrients are made up of vitamins, minerals, and phytochemicals.

4. GO LOW ON GLYCEMIC LOAD

Carbohydrates are found in foods like fruits, vegetables, cereal, oatmeal, pasta, noodles, rice, bread, cake, pie, cookies, crackers, juice, soda, and candies. Carbohydrates are essential to fetal development, and that is why I am usually not in favor of low-carb diets for pregnant women, or women who are planning to get pregnant (see Box 2.1).

box 2.1: low-carb diet for pregnancy?

I get asked frequently whether it is healthy for pregnant women, or women who are planning to get pregnant, to start or continue on a low-carb diet. I am not in favor of starting a low-carb diet just before or during pregnancy for the following reasons:

- Carbohydrates—I'll call them carbs here—are vital to fetal development. Glucose from carbs is the preferred fuel for the baby's developing brain and nervous system. Carbs, in the forms of glycoprotein and proteoglycan, are integral components of cell structure and play important roles in cell functions;
- Carbs are a primary source of energy for your body. Without carbs your body will burn protein and fat for fuel. Burning fat releases ketones, which can cross the placenta and destroy fetal brain cells and alter the delicate acid-base balance of the fetal system;
- Carbs are an important source of folic acid. Folic acid is needed to grow the baby's brain and nervous system. Since 1996, the Food and Drug Administration has required that folic acid be added to flour, bread, and grain products such as pastas and rice in order to reduce the risk of neural tube defects in babies. Many fortified breakfast cereals also contain folic acid. Folic acid is also found naturally in legumes, nuts, leafy green vegetables, and some fruits;
- Carbs contain lots of fiber, which can prevent constipation and possibly some cancers.
- Some low-carb diets restrict dairy products and calcium-fortified juices because of their carbohydrate content, which can deprive mothers (and their babies) of some of the best sources of calcium;   (continued)

- Most low-carb diets recommend high protein intake. In excess of 25 percent of total calories, high protein intake has been shown to be associated with increased risk of very early premature births and neonatal deaths.

For all these reasons, I do not recommend starting a low-carb diet when you are planning to get pregnant. If you are on the maintenance phase of a low-carb diet (e.g., Phase 3 of South Beach) already, you should see a registered dietician who can help you modify your diet in preparation for pregnancy.

Instead of a low-carb diet, I recommend that you eat a diet low in glycemic index or glycemic load. **Glycemic index** (GI) is a measure of *how fast* a particular carbohydrate gets into the bloodstream and raises your blood sugar level. When you consume foods that are high in GI, your blood sugar spikes up rapidly and sends you on a sugar high. The high blood sugar triggers an insulin response, which quickly drops your blood sugar level. Thus eating foods with high GI sends your blood sugar on a roller-coaster ride. When you consume foods that are low in GI, your blood sugar rises and falls more steadily.

A related concept is **glycemic load** (GL). Whereas glycemic index describes *how fast* a particular carbohydrate raises your blood sugar level, glycemic load takes into account *how much* carbohydrate a particular food contains. A food's glycemic load is determined by multiplying its glycemic index by the amount of carbohydrate it contains. This is important because some foods, like watermelon, have a high GI, but because they contain only a small amount of carbohydrate per serving, their GL is low and their impact on blood sugar levels is limited. For simplicity's sake (so I don't have to keep saying GI *and* GL), I will talk mostly about GI for the rest of the book. But in choosing a carbohydrate, it is useful to know both its GI and GL.

Generally speaking, GIs of 55 or below are considered low and 70

or above are considered high. GLs of 10 or below are considered low and 20 or above are considered high.

When you eat high-GI foods, your blood sugar rises rapidly. Blood sugar crosses the placenta easily. High-GI foods, therefore, can spike your baby's blood sugar. Beginning at about ten weeks after conception, the baby's pancreas starts to produce insulin, which keeps blood sugar in check. However, if the baby is constantly bombarded with high blood sugar, he or she will produce excess amounts of insulin. During critical periods of fetal development, all this excess insulin can do three things to the baby: 1) it can cause an overgrowth of fat cells, 2) it can program insulin resistance, and 3) it can program leptin resistance. You know about insulin resistance, but what does leptin resistance do? Leptin is a satiety hormone; it tells your brain to stop eating when you are full. So if your baby is born with leptin resistance in the brain, she is going to keep on eating even when she is full. Leptin also tells the pancreas to stop producing insulin; so if your baby has leptin resistance in the pancreas, she is going to produce more insulin, which is going to lay down more fat cells. So by the time the baby is born, she is predisposed to lifelong struggles with overweight, obesity, and early-onset type 2 diabetes because of all the excess fat cells and programmed insulin and leptin resistance.

But why worry before pregnancy? When your blood sugar goes up, your pancreas produces insulin, which shuttles blood sugar from the bloodstream into the cells for storage. But if you keep eating high-GI foods you keep bombarding your body with high blood sugar and challenging your body's insulin response. Over time your body becomes relatively insensitive or even resistant to the actions of insulin and can no longer take up glucose from the bloodstream efficiently. This is how a high-GI diet, over time, can create a state of insulin insensitivity or resistance in susceptible individuals.

Pregnancy itself is an insulin-resistant state. This is designed to keep maternal blood sugar higher so that more of it becomes available to the fetus. But if your body is already insulin-insensitive going into the pregnancy, you will become even more insulin resistant and flood the baby with too much blood sugar. To optimize fetal programming you need to go into your pregnancy with high-functioning insulin response and metabolic system; this is why you need to start eating healthily *before* pregnancy.

So how do you look up the GI of the foods you eat? A useful website is www.glycemicindex.com. You'll find some surprises when you start looking up GIs. For example, that plain bagel you had for breakfast probably has higher GI than table sugar. How can that be? There are a number of factors that influence how quickly carbohydrates in food raise your blood sugar, including

- *Fiber content.* Fiber shields the starchy carbohydrates in food from immediate and rapid attack by digestive enzymes. This slows the release of sugar molecules into the bloodstream. Foods high in fiber content usually have low GI, and vice versa.
- *Type of starch.* Starch comes in many different configurations. Some are easier to break into sugar molecules than others. The starch in potatoes, for example, is digested and absorbed into the bloodstream relatively quickly.
- *Fat content and acid content.* The more fat or acid a food contains, the more slowly its carbohydrates are converted to glucose and absorbed into the bloodstream.
- *Physical form.* Finely ground grain is more rapidly digested, and so has a higher GI, than more coarsely ground grain. Thus refined flour has a much higher GI than whole grain products.

This is why that plain bagel made of refined flour, or that puffy rice cake with all its surface area for rapid digestion, has a higher GI than even table sugar.

Here are some recommendations for choosing carbohydrates:

- **How many carbs do I need?** You should eat 5 to 7 servings of whole grains, 5 servings of fruits and vegetables, and ½ to 1 cup of legumes a day. If you are counting calories, you should eat

40 to 50 percent of your total daily calories as carbs. On a 2,000-calorie diet, this means you need to eat 800 to 1,000 calories of carbs a day. In terms of grams, this translates to 200 to 250 grams of carbs per day; check the product label to see how many grams of carbs each food product you eat contains.

- **Go low on glycemic load.** Try to choose, as much as you can, carbs with a **GI below 70** or a **GL below 20.**

If this whole business of counting GI or GL is too much for you, you can also just follow these few simple guidelines to choosing carbohydrates:

- **Start the day off with whole grains.** Choose breakfast cereals made from whole grains like oats, bran, or barley. If you prefer to start the day with toast or a bagel, choose those made from coarse, whole grains rather than refined carbohydrates. Make sure "whole grain" is **first** on the ingredient list. Don't be fooled by terms like "multi-grain" or the color; "multi-grain" can be highly refined, and the color may come from color additive.
- **For lunch sandwiches, use bread made from whole grains** instead of soft, white, fluffy bread (e.g., Wonder Bread Classic).
- **For dinner, pick up some whole-wheat pasta.** If whole grain products are just too chewy for you, look for those that are made with half whole-wheat flour and half white flour. If you are going to cook pasta for dinner, go **al dente**! Cooking spaghetti for 5 minutes instead of 20 reduces its GI from 61 to 38. Undercooking makes the food chewier and harder to digest, which results in slower release of glucose into your bloodstream. If you are eating rice, choose the harder, coarser brown rice, or even "newer" whole grains like bulgur, wheat berries, millet, or

hulled barley, over white rice (especially short-grained, sticky white rice). Avoid overcooking.

- **Go for high fiber.** In choosing your carbs, read product labels for fiber content. The higher the fiber content, the less processed and refined the food. Choose cereals and other whole grain products with a fiber content of 3 grams or higher per serving.

- **Lose the potatoes.** Potatoes contain starch that is digested and absorbed into the bloodstream relatively quickly. Limit your consumption to no more than once a week, and try to find healthier substitutes like sweet potatoes or yams.

- **Always add protein to your snacks.** Protein reduces the overall GI of your snack. Have a yogurt with your berries. If you are craving something sweet, try yogurt-covered raisins.

- **Choose fresh fruits over fruit juices and avoid punch or fruit rolls.** A fresh orange has a GI of 48; orange juice reconstituted from frozen concentrate, 57; Fanta orange soda, 68; and orange-flavored Gatorade, 89. A fresh orange also has a lot more vitamin C and other micronutrients than orange juice; orange soda and Gatorade have minimal nutritional values and lots of empty calories. Avoid soda, Gatorade, punch, fruit rolls, or anything with lots of added sugar or corn syrup.

- **Use vinaigrette dressing on your salads and vegetables.** Vinegar slows the breakdown of sugars and absorption of glucose into the bloodstream.

- **Mix it up.** If you are eating carbs with high GI, mix it with foods of low GI. For example, if you are not ready to give up those sweet frosted corn flakes just yet, mix them up with some whole grains like bran to bring down the overall GI of your breakfast cereal.

Now you know what carbs to eat, let's turn our attention to fats.

———

5. LOAD UP ON SMART FATS

Fats are not all created equal. When it comes to fats, there are smart fats, and then there are dumb fats. Smart fats are omega–3 fatty acids found in fish and some eggs, seeds and nuts (flax, pumpkin, and walnuts), oils (canola and soy), and dark leafy greens. Dumb fats are saturated fats found in red meat, poultry skin, butter, cream, cheese, and other dairy products made from whole milk, and palm and coconut oils. I also include *trans* fats and partially hydrogenated oils in the list of dumb fats. To make a smart and healthy baby, you need to eat more smart fats and less dumb fats. Remember, fats get stored in the body; the fats you eat today could be the building blocks for your baby's brain a few months from now.

Smart fats are fats that make your baby smart and healthy. A growing body of evidence suggests that omega–3 polyunsaturated fatty acids, especially docosahexaenoic acid (DHA) and eicosapentaenoic acid (EPA), may play a vital role in fetal brain and visual development. In one study, researchers randomly assigned pregnant women to receive a daily supplement consisting of 10cc of cod liver oil rich in DHA and EPA, versus 10cc of corn oil with minimal omega–3 fatty acids, and conducted intelligence testing on their children at age four. The study found that children whose mothers received cod liver oil supplementation during pregnancy performed significantly better on intelligence testing than those whose mothers received corn oil supplementation.

In addition to building a smart and healthy brain, omega–3 fatty acids do many other things in pregnancy that contribute to making a smart and healthy baby. Omega–3 fatty acids are anti-inflammatory. As I will discuss in Chapter 5, inflammation has been implicated in a whole host of pregnancy complications, including preterm birth. Several studies have demonstrated the benefits of fish oil (rich in omega–3 fatty acids) supplementation during pregnancy in reducing the risk for preterm birth. In a large European study, maternal supplementation with fish oil beginning at 20 weeks' gestation among women who had a previous preterm birth reduced the risk of repeat preterm birth by about half.

Another study found that maternal cod liver oil supplementation during pregnancy was associated with reduced risks of childhood diabetes, whereas cod liver oil consumption that began in infancy was not associated with reduced diabetes in childhood, suggesting a role for omega–3 fatty acids in fetal programming of insulin sensitivity. Some researchers have even postulated that babies with an insufficiency of omega–3 fatty acids during fetal development may be at greater risk for cardiovascular diseases later in life. In sum, a growing body of evidence now suggests that omega–3 fatty acids, especially DHA and EPA, may reduce the risk of preterm birth and possibly other pregnancy complications, improve fetal brain and visual development, and possibly avert childhood diabetes or even adult cardiovascular diseases. That's why I call them smart fats.

You can get DHA and EPA two ways. One way is by eating foods containing alpha-linolenic acid (LnA), such as flaxseeds, pumpkin seeds, walnuts, soy, canola and flaxseed oils, and dark leafy greens, which we don't get nearly enough of in the typical American diet. LnA then gets converted into DHA and EPA inside our body. However, too much omega–6 fatty acids and *trans* fats can interfere with the absorption and conversion of LnA. Omega–6 fatty acids are found in red meat, poultry, fried or fast-foods, all the polyunsaturated vegetable oils (including corn and peanut oils) on the market and all the baked goods made with them. *Trans* fats are found in commercially prepared baked goods, margarines, snack foods, fast-foods, and processed foods. So we don't get enough LnA in the typical American diet, and what little LnA we get doesn't get absorbed or converted to DHA and EPA well because we eat too much omega–6s and *trans* fats in our diet.

The second way to get our omega–3s is by directly eating preformed DHA and EPA. By far fish, especially coldwater fish, is the richest source of this kind of DHA. Fish like salmon and sardines get DHA by eating algae in the ocean. Unfortunately, as I will discuss later, concerns about methylmercury contamination has led the FDA/EPA to issue an advisory to pregnant women, and women who are planning to get pregnant, to limit their consumption of fish and seafood. Chickens in the wild can find plant sources of omega–3s and store them as DHA in the yolk of their eggs; however, chickens confined to cages eating standard feed will not produce eggs that have anywhere near the DHA content of eggs of free-ranging chickens that scratch and peck the ground for food. Similarly, animals that feed on wild grass will have higher levels of DHA in their body fat than animals fed on standard feeds.

So how can you be sure that you are getting enough smart fats in your diet? Here are a few recommendations:

- **How much smart fat do I need?** You should consume 220 mg of DHA a day before pregnancy, and 300 mg of DHA per day during pregnancy. Unfortunately, the typical American diet is quite deficient in DHA, and the recommended restrictions on fish consumption as well as current practices for raising chicken and cattle do not help the matter. The average daily intake of DHA for U.S. women of childbearing age is about 50 mg, significantly less than the 220 mg daily amount recommended by the International Society for the Study of Fatty Acids and Lipids. Among pregnant women, the average daily intake is 51 mg, far below the daily intake of 300 mg recommended by the Institute of Medicine. It's really not that hard to get 220/300 a day; one DHA-fortified egg can give you 300 mg of DHA, and one 4-oz fillet of steamed or poached wild Alaskan salmon contains 830 mg of DHA.
- **Eat more LnA and less omega–6 and *trans* fats.** To get more LnA from your diet, you need to eat more nuts, seeds, oils, and dark greens (e.g., flaxseeds, pumpkin seeds, walnuts, soybeans, canola oil, and purslane). Remember omega–6s and *trans* fats interfere with absorption and conversion of LnA, so you need to cut down on omega–6s and *trans* fats in your diet.
- **Eat wild coldwater fish.** You can eat up to 12 oz of wild (not farm-raised) coldwater fish a week. I'd recommend eating wild

Alaskan salmon, which has been found to contain minimal amount of methylmercury. One 4-oz fillet of steamed or poached wild Alaskan salmon contains 830 mg of DHA and 136 mg of EPA. However, eating wild coldwater fish can get expensive so look for them in freeze packs or in a can.

- **Take fish oil.** You can take fish oil. Most fish oil come in 1,000 mg capsules but you should read the label to make sure you are getting at least 220 mg of DHA (and a total of at least 650 mg for DHA plus EPA). Fish oil may be contaminated with methylmercury and PCB; you can go to the website for Environmental Defense Fund at www.edf.org to see which brands are purifying their fish oil and meeting the strictest standards for safe levels of contaminants.

- **Take microalgae DHA supplement.** You can also take DHA supplements made from non-fish sources. DHA produced by microalgae are now being marketed as supplements in the United States; read the product label to make sure you are getting at least 220 mg of DHA a day. DHA has also been added to a few prenatal vitamins, which is what I recommend to my patients who are planning to get pregnant.

- **Eat DHA eggs.** You can eat eggs from hens fed on DHA-producing microalgae. These eggs are a good source of DHA, without worries about methylmercury and PCB. In addition, they are rich in high-quality protein, vitamins, and minerals including vitamin A; vitamins B2, B6, B7, B9, D, and E; calcium; iron; chromium; phosphorous; and zinc. Studies have shown eating one or two such eggs a day for up to 24 weeks results in a significant increase in DHA but will not adversely affect your cholesterol levels. Look for "DHA" or "Omega–3" on the packaging, and compare product labels to see how much DHA you are getting per egg (several brands provide 300 mg of DHA per egg). I recommend eating one DHA egg at least every other day before and during pregnancy.

6. DUMP THE DUMB FATS

Now on to dumb fats. Dumb fats are fats that can make your baby, well, not so smart and healthy. A good example is saturated fats. Saturated fats come mostly from animal fats found in red meat, poultry skin, butter, cream, cheese, and other dairy products made from whole milk, but also a few plant sources (most notably two oils—palm and coconut oils). Saturated fats are dumb fats for three reasons.

- First, saturated fats increase LDL cholesterol, which can clog up placental blood vessels (the same way it can cause atherosclerotic plaques in older adults) and reduce placental blood flow and delivery of oxygen and nutrients to the baby.
- Second, LDL cholesterol can cross the placenta and get deposited in fetal blood vessels as fatty streaks; the long-term effects of these fatty streaks are presently not known but are feared to have adverse consequences on the baby's cardiovascular health later in life.
- Third and probably most important, LDL cholesterol oxidation can cause inflammation in the placenta and in fetal blood vessels and organs, and as we will discuss in Chapter 5, inflammation can cause permanent damage to the baby's vital organs, including the brain.

There is another fat that is probably dumber than saturated fats. *Trans* fats come from heating vegetable oils, which converts fatty acids from their natural state to an unnatural *trans* configuration. Starting in the 1950s, doctors were urging patients to make a switch from saturated fats to polyunsaturated vegetable oils, in the belief that vegetable oils were healthier. We were wrong. The problem with cooking with vegetable oils is that they are particularly susceptible to oxidation under heat. We now know that oxidized oils promote inflammation in the body, and they can generate free radicals that can cause "oxidative stress" to the placenta and fetal vessels and organs.

Most of the *trans* fats in the American diet are found in commercially prepared baked goods, margarines, snack foods, and processed foods. Fast-foods, especially those that are deep-fried, like French fries and onion rings, also contain a good deal of *trans* fat. What makes the matter worse is that most fast-food restaurants will reuse the oil in deep fryers over and over again and the oxidized fats will accumulate. So before you bite into a cheeseburger or fried chicken from a fast-food joint, think about all the oxidized *trans* fats you are about to deposit into your body's fat stores, where they can cause chronic inflammation. When you become pregnant, these fats can cross the placenta and create a great deal of oxidative stress and inflammation in the placenta and fetal organs. Moreover, these fats—what some dieticians call "funny fats"—are going to be the building blocks for your future baby's brain and other vital organs. Then go find yourself some smart fats to bite into instead.

One particular form of *trans* fat is partially hydrogenated oil. Partially hydrogenated oil is made by heating oil to high temperatures of 248 to 410 degrees Fahrenheit with hydrogen gas under pressure, usually in the presence of some metal catalysts. The end result is a complex mixture of compounds that include an abundance of *trans* fats. The purpose of hydrogenating oils is to harden them to improve their spreadability, mouth feel, baking qualities, and, especially, to extend the shelf life of products made from them. Margarine is made this way, with a high content (30 to 40 percent) of *trans* fats. Read the label of almost any brand of cookie, cracker, chip, or snack food you pick up in the supermarket and you will find "partially hydrogenated oil" high on the list of ingredients. Often the particular oil or oils are specified, such as "partially hydrogenated soybean oil" or "partially hydrogenated cottonseed and/or corn oil." Whatever the oils, they contain a lot of *trans* fats and can promote a great deal of inflammation in your (and your future baby's) body.

So here are a few suggestions on how you can reduce your (and your future baby's) exposure to "dumb fats":

- **Get no more than 30 percent of your total daily calories from fat, and no more than 5 percent from saturated fat.** For a 2,000-calorie diet, this translates to no more than 600 calories, or 67 grams, of total fat per day, and no more than 100 calories or 11 grams of saturated fat per day. Considering that a Burger King Whopper with cheese has 64 grams of total fat and 30 grams of saturated fat, and that a scoop of Ben and Jerry's Chunky Monkey Ice Cream in a chocolate-dipped waffle cone contains 30 grams of saturated fat, you actually have to work pretty hard to keep your exposure to dumb fats below the limit.

- **Go non-fat on dairy.** You can reduce the amount of saturated fat in your diet by cutting back on butter, cream, whole milk, yogurt, and especially cheese made from whole milk. If you like dairy products, go non-fat if you can. If you don't like the taste, try mixing non-fat and low-fat milk for one week. This might help transition your taste buds to non-fat. Eat cheese and other dairy products made from part-skim milk.

- **Minimize red meat and unskinned poultry.** You should also cut back on red meat and unskinned poultry to reduce your intake of saturated fats. Also minimize the use of coconut and palm oils, the only two oils with high concentrations of saturated fats. If you are going to eat chicken, choose drug-free, hormone-free, free-range chicken and remove the skin and fat before cooking. If you are going to eat beef, choose the leanest cut of hormone-free beef from free-range, grass-fed cattle.

- **Avoid cooking with polyunsaturated vegetable oils** (e.g., safflower, sunflower, sesame, corn, soy, cottonseed) and products made from them as much as you can. Heating turns them into *trans* fats and increases oxidation. Olive oil should be your principal dietary oil, but it also has a relatively lower smoke point and is therefore not suitable for stir-frying or deep-frying. As an alternative, you can use organic, expeller-pressed canola oil in moderation as cooking oil.

- **Avoid deep-fried foods in restaurants.** Do not eat deep-fried foods in restaurants, especially in fast-food restaurants. If you deep-fry foods at home (which you are better off not doing much of), throw out the oil after cooking each time rather than saving it for reuse.
- **Substitute natural vegetable oil spreads for butter and margarine.** Avoid butter, margarine, and vegetable shortening and products made from *trans* fats and partially hydrogenated oils. Substitute with non-dairy, *trans* fat-free spreads made from natural vegetable oils.
- **Go *trans* fat-free and avoid partially hydrogenated oils.** Avoid as much as you can all products containing *trans* fats and partially hydrogenated oils of any kind. Read food labels carefully; some *trans* fat-free products may contain higher amounts of saturated fats for taste, so be careful what you buy.

Now that you know about what smart fats to eat and what dumb fats to avoid, let's turn our attention to protein.

7. EAT HIGH-QUALITY PROTEINS

Protein comes from two sources—animals and plants.

Animal sources of protein include meat from cows, pigs, sheep, chicken and other poultry, fish and shellfish, eggs (mostly from chickens), and milk (mostly from cows) and products derived from it. They are considered "complete" proteins because they contain all the essential amino acids that the body cannot make on its own and must obtain from the food we eat. They are also rich in several micronutrients, including iron, vitamin B12, and zinc, that are not easily obtained from a plant-based diet. Thus animal protein provides all the essential amino acids and important micronutrients that your future baby will use as building blocks for growth and development.

There are, however, two major problems with animal protein. First, most animal meat comes with lots of saturated fat. Beef is the worst—in most cuts, more than half of their fat content is saturated fat, and even in the leanest cuts, 40 percent of their total fat is saturated fat. Pig fat, or lard, has 41 percent saturated fat. Even chicken has 30 percent saturated fat, mostly under the skin and external to the muscles. Chicken wings and thighs have a lot more saturated fat than breasts and legs.

Second, most animal meat is now contaminated; some of the contaminants are known reproductive toxins. As discussed earlier in the chapter, dioxins are potent endocrine disruptors that can interfere with fetal brain and immune development. Dioxins accumulate in animal fat; the fattier the cut of meat you eat, the more dioxins you accumulate in your body fat and the more dioxins your future baby will be exposed to. The current animal husbandry practice of feeding animal fat to cows, pigs, and other animals to fatten them up certainly does not help the matter. In 2003, a panel of scientists convened by the Institute of Medicine concluded that the only practical way to reduce dioxins exposure in fetuses and breast-feeding infants is by minimizing girls' and young women's intake of dioxins during the years before pregnancy. This means reducing fat intake in foods and milk (e.g., eating less red meat and drinking low-fat milk). The panel of experts also urged the government to do something about curtailing the recycling of dioxins that occurs when contaminated animal fats are included as ingredients in animal feed.

Fish used to be considered "brain food" for the developing fetus because of its high quality protein and high DHA content, but growing concerns over methylmercury contamination have led the FDA/EPA advisory to limit fish and seafood consumption for pregnant women, women who might become pregnant, nursing mothers, and young children (see Box 2.2). Methylmercury can interfere with your baby's brain development even at the earliest stages, by disrupting normal migration patterns of neurons.

box 2.2: what you need to know about mercury in fish and shellfish

2004 Environmental Protection Agency/Food and Drug Administration Fish Advisory for:

- Women who might become pregnant
- Women who are pregnant
- Nursing mothers
- Young children

1. Do not eat **shark, swordfish, king mackerel, or tilefish** because they contain high levels of mercury.
2. Eat up to **12 oz a week** of a variety of fish and shellfish that are lower in mercury.
   - Five of the most commonly eaten fish that are low in mercury are shrimp, canned light tuna, salmon, pollock, and catfish.
   - Albacore ("white") tuna, another commonly eaten fish, has more mercury than canned light tuna. So, when choosing your two meals of fish and shellfish, you may only eat up to 6 oz of albacore tuna per week.
3. **Check local advisories** about the safety of fish caught by family and friends in your local lakes, rivers, and coastal areas. If no advice is available, eat only up to 6 oz per week of fish you catch from local waters, but don't consume any other fish during that week.

Farm-raised fish is of particular concern because they have been found to contain higher levels of methylmercury, PCBs, dioxins, and organo-chlorine pesticides than wild fish. In my opinion, farmed fish should be consumed infrequently, or avoided altogether if you are getting ready to get pregnant. Many shellfish are scavengers and bottom-feeders and live in places where toxic pollutants accumulate. Their consumption before and during pregnancy should also be minimized.

If you eat animal protein, try to reduce your intake of saturated fat and environmental toxicants. Here are a few suggestions:

- **How much protein do I need?** This is somewhat controversial. The Institute of Medicine recommends that healthy adults get a *minimum* of 0.8 grams of protein for every kilogram body weight per day. That's about 51 grams for a 140-lb adult. Some health experts argue that in order to reduce your intake of carbs to 40 to 50 percent of your total daily calories, you will need to increase your intake of protein to 20 to 25 percent of your total daily calories (in order to keep your daily fat intake to under 30 percent). On a 2,000-calorie diet, this means you need to eat 100 to 125 grams of protein a day. Too much protein (in excess of 25 percent), however, has been linked to increased risk for premature birth and neonatal death. I think it's best to stay between **50 to 100 grams of protein a day.**

  Generally speaking, an ounce of meat or fish has approximately seven grams of protein; thus a four-ounce hamburger patty, chicken breast, or salmon fillet contains about 28 grams of protein. Here are a few more examples of high-protein foods and the amounts of protein (in grams) they contain:
  1 large egg—6 grams
  1 cup of milk—8 grams
  ½ cup of cottage cheese—15 grams
  1 cup of yogurt—8–12 grams
  ½ cup of tofu—20 grams
  1 cup of soy milk—6–10 grams
  ½ cup of most beans (black, pinto, lentils, etc.)—
      7–10 grams

½ cup of soybeans—14 grams

2 tsp of peanut butter—8 grams

¼ cup of almonds—8 grams

¼ cup of pumpkin seeds—19 grams

¼ cup of flax seeds—8 grams

- **Reduce consumption of beef.** If you eat beef, choose the leanest cut (which usually has "loin" or "round" contained within the description, such as sirloin, tenderloin, eye of round, or top round) of hormone-free beef from free-range, grass-fed cattle. Avoid cuts that are graded "prime" or "choice," or cuts that are well-marbled (e.g., "rib-eye"), because they contain the highest amounts of saturated fats (which, unfortunately, are what make a steak tender and juicy).

- **Drink non-fat milk (or low-fat) and eat cheese made from skim milk.** If you drink cow milk, choose non-fat (or 1 percent low-fat) or pasteurized, organic (hormone-free, antibiotic-free, pesticide-free) milk from free-range, grass-fed cows. If you like cheese or other dairy products, use those made from low-fat part-skim milk.

- **De-skin poultry.** If you eat chicken, choose drug-free, hormone-free, free-range chicken and remove the skin and fat. Or choose healthier poultry (e.g., turkey) with less saturated fat. You can make turkey even healthier by taking off the skin before eating.

- **Eat DHA eggs.** If you eat eggs, use omega–3 fortified, organically raised eggs from free-range chickens. Quality proteins are found in the egg whites.

- **Choose wild coldwater fish over farm-raised fish.** If you eat fish and shellfish, follow the EPA/FDA advisory. Avoid shark, swordfish, king mackerel, and tilefish. Do not eat more than 12 oz of fish per week. Choose wild ocean fish (e.g., Alaskan wild salmon) over farm-raised fish, and reduce consumption of shellfish, to avoid exposure to methylmercury, PCBs, dioxins, and other toxic environmental pollutants.

Plant protein comes primarily from nuts and seeds, particularly seeds of legumes (beans, peas, and lentils). There are several advantages to getting your protein from plant sources. They contain healthier fat (with the exceptions of coconut and palm nuts), as well as many micronutrients and fiber that are missing from animal protein sources. They are lower on the food chain and thus accumulate less environmental toxicants. They are cheaper and less perishable, and for some of you, their consumption may raise less ethical problems and environmental concerns than eating animal protein.

If you are a vegetarian but eat eggs or drink milk, nutritional deficiency is usually not a problem. Just follow the recommendations in this chapter, and you will be well prepared for pregnancy.

If you are a vegan, follow these guidelines to help you get ready for pregnancy.

- **Go see a registered dietician.** This is especially important if you are underweight. A registered dietician can help you create a vegan diet with adequate calories, protein, and other nutrients in preparation for pregnancy. Be sure to find someone who is knowledgeable about pregnancy and respectful of the vegan way.
- **Eat a variety of plant proteins.** Pay attention to quality because the quality of plant proteins varies. For example, soy protein can meet protein needs as effectively as animal protein, whereas wheat protein eaten alone contains 50 percent less usable protein than animal protein. Cereals tend to be low in lysine, an essential amino acid. Beans and soy have a much higher lysine content. Thus, the best thing to do to make sure you are getting complete proteins from a vegan diet is to eat a variety of plant proteins. Some dieticians have suggested combining proteins (e.g., rice with beans); these complementary proteins can be eaten over the course of a day and do not need be consumed in the same meal.
- **Eat smart fats.** You can get adequate amounts of smart fats by

increasing your intake of alpha-linolenic acid (LnA) from tofu, soybeans, walnuts, flaxseed, and their oils, or simply by taking DHA supplements made from microalgae.

- **Make sure you get enough iron.** Plant sources of iron include tofu, lentils, kidney and garbanzo beans, pumpkin and squash seeds, cream of wheat and oatmeal, spinach, apricots, and mushrooms. Plant foods contain only non-heme iron, which is not absorbed as well as heme iron from animal sources; thus iron intake for vegans needs to be twice that of non-vegans because of lower bioavailability of iron from a plant-based diet. Absorption of non-heme iron is inhibited by calcium, phytate in teas, coffee, cocoa, and fiber, so don't drink coffee or tea with your meals. Absorption is enhanced by vitamin C, so eating fruits and vegetables can increase your iron absorption from plant sources.

- **Make sure you get enough vitamin B12.** Look for cereals or veggie "meat" fortified with B12, or take a multivitamin supplement that includes an adequate amount of B12 (2.6 micrograms a day).

- **Pay attention to other micronutrients.** Zinc deficiency can be avoided by ensuring adequate intake of tofu, legumes, nuts and seeds, and fortified cereals, and reducing simultaneous intake of phytate. Calcium and vitamin D deficiency can be prevented by consuming adequate amounts of fortified cereal and soymilk, tofu, almonds, figs, oranges and orange juice, collard greens, and turnip greens. There are plenty of vegan foods that provide a good amount of riboflavin, including asparagus, bananas, beans, broccoli, figs, kale, lentils, peas, seeds, sesame tahini, sweet potatoes, tofu, tempeh, wheat germ, and enriched bread. All preformed vitamin A comes from animal sources, and so vegans need to ensure adequate intake of vegetables rich in beta-carotene, which then gets converted in the body to vitamin A. Iodine deficiency is not a problem if you eat plenty of sea vegetables (e.g.,

seaweed), or use one-half teaspoon of iodized table salt
daily.

In sum, you can get complete protein from a plant-based diet, but
only if you eat a variety of plant proteins and pay attention to meeting
your daily energy and micronutrient requirements, particularly iron, vitamin B12, calcium, and zinc.

8. EAT A RAINBOW OF FRUITS AND VEGETABLES

Carbohydrates, fats, and proteins make up the macronutrients, while vitamins, minerals, and phytochemicals make up the micronutrients. Micronutrients are critically important for fetal development. For example,
maternal vitamin B9 (folic acid) and B12 deficiencies have been linked
to fetal neural tube defects, and deficiencies in B-vitamins, vitamin K,
magnesium, copper, and zinc have also been linked to other birth defects. In animal studies, maternal zinc deprivation has also been shown
to cause immune deficiency in the offspring. Some phytochemicals contain powerful antioxidants that can neutralize the oxygen radicals that
cause general oxidative stress—the primary force behind inflammation.

How do you ensure that your future baby will get adequate amounts
of micronutrients? One simple answer—get into a habit of eating a rainbow of fruits and vegetables. With few exceptions, you can get almost all
the vitamins, minerals, and phytochemicals you and your baby need by
eating a variety of fruits and vegetables. The exceptions are vitamin B12
(meat, seafood, and milk), vitamin D (cereals, seafood, and milk), iodine
(iodized salt, breads, seafood, and milk), phosphorous (beef and milk), and
selenium (whole grains, beef, and seafood).

Here are my recommendations for choosing fruits and vegetables:

- **Eat five a day.** You should eat five servings of fruits and
  vegetables a day.
- **Think ROYGBIV.** In choosing your fruits and vegetables,

think about the colors of the rainbow. Get into the habit of shopping for your fruits and vegetables by colors. Here are some fruits and vegetables that will give you the biggest bang for your buck.

- **Think Red.** Red fruits and vegetables are packed with antioxidants. Most red fruits contain anthocyanins, which give them their red color; red bell peppers and beets also contain beta-carotene. Tomatoes are packed with lycopene, and cranberries with flavonoids. The six red fruits and vegetables with the highest antioxidant capacity are strawberries, raspberries, red grapes, pink grapefruit, beets, and red bell peppers. Honorable mentions include cherries and pomegranates.

- **Think Orange.** Orange tops the list of orange fruits and vegetables in terms of its antioxidant capacity. In addition to beta-carotene (which gives orange foods its color), it also contains potent antioxidants, cryptoxanthin, and flavonoids. Orange is also loaded with vitamin B1 (thiamin), B9 (folic acid), and vitamin C. Other great sources of beta-carotene include apricots, orange bell peppers, carrots, oranges, papayas, peaches, sweet potatoes, and yams. Honorable mentions include cantaloupes, peaches, mangoes, and pumpkins.

- **Think Yellow.** Corn tops the list of yellow fruits and vegetables in terms of its antioxidant capacity. It is packed with both lutein and zeaxanthin. The latter is an antioxidant that gives these vegetables their yellow color. Honorable mentions include yellow bell pepper, squash, banana, lemon, pineapple, plantain, and star fruit.

- **Think Green.** There are plenty of green fruits and vegetables to choose from, including dark, leafy greens such as spinach, kale, collards, Brussels sprouts, and cruciferous vegetables such as broccoli, cauliflower, and cabbage, as well as other fruits and vegetables such as green beans, peas, avocadoes, kiwifruits, lime, green grapes, and green apples. Generally speaking, dark, leafy greens are packed with the antioxidant lutein, while cruciferous vegetables are packed with super antioxidant indoles and glucosinolates. Spinach and broccoli deserve special mention because they are rich in magnesium, manganese, vitamins B2 (riboflavin), B9 (folic acid), and vitamin K. Spinach is also full of iron, vitamins A and E, while broccoli is full of calcium, chromium, and vitamin C.

- **Think Blue, Indigo, and Violet:** Prunes, raisins, blueberries, and plums top the list of blue, indigo, and violet fruits and vegetables in terms of their antioxidant capacity. Prunes and raisins also offer more dietary fiber per serving than any other fruits. Honorable mentions include açaí, blackberries, purple grapes, purple cabbage, and eggplant.

- **Buy organic and wash thoroughly.** Some fruits and vegetables consistently carry much higher levels of pesticides than others, even after washing. The Environmental Working Group (EWG) has come up with the "dirty dozen" of fruits and vegetables with the highest pesticide load, with peaches topping the list (worst):

1. Peaches
2. Apples
3. Sweet bell peppers
4. Celery
5. Nectarines
6. Strawberries
7. Cherries
8. Lettuce
9. Grapes—imported
10. Pears
11. Spinach
12. Potatoes

In contrast, onions, avocados, frozen sweet corn and peas, pineapples, mangoes, asparagus, kiwis, bananas, cabbage, broccoli, and eggplant generally have minimal pesticide residue and therefore do not need to be organic. Regardless of what you buy, wash or immerse in clean water thoroughly just before preparation or eating; scrub with a brush when appropriate (even if they are "pre-washed"—see Chapter 5 on food safety).

9. TAKE A DAILY MULTIVITAMIN CONTAINING FOLIC ACID

Taking an adequate amount of folic acid daily is probably one of the best things you can do to prepare yourself for pregnancy. Folic acid is required for DNA synthesis; folic acid deficiency just before or during early pregnancy has been linked to birth defects, in particular neural tube defects (mostly spina bifida and anencephaly). In four studies involving over 6,000 women who were randomized to receive folic acid supplements versus a placebo, folic acid supplementation just before and during early pregnancy was associated with an average 72 percent reduction in the risk of neural tube defects. Folic acid intake that began four weeks after conception showed no benefit, probably because the neural tube was already completely formed. These findings led the Centers for Disease Control and Prevention (CDC) to recommend in 1992 that **all women of childbearing age who are capable of becoming pregnant should consume 400 micrograms of folic acid every day.**

While a number of fruits and vegetables contain an abundance of folic acid (e.g., oranges, asparagus, broccoli, spinach, beets, and romaine lettuce), the natural form of folic acid is not as well absorbed as the synthetic form. Therefore, since 1996, the FDA has required that all grain products be fortified with synthetic folic acid; while this requirement has significantly raised the blood level of this vitamin in the U.S. population, for many women both their dietary intake and blood levels of folic acid are still too low (especially if they are on a low-carb diet). I usually don't like to push pills, but a daily multivitamin with folic acid is one supplement I strongly recommend that you take if you are getting ready to get pregnant.

You can take folic acid by itself, or as part of a multivitamin. Besides folic acid, deficiencies in other B-vitamins, vitamin K, magnesium, copper, and zinc have also been linked to birth defects. Several minerals, such as iodine, choline, and zinc, may also play critical roles in fetal brain development. Selenium and manganese are needed by the body's enzymes that destroy free radicals. One recent study found that women who took a multivitamin *before* pregnancy were half as likely to deliver preterm as women who did not. For all these reasons, I would recommend that you take a daily multivitamin containing at least 400 micrograms of folic acid. The following table (Table 2.2) summarizes the recommended daily intake (from both food sources and supplements) for vitamins and minerals before and during pregnancy.

Make sure you are meeting the recommended daily intake for these micronutrients. Several national surveys found more than half of pregnant women failed to meet their recommended daily intake for iron, iodine, magnesium, zinc, vitamins A, B6, B9, E, and K, and a substantial proportion did not get adequate amounts of calcium, vitamins B1, B2, B3, and C from food sources. For these women, taking a daily multivitamin before and during pregnancy is a good insurance policy.

Here are some tips for taking multivitamins:

- **In choosing a multivitamin**, make sure the multivitamin you choose meets your nutritional needs. For example, if you are a vegan, you need to make sure that the multivitamin you choose contains adequate amounts of iron and B12 (along with calcium, vitamin D, phosphorous, iodine, and zinc) to make up for any dietary deficiencies.
- **Get adequate folic acid.** Make sure the multivitamin you take contains at least **400 micrograms** of folic acid. Most

table 2.2: recommended daily intake of micronutrients before & during pregnancy

Micronutrient	Recommended Daily Intake Before Pregnancy	Recommended Daily Intake During Pregnancy
Calcium	1,000 mg/d	1,000 mg/d
Copper	900 µg/d	1,000 µg/d
Iodine	150 µg/d	220 µg/d
Iron	18 mg/d	27 mg/d
Magnesium	310 mg/d	350 mg/d
Manganese	1.8 mg/d	2.0 mg/d
Molybdenum	45 mg/d	50 mg/d
Phosphorus	700 mg/d	700 mg/d
Selenium	55 mg/d	60 µg/d
Zinc	8 mg/d	11 mg/d
Vitamin A	700 ug/d	770 µg/d
Vitamin B1 (Thiamin)	1.1 mg/d	1.4 mg/d
Vitamin B2 (Riboflavin)	1.1 mg/d	1.4 mg/d
Vitamin B3 (Niacin)	14 mg/d	18 mg/d
Vitamin B4 (Choline)	425 mg/d	450 mg/d
Vitamin B5 (Panththenic Acid)	5 mg/d	6 mg/d
Vitamin B6 (Pyridoxine)	1.3 mg/d	1.9 mg/d
Vitamin B7 (Biotin)	30 ug/d	30 ug/d
Vitamin B9 (Folate)	400 ug/d	600 µg/d
Vitamin B12 (Cobalamine)	2.4 ug/d	2.6 µg/d
Vitamin C	75 mg/d	85 mg/d
Vitamin D (Calciferol)	5 ug/d	5 µg/d
Vitamin E (alpha-Tocopherol)	15 mg/d	15 mg/d
Vitamin K	90 ug/d	90 µg/d

multivitamins come with 800 or 1,000 micrograms of folic acid, which are okay to take. You should avoid taking too much folic acid (more than 1,000 micrograms per day) unless directed by your doctor to do so; too much folic acid can, in rare cases, mask symptoms of pernicious anemia or vitamin B12 deficiency. However, if you have had a prior pregnancy affected by neural tube defect, then you should take 4,000 micrograms of folic acid a day (ten times the amounts recommended for women without such a history).

- **Avoid excess.** More isn't always better. Some vitamins and minerals are toxic in high doses for women and their developing babies. Examples are iron, chromium, selenium, and vitamins A and D. Large doses of vitamin A (in excess of 10,000 IU) and vitamin D (in excess of 4,000 IU) can cause birth defects. Large doses of vitamin C can interfere with vitamin B12 absorption; large doses of vitamin B6 can interfere with vitamin B2 absorption, and large doses of vitamin D and E can interfere with vitamin A absorption (and vice versa). Bottom line—avoid excess; don't take more than you have to.

  For vitamin A, it is preferable to choose a vitamin supplement that has all or the vast majority of its vitamin A in the form of beta-carotene. The body can form vitamin A from beta-carotene as needed, and beta-carotene is not toxic even at high levels of intake.

- **When is the best time to take your multivitamin?** Morning or evening? It really doesn't matter when you take it, as long as you can be consistent about taking it. With or without food? Some vitamins (e.g., fat-soluble vitamins) and minerals are better absorbed with food; some are better on an empty stomach. I usually recommend my patients take their multivitamin with food simply because several vitamins and minerals, such as B-vitamins, iron, and zinc, can cause nausea and stomach upset when taken on an empty stomach.

- **Do's and don'ts with iron supplements.** If you are taking iron supplements to correct anemia, here are some do's and don'ts. Vitamin C enhances iron absorption, so you should wash down your iron pill with juice. Calcium can interfere with iron absorption. If you are taking a multivitamin that contains both iron and calcium, you will lose a little bit of iron but will still absorb enough. If you are taking large doses of iron and calcium supplement, take the iron at least two hours apart from the calcium supplement and on an empty stomach, if tolerable. Tannin in tea and coffee, phytate in some grains including soy, and phosphates in cola drinks interfere with iron absorption. Tea reduces iron absorption by 60 percent, and coffee decreases iron uptake by 50 percent; therefore, don't take your iron supplement or multivitamin with tea or coffee.
- **Healthy nutrition comes first.** A multivitamin supplement is just that—a supplement; it does not replace healthy nutrition. A standard multivitamin supplement doesn't come close to making up for an unhealthy diet. Most multivitamins provide about 20 or so vitamins and minerals known to maintain health, a mere shadow of what's available from eating plenty of fruits, vegetables, and whole grains. Instead, think of a daily multivitamin supplement as a sort of nutritional safety net.

You can go to the March of Dimes website at www.marchofdimes.org or the Harvard School of Public Health website at www.hsph.harvard .edu for more information on choosing a multivitamin that is right for you before and during pregnancy.

10. EAT MORE BRAIN FOODS AND LESS TOXIC FOODS

Some foods are packed with nutrients. These nutrient-dense foods are sometimes called "superfoods," a concept popularized by such books as *Superfoods Rx*, by ophthalmologist Dr. Steven Pratt and his co-writer Kathy Matthews, and the *Perricone Promise*, by dermatologist Dr.

Nicholas Perricone. These books cast a spotlight on a dozen or more foods that can ward off conditions ranging from macular degeneration to skin wrinkles. No, these superfoods are not the nutritional equivalent of a fountain of youth, and will not save you from cancer, heart disease, diabetes, and every other scourge of good health, as some superfoods enthusiasts and manufacturers would like you to believe. But that doesn't mean superfoods should be dismissed. They still deliver good nutrition— many made the list because they are antioxidant powerhouses that can reduce oxidative stress and inflammation; others made the list because they contain complex carbohydrates with high fiber and low glycemic load and can improve insulin sensitivity; still others made the list because they deliver high-quality protein without a whole lot of saturated fats.

To help get you ready for pregnancy, I came up with a list of "brain foods" that are designed to counteract some of the biggest threats to a healthy pregnancy in the typical American diet—too much sugar, too much saturated fats, and too much inflammation. These brain foods include beans, eggs, nuts and seeds, olive oil, Alaskan wild salmon, yogurt and kefir, whole grains, spinach, collards, kale, broccoli, prunes, raisins, blueberries, oranges, red bell peppers, and tomatoes. In preparation for pregnancy, you should eat more brain foods as part of a balanced diet.

Some foods contain high levels of chemicals that can affect your future baby's development. And although you are not pregnant right now, toxicants like methylmercury and dioxins can accumulate in your body and affect your future pregnancy. Other foods put you at risk for an infection that may persist into pregnancy, or they may cause an infection if you consume them during pregnancy. Still other foods can cause wear and tear (allostatic overload) on your body's metabolic functions, creating an internal milieu of high sugar, high fat, insulin resistance, and chronic inflammation. I called them "toxic foods" because they are unhealthful and can cause harm to your future baby. They include swordfish, shark, king mackerel, and tilefish, soft cheeses and unpasteurized milk, hot dogs, luncheon meats, deli meats, raw or smoked seafood, raw or undercooked meat, unwashed vegetables, raw vegetable sprouts,

unpasteurized juices, liver, saturated fats, *trans* fats, partially hydrogenated oils, added sugars including high-fructose corn syrup, refined flour,
and herbal preparations. To get yourself ready for pregnancy, you should
avoid these toxic foods as much as possible.

Because these foods are so important for making a smart and healthy
baby, I will devote the entire next chapter to discussing these brain foods
and toxic foods in greater detail.

brain foods and toxic foods

"Let food be thy medicine," the ancient Greek physician Hippocrates declared over 2,000 years ago. *"And thy medicine shall be thy food."* In this chapter I will feature ten brain foods for making a smart and healthy baby, and ten toxic foods you should avoid before and during pregnancy.

Let's start with brain foods. First, let me say a word about how these brain foods were chosen. There are certainly more than ten brain foods; indeed, there is an abundance of foods that are good for you and your baby before and during pregnancy. I chose to spotlight these ten brain foods because they represent the cream of the crop. They are some of the most nutrient-dense foods per calorie of food intake; they deliver the highest quality protein, the best glycemic profile, the greatest amounts of smart fats and the lowest amounts of dumb fats, and the most antioxidant capacity. These brain foods were chosen specifically to counteract some of the biggest threats to a healthy pregnancy in the typical American diet— too much sugar, too much dumb fats, and too much inflammation.

These ten brain foods were also chosen because they are safe. A number of popular "superfoods" did not make my list because of concerns about their safety during pregnancy. Despite their high antioxidant capacity, raw sprouts (e.g., alfalfa) were kept off my list because of concerns about foodborne illnesses stemming from the bacteria Salmonella and *E. coli*. Herbs and spices were kept off my list because there is still too much we don't know about their actions in early pregnancy. Instead of recommending exotic superfoods whose safety during pregnancy has not been established, I stuck with common foods known to be safe for pregnancy.

Lastly, these ten brain foods were chosen because they are widely available, affordable, and accessible. Indeed, açaí and pomegranate are power packs of antioxidants, but açaí is hard to find (and even harder to pronounce), and pomegranates and pomegranate juice are just too expensive to buy on a regular basis for many of my patients. Instead, I went with common, inexpensive foods such as beans, eggs, nuts, yogurt, whole grains, spinach, prunes, and red bell peppers that I don't think we eat enough of in the typical American diet. These brain foods were chosen to give you the biggest bang for your buck.

top ten brain foods

Here is my top-ten list of brain foods for making smart and healthy babies:

Brain food #1: Legumes
Brain food #2: Eggs
Brain food #3: Nuts and seeds
Brain food #4: Olive oil
Brain food #5: Alaskan wild salmon
Brain food #6: Yogurt and kefir
Brain food #7: Whole grains
Brain food #8: Spinach, collards, kale, and broccoli
Brain food #9: Prunes, raisins, and blueberries
Brain food #10: Oranges, red bell peppers, and tomatoes

I will now describe the health benefits of each of these ten brain foods, for you and your future baby.

BRAIN FOOD #1: LEGUMES

Legumes are a family of pod-bearing plants that include beans, peas, and lentils. Legumes top my list of brain foods because they offer all of the following:

- **High quality protein.** Beans, peas, and lentils are an excellent source of protein. When combined with rice, barley, or oats, they offer all the essential amino acids your body (and your future baby) needs.
- **Complex carbohydrates with low glycemic load.** Beans are also high in complex carbohydrates with low glycemic load. However, not all beans are created equal. The glycemic indices of garbanzo beans, kidney beans, and navy beans run between 50 and 80, while those of lima beans and dried kidney beans run between 30 and 50, and that of soybeans is under 30.
- **Low-fat.** Most beans are low-fat. While many contain a small amount of omega–6 fatty acids, soybeans are rich in omega–3 fatty acids, which are quite anti-inflammatory and play an important role in your future baby's brain and visual development.
- **High fiber.** Beans offer lots of fiber; one cup of cooked beans can provide as much as 15 grams of fiber.
- **Folic acid.** Dry beans are an excellent source of folic acid. One cup of cooked dry beans provides about 264 micrograms of folate. Periconceptional consumption of folate has been shown to substantially reduce the risk of neural tube defects in babies.
- **Antioxidants.** Beans contain flavonoids and flavonals, which are potent antioxidants. They soak up oxygen radicals and protect your body against oxidative stress and chronic inflammation. Their antioxidant activities are 50 times greater than vitamin E. They are also among the richest food sources of saponins, chemicals that help prevent undesirable genetic mutations.

Here is some more food for thought about legumes:

- **Which is the healthiest of all beans?** Because so many beans are beneficial, it is hard to narrow it down to just one. The cream of the crop includes black beans, kidney beans, pinto beans, navy beans, lima beans, and soybeans.
- **What you need to know about soybeans.** Soy isoflavones can potentially cause fetal goiter in women who are iodine deficient, so make sure you are getting enough iodine (150 micrograms a day) from food sources (e.g., iodized salt) or a multivitamin. Soybean products contain a plant estrogen called genistein, which can act like an endocrine disruptor (see Chapter 6). While soy consumption has not been linked to birth defects in humans, it may be advisable to limit your daily soy consumption to no more than 30 grams (approximately one ounce) before and during pregnancy, and for your man to minimize his soy consumption starting three months before attempting to conceive.
- **Peas and lentils.** Legumes also include peas and lentils. Peas and lentils offer many of the same health benefits as beans (they provide high quality protein and low-glycemic carbohydrates, are low in fat, and are rich in antioxidants). Lentils cook quickly and do not require pre-soaking; they are a mainstay of Indian cuisine. Hummus, made from pureed chickpeas and sesame and flavored with fresh lemon juice, olive oil, and garlic, can be served as a tasty appetizer.

I recommend eating ½ to 1 cup of legumes a day before and during pregnancy.

BRAIN FOOD #2: EGGS
Eggs are a nutrient-dense food that offers all of the following benefits:

- **Complete protein.** Egg white is pure protein of the highest quality; it contains all the essential amino acids your body (and your future baby) needs, without all the saturated fats that typically accompany animal proteins (an egg has only 2 grams of saturated fatty acids, whereas a quarter-pound hamburger has four times the amount of saturated fats).

- **Smart fat.** Egg yolk is high in essential fatty acids. Recently a new egg has appeared on the American market, one that is high in the omega–3 fatty acid DHA. This "designer egg" comes from hens fed a micro-algae diet high in omega–3 content; the omega–3 fatty acids get stored in the yolk. You can find these DHA-fortified eggs in many high-end supermarkets; look for "DHA" or "Omega–3" on the packaging, and compare product labels to see how much DHA each egg contains. These eggs are a little more expensive but totally worth the price. They offer an important source of omega–3 fatty acids without worries about mercury contamination associated with seafood or fish oil.

- **Vitamins and minerals.** Eggs are an important source of vitamins and minerals including vitamin A, vitamins B2, B6, B7, B9, D, and E, calcium, iron, chromium, phosphorous, and zinc.

- **Low calorie.** One egg can pack in 6 grams of protein (with only 2 grams of saturated fats), 300 milligrams of DHA, and all those vitamins and minerals into a mere 75 calories. Eggs epitomize a nutrient-dense power pack.

- **What about all the cholesterol?** Eggs have gotten a bum rap because of their high cholesterol content. It turns out that most people's cholesterol levels probably have more to do with their dietary intake of saturated fats and carbohydrates (which in excess get converted into fats) than their dietary intake of cholesterol. Eating an egg a day should not raise your cholesterol much.

Here are a few food safety tips for eggs:

- **Egg safety tips.** Remember that eggs can carry Salmonella bacteria, which can make you very sick. To avoid illness from eggs, you should never eat raw eggs. Beware that some home-made Caesar dressings, mayonnaise, homemade ice cream or custards, and Hollandaise sauces may be made with raw eggs (commercially manufactured ice cream, dressings and eggnog, and Hollandaise sauce or dressings served in restaurants should be made with pasteurized eggs and do not increase the risk of Salmonella). You should buy only eggs kept in a refrigerator or refrigerator case. Open the carton and make sure that the eggs are clean and the shells are not cracked. Refrigerate promptly in their original carton and use them within three weeks for best quality. Thorough cooking is perhaps the most important step in making sure eggs are safe. Cook eggs until both the yolk and the white are firm. Scrambled eggs should not be runny. Casseroles and other dishes containing eggs should be cooked to 160°F (72°C) (use a thermometer to be sure). You should serve cooked eggs (including hard-boiled eggs) and egg-containing dishes immediately; they should not sit out for more than two hours. Leftover egg dishes that are promptly refrigerated can be kept for three to four days; make sure they are thoroughly reheated to 165°F (74°C) before serving. You can find more information about food safety for eggs on the Food and Drug Administration website at www.fda.gov.

I recommend eating one DHA-fortified egg, from drug- and hormone-free, uncaged chickens, at least every other day.

BRAIN FOOD #3: NUTS AND SEEDS

Nuts and seeds are great for snacking and a lot healthier than candies, potato chips, or most other snack foods. You can also add a tablespoon of chopped almonds to your oatmeal or walnuts to your salad to get more nuts in your daily intake. Nuts and seeds offer all the following health benefits:

- **High quality protein.** Some nuts (almonds, walnuts, and hazelnuts) and seeds (sesame, sunflower) are particularly rich in protein. Most nuts are high in arginine, an amino acid that is a precursor to nitric oxide. Nitric oxide is thought to play major roles in the processes of human reproduction, including ovulation, implantation, pregnancy maintenance, labor, and delivery.

- **Smart fat.** Several nuts, seeds, and their oils contain omega–3 fatty acids, including walnuts and walnut oil, flaxseeds and flax oil, pumpkin seeds and pumpkin seed oil. Flax oil has about 55 percent omega–3s, and walnut oil has about 10 percent omega–3s.

- **Vitamins and minerals.** Nuts are also a good source of vitamin E and folate, as well as minerals such as calcium, magnesium, potassium, and selenium. According to a national nutritional survey, most American women (more than 95 percent) do not consume sufficient amounts of vitamin E and folate during pregnancy, and a substantial proportion fail to meet the daily recommended amounts for calcium and magnesium. Snacking on nuts and seeds will add a good measure of these vitamins and minerals to your diet.

- **Antioxidants.** The coating of all nuts and seeds, such as the thin, brown papery layer coating almonds and peanuts, contains the antioxidant polyphenols (another reason to choose raw nuts and seeds in the shell, rather than processed nuts and seeds that are denuded of their coatings). Walnuts contain ellagic acid, which is a strong antioxidant also found in pomegranates and raspberries. Most nuts also contain phytic acid and phytoesterols, which can also help reduce oxidative stress and inflammation.

There are few things you need to know about nuts and seeds (before you go nuts on them):

- **What you need to know about nuts and seeds.** Nuts oxidize very quickly when exposed to light and heat. Nuts and seeds should be bought in small quantities and stored in their shells in the refrigerator. Discard any shells with cracks, and any nuts or seeds that are discolored, rubbery, moldy, shriveled, or have a rancid, stale taste. You should buy raw, natural, unsalted nuts and seeds rather than salted, oiled, or roasted ones. Once the nuts are roasted and chopped, the oils in them will oxidize quickly. If you like cooked nuts, you can dry-roast them yourself in the toaster oven or toss them in a hot skillet. Nut oils should never be heated because they are particularly susceptible to oxidation. Flax oils can be used in salad dressing; they need to be refrigerated in opaque bottles and used quickly. You can also eat freshly ground flax meal by grinding up flaxseeds (in a coffee grinder). Generally speaking, eating nuts and seeds is better than using their oils. Nut butters are also great in moderation. Try using almond, cashew, and macadamia nut butters rather than peanut butter because peanut butter has higher content of saturated fat and is more likely to contain traces of aflatoxin, a toxic metabolite produced by a mold.

- **Peanuts and allergies.** There is growing concern that if a woman consumes peanuts (or peanut butter) during pregnancy, her fetus may become sensitized to peanut allergens and predisposed to developing a peanut allergy in childhood. While the research is still quite inconclusive, it may be advisable for women with any type of allergy (certainly nut allergies, but also asthma, eczema, or even "hay fever") to avoid peanut consumption during pregnancy.

I recommend eating a small handful of raw, natural, unsalted, or lightly salted nuts or seeds everyday.

BRAIN FOOD #4: OLIVE OIL

Olive oil offers a great deal of health benefits before and during pregnancy:

- **Monounsaturated fat.** Olive oil has the highest content of monounsaturated fat of any of the edible oils. It contains

77 percent of a monounsaturated fatty acid called oleic acid. Unlike saturated fats, which can increase your LDL cholesterol and cause oxidative stress and inflammation in the placenta and possibly fetal organs, as a monounsaturated fat olive oil actually decreases your LDL cholesterol while raising your HDL (good) cholesterol. And unlike polyunsaturated fats, which have many reactive sites and can oxidize easily to cause oxidative stress and inflammation, as a monounsaturated fat (which has only one reactive site) olive oil is very stable. Thus olive oil is considered one of the most powerful anti-inflammatory foods in existence. Olive oil does not need to be refrigerated but should be stored in a dark, cool place.

- **Antioxidants.** Olive oil also contains antioxidants, including beta-carotene, and polyphenols, including hydroxytyrosol, with powerful antioxidant and anti-inflammatory properties.
- **Cancer prevention.** Several intriguing animal studies have shown that feeding the mother a diet high in olive oil before and during pregnancy and lactation may have a protective effect against future development of breast cancer (as well as spleen and colon tumors) in the female offspring. While the studies remain to be confirmed, they raise the possibility that olive oil may have beneficial effects on fetal programming of the developing immune system.

My recommendations are to

- **Make olive oil your principal dietary oil** for all the health benefits I just described.
- **Buy extra virgin.** The best olive oil, called "extra virgin," comes from the first, gentle pressing of olives. It has the highest amounts of monounsaturated fatty acids and antioxidants. With each subsequent pressing, some fatty acids and

antioxidants are lost. Olive oils are labeled "virgin" if they are extracted by means of pressure from the millstones; heat and chemical extraction reduces much of the health benefits. Bottom line: Go virgin, extra virgin if you can.

- **Use canola oil for frying.** Olive oil has a relatively lower smoke point than most other oils and is therefore not suitable for stir-frying or deep-frying. Canola oil has the second highest content of monounsaturated fatty acids (59 percent) and is considered best for cooking and frying. Extra virgin olive oil has a strong taste, whereas canola oil has a more neutral taste, which may be more appropriate for certain dishes (e.g., Asian stir-fry).

BRAIN FOOD #5: ALASKAN WILD SALMON

I recommend Alaskan wild salmon for all the following benefits:

- **High quality protein without saturated fat**. One 4-oz fillet gives you about 28 g of high-quality, complete protein with less than 1 g of saturated fatty acids.
- **Smart fat.** One 4-oz fillet of steam or poached wild Alaskan salmon contains 830 mg of DHA and 136 mg of EPA. Recall the recommended dietary intake for DHA is 220 mg per day for non-pregnant women and 300 mg per day for pregnant women, and so two 4- to 6-oz fillets come close to covering your nutritional requirements for smart fats for the week.
- **Micronutrients.** Alaskan wild salmon is also rich in several micronutrients, including selenium, niacin, cobalamine, and, perhaps most important, astaxanthin. Astaxanthin is a potent antioxidant that gives salmon its pink color. One 4-oz fillet provides 4.5 mg of astaxanthin, with an antioxidant capacity ten times more potent than other carotenoids and 100 times stronger than vitamin E.

box 3.1: go wild on salmon

Wild salmon is a lot healthier than farm-raised salmon. Generally speaking, farm-raised salmon contains lower levels of omega–3 fatty acids and astaxanthin, and higher levels of PCBs, dioxins, methylmercury, and organochlorine pesticides. As a rule of thumb, the vast majority (greater than 99 percent) of "Atlantic salmon" available in the world's market is farmed, whereas the majority (greater than 80 percent) of "Pacific salmon" is wild-caught. I recommend Alaskan wild salmon because it is the least contaminated; it is more expensive but may be well worth the price. Canned Alaskan wild salmon may be more affordable, and has a lot less contaminants than most other canned fish. One FDA study found that the average methylmercury level of canned albacore tuna (so-called "solid white tuna") was 35 times higher than that found in canned wild salmon.

I recommend eating a 4- to 6-oz fillet of wild Alaskan salmon twice a week. This can get expensive so look for them in freeze packs or in a can for the same health benefits.

BRAIN FOOD #6: YOGURT AND KEFIR
Both yogurt and kefir are made from fermented milk. Kefir is a yogurt-like drink made from sheep, goat, cow, and soy milk, with a mildly sweet and tart taste. I recommend yogurt and kefir for all the following benefits:

- **Probiotics.** Probiotics are live organisms; when taken in adequate amounts, they confer a health benefit to the host. One probiotic organism that has been shown to confer a health benefit during pregnancy is *Lactobacillus rhamnosus* GG. A 2001 *Lancet* article showed that this strain could be

used safely in pregnant women and halved the episodes of
atopic dermatitis in their babies. Other *Lactobacillus* species
have also been shown to reduce the risk of bacterial vaginosis,
an important risk factor for preterm labor. These probiotics
work by promoting growth of normal bacteria and inhibiting
growth of pathogenic bacteria in the vagina, as well as
enhancing the actions of anti-inflammatory cytokines to
suppress local inflammation.

Not all yogurt and kefir contain probiotics; in fact, many
brands of yogurt and kefir, as well as so-called probiotic
preparations that are commercially available, have dead or
unreliable contents. In choosing yogurt and kefir, look for the
"Live Active Culture" seal on the package. The seal requires
that the product contain at least 108 viable lactic acid bacteria
per gram for refrigerated products and 107 for frozen products.
Then look for probiotics that have been proven to confer a
health benefit, such as *Lactobacillus* or *Bifidobacterium*.
Lifeway Foods Kefir contains among its ten live active cultures
Lactobacillus rhamnosus GG, and Stonyfield and Horizon
Organic Yogurts also contain several species of *Lactobacillus* as
well as *Bifidobacterium*. For probiotics from dietary supplements, try VSL#3, which contain eight active cultures,
including *Lactobacillus* and *Bifidobacterium* species, or
Culturelle, which contains *Lactobacillus rhamnosus* GG.

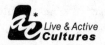

- **High-quality protein.** Yogurt and kefir are made from
  fermented milk, which contains high-quality protein (especially if made from organic milk). One 6-oz container of
  low-fat yogurt provides 7 grams of protein with only
  1 gram of saturated fat (or less if you get the non-fat variety).

- **Micronutrients.** Yogurt is also rich in many vitamins and minerals, including vitamins B2, B12, calcium, magnesium, phosphorus, and zinc. On average, one 6-oz container of low-fat yogurt of fruity variety provides more than 25 percent of recommended daily intake of calcium and phosphorous and more than 10 percent of daily value for zinc.

I recommend 6–8 oz of yogurt or kefir once or twice a day.

BRAIN FOOD #7: WHOLE GRAINS

What makes a grain whole is that it contains all three parts of the entire grain kernel—bran, germ, and endosperm. In contrast, refined grains have been milled, a process that removes the bran and germ. This is done to give grains a finer texture and improve their shelf life, but it also removes dietary fiber, iron, and many B-vitamins. Some examples of whole grain and refined grain products are:

Whole grains

- whole-wheat flour, pasta, tortilla, or bread
- bulgur (cracked wheat)
- buckwheat
- hulled whole grain barley
- whole rye
- oatmeal
- whole cornmeal
- brown, basmati, or wild rice
- popcorn

Refined grains

- white flour

(continued)

- degermed cornmeal
- white bread
- white rice
- pretzels
- grits

Most tortillas, noodles, pasta, pitas, and ready-to-eat breakfast cereals (e.g., corn flakes) are made from refined grains, though some may be made from whole grains. Read product labels to make sure that whole grain is the **first** ingredient listed.

I recommend switching to whole grains for the following reasons:

- **Low glycemic index.** Here are some side-by-side comparisons of some common whole grain foods and their refined grain counterparts with respect to their glycemic index (Table 3.1).

   Remember lower GI means lower and slower rise and fall in blood sugar and insulin, and possibly lower risk for diabetes and obesity for you and your future baby.

table 3.1: glycemic indices of whole grain and refined grain foods

Whole Grain Foods	GI	Refined Grain Foods	GI
Brown rice	55	White rice, short grain	72
100 percent whole grain bread	51	Wonder Bread Classic	73
Oatmeal	58	Grits	69
Kellogg's All Bran	51	Kellogg's Corn Flakes	84

- **High fiber.** Whole grains have high fiber content. Barley, bulgur, whole grain wheat flour, oat bran, and whole buckwheat groat are among the top 20 foods in terms of their fiber content (the others on the top 20 list are all beans, peas, and lentils). Refined white wheat flour contains 3.4 grams of dietary fiber in a cup, while a cup of whole grain wheat flour contains 14.6 grams of dietary fiber. Refined flour may be enriched with iron and a few B-vitamins (which are lost in the refining process), but fiber is usually not added back.
- **Micronutrients, including folic acid.** Most of you are well aware that fruits and vegetables are a rich source of micronutrients, but you may not realize that whole grains are often an even better source. Much of the micronutrients are found in the germ and the bran of a grain, which are lost in the refining process. Whole grain flour has two to three times higher iron, calcium, zinc, and B-vitamins than refined grain flour. As a percent of weight, whole grain flour offers 7 times the folic acid and 25 times the vitamin E as refined grain flour; enrichment does not come close to putting back in the nutrients lost in the refining process.

How do you get more whole grains in your diet? Here are some recommendations:

- Replace white bread with whole grain bread.
- Have a serving of whole grain breakfast cereal in the morning.
- Eat oatmeal with nuts or fresh fruits for breakfast.
- Can't really give up your favorite frosted cereal? Mix in some high fiber whole grain cereal as well as fresh fruit with your frosted cereal.
- Substitute half the white flour with whole-wheat flour in your regular recipes for cookies, muffins, quick breads, and pancakes.
- Add brown rice, wild rice, or barley in your vegetable soup.

Barley. I want to draw your attention to one particular whole grain: barley. Barley is loaded with fiber and micronutrients and has the lowest GIs among whole grains. One cup of pearled barley contains 31 grams of dietary fiber and 46 micrograms of folate, with a GI of only 22. Hulled barley is less processed than pearled barley, and has an even higher fiber content with a lower GI. Here are some recommendations on how to increase your daily intake of barley:

- Add barley to stews and soups or other dishes, such as risotto, to enhance texture.
- Mix barley flour with wheat flour to make breads and muffins.
- Use cracked barley or barley flakes to make hot cereal.
- Toss chilled, cooked, hulled barley into salads.

You can get more advice on how to increase whole grains and barley in your diet from the website www.healthcastle.com.

- **Read food label.** Look for the words "whole grain" **first** on the ingredient list; if they are not there, it is probably not whole grain. You can also look for the following "Whole Grain" stamps on foods that are a good or excellent source of whole grain.

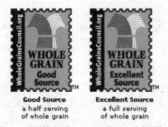

Courtesy of Oldways Preservation Trust and the Whole Grains Council (*www.wholegrainscouncil.org*).

The 2005 Dietary Guidelines for Americans, issued by the Department of Health and Human Services and the USDA, recommends that all adults eat half of their grains as whole grains—that's at least three servings a day. I'd recommend that most of the grains you eat should be whole grains—that's five to seven servings a day. On a 2,000-calorie diet, you should eat at least 100 to 150 grams of whole grains a day.

BRAIN FOOD #8: DARK GREEN VEGETABLES: SPINACH, KALE, COLLARDS, AND BROCCOLI

These are stand-outs among green foods for the following reasons:

- **Spinach.** Spinach is rich in folate; one cup of cooked spinach provides 263 micrograms of folate. It is also loaded with vitamin K; one cup of cooked spinach provides 888 micrograms of vitamin K. Popeye made us aware of the iron content of spinach, which gave him strength. One cup of cooked spinach contains 6.4 mg of non-heme iron, about a third of recommended daily allowance. However, because spinach contains oxalic acid, which interferes with absorption of non-heme iron, it should be eaten with foods containing iron absorption enhancers such as meat, orange juice (or any fruit or fruit juice with high vitamin C content), and broccoli. Spinach is also an excellent source of manganese, magnesium, calcium, potassium, vitamins A, B2, B6, C, and dietary fiber.
- **Kale and collards.** Kale and collards rank number one and two in vitamin K content; one cup of cooked kale contains 1,147 micrograms of vitamin K; one cup of cooked collard greens, 559 micrograms. They are also an excellent source of vitamins A and C and manganese. One cup of cooked collards has 118 micrograms of folate.
- **Broccoli.** Broccoli is loaded with vitamins A, C, K, folate, and dietary fiber. One cup of cooked broccoli contains 120 micrograms of vitamin A, 100 milligrams of vitamin C, 219 micrograms of vitamin K, and 168 micrograms of folate. It is also an excellent source of dietary fiber.

- **Antioxidants.** The most important reason I am recommending these green vegetables as brain foods is because of their antioxidant capacity. Among vegetables, kale tops the Oxygen Radical Absorbance Capacity (ORAC) chart, followed by spinach in second place and broccoli flowers in fourth place. They are rich in beta-carotene, lutein, and zeaxanthin. There are over 11,000 micrograms of beta-carotene in one cup of cooked spinach, over 10,000 in one cup of cooked kale, and over 9,000 in one cup of cooked collards. For lutein and zeaxanthin, kale, spinach, and collards again top the list. There are over 23,000 micrograms of lutein and zeaxanthin in one cup of cooked kale, over 20,000 in one cup of cooked spinach, and nearly 15,000 in one cup of cooked collards. One cup of cooked broccoli also has over 1,000 micrograms of beta-carotene, lutein, and zeaxanthin. Remember, antioxidants neutralize oxygen radicals and reduce oxidative stress and inflammation.

I recommend 1 to 2 cups of cooked or raw spinach, kale, collards, or broccoli at least once a day. Be sure to buy organic and wash them well if you are going to eat them raw.

BRAIN FOOD #9: DARK PURPLE FRUITS: PRUNES, RAISINS, AND BLUEBERRIES

I recommend these dark purple foods primarily for their antioxidant capacity and dietary fibers:

- **Antioxidants.** Among fruits, prunes, raisins, and blueberries top the ORAC chart, in that order. Prunes score a whopping 5,770 on the ORAC scale, raisins 2,830, and blueberries 2,400 (compared to, for example, red grapes at 739). They are rich sources of a potent antioxidant called anthocyanins; in addition, prunes also contain beta-carotene, cyrptoxanthin, and lutein.

- **Fiber.** Prunes, raisins, and blueberries are also excellent sources of dietary fiber. One cup of dried prunes contains 3 grams of dietary fiber; this is why your doctor tells you to eat prunes or drink prune juice when you are constipated. There are 1.5 grams of fiber in a small box (43 g) of raisins, and 1.7 grams of fiber in ½ cup of blueberries.
- **Iron.** Prunes and raisins are also rich in iron. Four oz of raisins gives you as much iron (albeit non-heme) as 4 oz of veal, and 8 oz of prune juice gives you more iron than a quarter-pounder.

I recommend one serving of prunes, raisins, or blueberries once a day. That would be about 1 cup of prunes, a small box (43 grams) of raisins, or ½ cup of blueberries every day.

BRAIN FOOD #10: ORANGE/RED FRUIT AND VEGETABLES: ORANGES, RED BELL PEPPERS, AND TOMATOES

These orange/red foods are packed with micronutrients and dietary fiber.

- **Oranges.** Oranges are known for their vitamin C; just one medium-size orange delivers 70 mg of vitamin C (116 percent of daily value). They are also a good source of folate; one orange gives you about 40 micrograms of folate. They are rich in dietary fiber, vitamins A and B1, potassium, and calcium. One 8-oz glass of orange juice actually delivers more vitamin C (about 100 mg), but it is also high in sugar (24 grams) and lower in dietary fiber. Many of the antioxidants are found in the peel and the inner white pulp of oranges, and are often lost when oranges are processed into juice.
- **Red bell peppers.** Red bell peppers are one of my favorite foods, and they are packed with micronutrients. They rank number two (behind frozen concentrate orange juice) in their vitamin C content; one medium-size red bell pepper delivers 283 mg of vitamin C (about 460 percent of daily value). They

are also an excellent source of vitamin A and B6, and a good source of folate, vitamin K, manganese, molybdenum, and dietary fiber. B6 and folate have been shown to reduce the level of homocysteine; elevated levels of homocysteine are associated with greater risk for neural tube defects and other pregnancy complications in susceptible individuals.

- **Tomatoes.** Tomatoes are also an excellent source of vitamin C, vitamins A and K, and a very good source of vitamin B1, manganese, molybdenum, chromium, potassium, and dietary fiber.

- **Antioxidants.** Most important, these foods were chosen because of their antioxidant capacity. Tomatoes, both raw and canned, are packed with lycopene. One can of tomato paste delivers over 75,000 micrograms of lycopene, while one fresh tomato delivers nearly 5,000 micrograms of lycopene. Cooking releases more lycopene from tomatoes, and so cooked tomatoes will deliver more antioxidant capacity than raw tomatoes. Tomatoes are also rich in beta-carotene. Oranges are also packed with antioxidants, including citrus flavanones (which include hesperedin, which has powerful antioxidant and anti-inflammatory properties), anthocyanins, beta-carotene, and a variety of polyphenols. These, in combination with vitamin C, make oranges an antioxidant power pack; oranges rank seventh among fruits in ORAC score. Sweet red bell peppers are rich in cryptoxanthin, beta-carotene, and flavonoids. Indeed, sweet red bell pepper ranks second among all foods in its cryptoxanthin content; one medium-size red bell pepper delivers 2,817 micrograms of beta-cryptoxanthin cooked, and 730 micrograms raw. Cryptoxanthin is a powerful antioxidant in the carotenoids family and has been shown to prevent cancers of the female genital tract.

- **Buy organic** if you can. Oranges and red bell peppers are among the foods most frequently found to have pesticide residues. These foods also deliver more antioxidants when they are organically grown.

I recommend eating one organic orange, red bell pepper, or tomato, at least once a day.

top ten toxic foods

> *Part of the secret of success in life is to eat what you like and let the food fight it out inside.*
> — MARK TWAIN

> *McDonald's announced it's considering a more humane way of slaughtering its animals. You know they fatten them up and then kill them. You know, the same thing they do to their customers, isn't it?*
> — JAY LENO

There is some truth to the humor of Mark Twain and Jay Leno. Some foods do fight it out inside. They can cause infection inside the digestive tract or inflammation inside blood vessels, fat cells, and even the brain. During pregnancy the battle line could be moved across the placenta, making the baby a casualty. McDonald's may not be as bad as Jay Leno's joke makes it out to be, but all the saturated fats, *trans* fats and partially hydrogenated oils that fast-food joints serve up can slowly clog up your arteries. They could do the same to placental vessels during pregnancy. The dioxins and cholesterol from all these fats can also cross the placenta to cause inflammation and damage to the baby's vital organs, including the brain. Some foods you eat before pregnancy can cause wear and tear on your body's systems, creating an internal environment of high sugar, high fat, insulin resistance, and chronic inflammation. If you enter pregnancy in this state, you are not going to get good fetal programming.

Here is my top-ten list of "toxic foods" you should try to avoid, before and during pregnancy. I call them toxic foods because they are unhealthful and can cause harm to your future baby.

Toxic food #1: Swordfish, shark, king mackerel, and tilefish
Toxic food #2: Soft cheeses and unpasteurized milk
Toxic food #3: Hot dogs, luncheon meats, deli meats, raw or smoked seafood
Toxic food #4: Raw or undercooked meat
Toxic food #5: Unwashed vegetables, raw vegetable sprouts, and unpasteurized juices
Toxic food #6: Liver
Toxic food #7: Saturated fats, *trans* fats, and partially hydrogenated oils
Toxic food #8: Added sugars
Toxic food #9: Refined flour
Toxic food #10: Herbal preparations

TOXIC FOOD #1: SWORDFISH, SHARK, KING MACKEREL, AND TILEFISH

These predatory fish can contain high levels of methylmercury, which can accumulate in your body and get transferred across the placenta when you become pregnant. Methylmercury disrupts mitosis and migration of neurons in the developing brain, and can cause developmental delays in children. Please see Box 2.2 for the FDA/EPA joint advisory on seafood for pregnant women, or women who are planning to get pregnant.

TOXIC FOOD #2: SOFT CHEESES AND UNPASTEURIZED MILK

Soft cheeses, such as feta, Brie, and Camembert; blue-veined cheeses; or Mexican-style cheeses, such as queso blanco, queso fresco, and Panela can carry *Listeria monocytogenes*, the bacterium that causes listeriosis. Unpasteurized milk can also be contaminated with *Listeria*. Listeriosis in pregnancy can cause miscarriage or stillbirth, premature delivery, or infection of the newborn. So make a habit of avoiding soft cheeses, unless they have labels that clearly state they are made from pasteurized milk.

TOXIC FOOD #3: HOT DOGS, LUNCHEON MEATS, DELI MEATS, RAW OR SMOKED SEAFOOD

These meats can also be contaminated with *Listeria*. You should get into the habit of avoiding hot dogs, luncheon meats, or deli meats (e.g., ham, turkey, salami, and bologna), unless they are reheated until steaming hot. Avoid getting fluid from hot dog packages on other foods, utensils, and food preparation surfaces, and wash your hands after handling hot dogs, luncheon meats, and deli meats. Do not eat refrigerated pâtés or meat spreads. Canned or shelf-stable pâtés and meat spreads may be eaten. You should avoid eating refrigerated smoked seafood, such as salmon, trout, whitefish, cod, tuna, or mackerel (often labeled as "nova-style," "lox," "kippered," "smoked," or "jerky")—so no more lox and bagel for breakfast when you are pregnant, or actively trying to get pregnant. They are commonly found in the refrigerator section or sold at deli counters of grocery stores and delicatessens. Canned or shelf-stable smoked seafood may be eaten, as well as smoked seafood contained in a cooked dish, such as a casserole. Avoid raw fish, shellfish, or any uncooked or undercooked seafood. This means no more sushi or sashimi just before or during pregnancy.

TOXIC FOOD #4: RAW OR UNDERCOOKED MEAT

Another parasite that can be carried by raw or undercooked meat is *Toxoplasma gondii*, the organism that causes Toxoplasmosis. *Toxoplasma* can cross the placenta and infect the baby; infected babies can be born with hearing loss, mental retardation, and blindness. Some children can develop brain or eye problems years after birth. *Toxoplasma* gets into your bloodstream about a week after ingestion; women who become infected can be treated with medications to clear up the infection, but some experts suggest waiting for six months after infection before attempting to get pregnant. So avoid eating raw or undercooked meat just before or during pregnancy, especially pork, lamb, or venison; in a restaurant ask for meat that is "well-done" and not "rare" or "medium rare." Cook all meat thoroughly; you can make sure that meat and poultry are thoroughly cooked by using a meat thermometer. Pork and ground beef should be cooked to at least 160°F (at which temperature no pink is usually visible); roasts and steaks to 145°F (slightly pink in the center); and whole poultry to 180°F. Do not taste meat before it is fully cooked. When preparing raw meat, wash any cutting boards, sinks, knives, and other utensils that might have touched the raw meat thoroughly with soap and hot water to avoid cross-contaminating other foods. Wash your hands well with soap and water after handling raw meat.

TOXIC FOOD #5: UNWASHED VEGETABLES, RAW VEGETABLE SPROUTS, AND UNPASTEURIZED JUICES

Wash your vegetables thoroughly in running tap water, especially those that are to be eaten raw (e.g., in your salad). Unwashed vegetables can carry and spread *Toxoplasma, E. coli,* and other disease-causing pathogens. Remove and discard the outermost leaves of a head of lettuce or cabbage. If you are buying packaged vegetables, go ahead and wash them again before serving raw, even if they have already been prewashed. They can be contaminated if they were irrigated or washed with water contaminated with animal manure or human sewage, or during the food-processing process. Raw vegetable sprouts (including alfalfa, clover, radish, and mung bean) and fresh (unpasteurized) fruit and vegetable juices are notorious for carrying disease-causing bacteria, such as Salmonella and *E. coli.* These infections generally cause mild gastrointestinal symptoms, though in some pregnant women they can cause severe illness and can be passed on to the fetus.

Check the label on the juices you buy; the FDA requires that packaged unpasteurized juices carry a label stating that they are not pasteurized. The juices you find with an extended shelf life that are sold at room temperature on store shelves (juice in cardboard boxes, vacuum-sealed juice in glass containers) have been pasteurized, although this is generally not indicated on the label. Juice concentrates have also been heated sufficiently to kill pathogens so they are safe to consume. Juices that are fresh-squeezed and sold by the glass, such as at farmer's markets, at roadside stands, or in some juice bars, may not be pasteurized or otherwise treated to ensure their safety. Warning labels are not required on these products; it's best to avoid them if you are planning to get pregnant.

TOXIC FOOD #6: LIVER

The major concern about liver is that it is the only food that contains very high amounts of vitamin A. According to the USDA, a 3-oz serving of beef liver may contain 30,000 IU (international units); chicken liver, 14,000 IU; and canned chicken pâté, 724 IU. A pregnant woman who eats liver regularly may consume enough vitamin A to pose a risk to her baby. A 1995 study found that women who took more than 10,000 IU of vitamin A daily in the first two months of pregnancy had more than double the risk of having a baby with birth defects, though this risk has not been consistently shown in other studies. The Institute of Medicine's Recommended Dietary Allowance (RDA) for vitamin A is 2,565 IU for pregnant women, which is far exceeded by a serving of beef or chicken liver. Thus, it is best to avoid eating liver altogether just before and during pregnancy, and to get your vitamin A mostly in the form of beta-carotene.

TOXIC FOOD #7: SATURATED FATS, TRANS FATS, AND PARTIALLY HYDROGENATED OILS

These are the dumb fats I talked about in Chapter 2. Saturated fats increase LDL cholesterol, which can clog up placental and fetal vessels. Saturated fats come mostly from animal fats (e.g., beef, butter, cream, and cheese from whole milk), which may also be contaminated with dioxins. Dioxins are toxic to fetal brain and immune development. *Trans* fats, so-called "funny fats," which are the unnatural forms of polyunsaturated fatty acids, can get incorporated into cell membranes and hormones. Most important, all these dumb fats can cause oxidative stress and inflammation in the body, which can potentially damage the placenta and fetal organs (including the developing brain). Fats get deposited in the body's fat stores for a long time; reduce your intake of saturated fats, *trans* fats, and anything made with partially hydrogenated oils now if you don't want to these dumb fats to be the building blocks for your baby's brain and other vital organs in the future.

TOXIC FOOD #8: ADDED SUGARS

Added sugars are ubiquitous to processed foods in the United States. They are added to regular soft drinks like Coke and Pepsi but also fruitaids and fruit punch, candy, cakes, cookies, pies, ice cream, sweetened yogurt and sweetened milk, and grain products such as sweet rolls and cinnamon toast. Just read the ingredients label on most processed foods and you will find added sugars, with **high-fructose corn syrup** being one of the most common added sugars. Added sugars are not all equally bad. Fructose, for example has a low glycemic index of about 20, whereas high-fructose corn syrup (which is a mixture of fructose and glucose) has a higher glycemic index of 60. The problem with added sugars is that they add empty calories without adding any nutritional benefits. Some scientists have attributed the growing epidemic of obesity in the United States to increasing consumption of added sugars in the past two decades, though this claim is still being hotly debated. In addition, the excessive intake of added sugars with a high glycemic index can cause insulin resistance in susceptible individuals. There is also a growing body of evidence that suggests that diets with lots of added sugars promote chronic, systemic inflammation. Thus all the added sugars in your foods can create an internal milieu of insulin resistance and chronic inflammation, and can cross the placenta and do the same to your baby when you become pregnant.

Here are some tips on how to reduce your intake of added sugars:

- **Drink water or diet sodas** instead of regular sodas. Regular, non-diet sodas are the number one source of added sugars in the American diet. Try mixing 100 percent juice (without added sugars) with sparkling water in 1:2 mix for a refreshing change.

- **Avoid saccharin** if you are going diet. Saccharin is found in Sweet'N Low that comes in pink packets. There has been some controversy surrounding the safety of saccharin, which was once listed (and then delisted) by the government as a carcinogen. Despite the fact that saccharin has not been shown to cause birth defects, I think it is best to be cautious. Watch out for diet sodas from fountain dispensers found in movie theaters and restaurants—diet versions of Coke and Pepsi in the bottle or can contain only aspartame, but may contain a blend of aspartame and saccharin in the fountain version.

- **Aspartame** (packaged as Nutrasweet or Equal) and **sucralose** (packaged as Splenda) **are considered safe for pregnancy**, though you should avoid aspartame if you have a rare genetic disorder called phenylketonuria (PKU). The FDA, the Council on Scientific Affairs of the American Medical Association, and a special task force of the American Pediatric Association have all concluded that pregnant women and nursing mothers can safely use aspartame in moderation. The acceptable daily intake of aspartame is about 2 grams a day, which is equivalent to drinking about 13 cans of diet soft drink daily (not that you should drink this much).

- **Eat fresh fruits** instead of drinking fruitaids and fruit punch. If you are going to drink juice, drink 100 percent fruit juice **without added sugars**.

- **Avoid high-fructose corn syrup.** Read food labels—try to avoid added sugars as much as you can, especially foods made with high-fructose corn syrup.

- **Substitute whole, natural foods for processed foods.** *This is probably the most important piece of nutrition advice in my book.* If you can substitute processed foods with whole, natural foods, you will eliminate a lot of added sugars, as well as *trans* fats and partially hydrogenated oils from your diet.

TOXIC FOOD #9: REFINED FLOUR

Refined flour is another invention of modern food technology and one of its unhealthiest creations, according to Dr. Andrew Weil, clinical professor of medicine at the University of Arizona and founder of the Foundation for Integrative Medicine. Refined flour is made from degerminated (embryo removed and discarded) and decoated (seed coat, or bran, removed) grain ground into a white fluff of pure, superfine particles with a huge surface area and a very high glycemic index. The refining process removes many of the vitamins, elements, and oils from the germ, fiber from the bran, and turns coarse whole grains with a low GI into white, fluffy starch with a high GI. Table 3.2 compares the nutritional contents of whole-wheat versus refined wheat flour.

Bread made from refined flour is so fine and fluffy that it is aptly named "Wonder Bread," but there is nothing wonderful about its nutritional content or glycemic index. Noodles, pastas, and tortillas made from refined flour are so popular that they have replaced their coarser counterparts made from whole grain as a main staple in many traditional diets; these are thought to have contributed significantly to the epidemic of obesity and diabetes in some ethnic communities in the United States. Refined flour is less than a shell of the nutritional whole grain it used to be. If you want a smart and healthy baby, you should reduce your intake of refined flour before and during pregnancy.

Here are two easy steps that you can take to reduce the amounts of refined flour in your diet:

- **Choose whole grains over refined flour.** Make an effort to replace white and fluffy bread with dense, chewy, grainy breads whenever possible. Similarly, choose other products made from stone-milled whole grains rather than highly processed refined flour. They may be coarser and chewier, but they are a lot better for you and your future baby.
- **Read food labels.** Choose foods that list whole grains **first** on

table 3.2: nutritional contents of whole-wheat vs. refined wheat flour

Major nutrients (% of weight)	Whole-wheat flour	Refined wheat flour
Dietary fiber	12.6	2.9
Protein	14.2	13.5
Carbohydrates	67.2	81.2
Sugar	2.7	1.6
Minerals		
Calcium (mg/g)	0.44	0.25
Phosphorus (mg/g)	3.8	1.3
Zinc (PPM*)	29.0	8.0
Copper (PPM*)	4.0	1.6
Iron (PPM*)	35.0	13.0
Manganese (PPM*)	30.5	2.8
Selenium (PPM*)	0.04	0.03
Vitamins		
Thiamin (mg/g)	5.8	2.2
Riboflavin (mg/g)	0.95	0.39
Vitamin B6 (mg/g)	7.5	1.4
Folic acid (mg/g)	0.75	0.11
Biotin (mg/g)	116.0	46.0
Niacin (mg/g)	25.2	5.2
Pantothenic acid (mg/100g)	0.37	0.18
Vitamin E (mg/100g)	2.05	0.08

* PPM=parts per million

their ingredient list; make sure the word **"whole"** appears in the ingredient list. Don't be fooled by terms like "multi-grain," "stone-ground," "100 percent wheat," "cracked wheat," "seven-grain," or "bran"; they are likely to contain mostly refined grains. Don't be fooled by the color; dark-colored rye

and "brown" wheat breads that are not labeled whole grain
may have color added to confuse you.

TOXIC FOOD #10: HERBAL PREPARATIONS

It is unfortunate we don't know more about the use of herbal preparations
before and during pregnancy. Many herbs are loaded with antioxidants,
and some may have potential medical benefits (e.g., cinnamon for
management of gestational diabetes). Unfortunately, there is just too
much that we don't know about the potential harms posed by herbal
preparations to the developing embryo and fetus, especially in early pregnancy. One recent animal study tested the effects of five plant essential
oils (sage, oregano, thyme, clove, and cinnamon) on growth and development of mouse embryo. These oils are known to have strong antimi-
crobial, anti-inflammatory, and antioxidative properties. The study found
none of the essential oils had any positive effect on embryo development,
but cinnamon and sage reduced cell numbers while oregano and clove
increased the incidence of cell death. Ginger is commonly recommended
for treatment of morning sickness, but in animal studies it has been
found to cause early embryo loss and induce apoptosis (cell death), which
may disrupt normal fetal brain remodeling in early pregnancy.

Presently there are no rigorous human studies of the safety of herbal
preparations during pregnancy, and serious concerns have been raised
regarding poor quality control in the production of many herbal preparations. While it is probably safe to use herbs and spices in small amounts
for cooking, seasoning, and in tea, I support the recommendations of the
American College of Obstetricians and Gynecologists and the Teratogen Society to avoid the use of herbal preparations in large quantities or
for medicinal purposes during pregnancy. If you are using herbal preparations as part of a fertility treatment, make sure you tell your doctor what
you are taking and quit taking them as soon as you become pregnant.

Now that you know about toxic foods, let's turn our attention to
something else that may be even more toxic to you and your future baby:
stress.

CHAPTER 4

stress resilience

Stress is one of the most important risk factors in pregnancy. It is also one of the most common. Life is stressful. Whether you are a high-power executive running a multinational corporation or a single mom juggling work and family, for many of you stress is a fact of life. From the moment you wake up in the morning to the moment you go to bed at night, you are bombarded with stress—from deadlines at work to problems at home, from bills to pay to worries about the future. In today's world stress is inescapable.

Stress is also something that you are unlikely to get much good advice about from your doctor. Most doctors aren't trained very well in helping their patients cope with stress. They wouldn't even know to whom they should refer you if you tell them that you are stressed out. Many therapists won't see you if you don't have a *DSM-IV* diagnosis. Many social workers won't help you unless you are in some kind of crisis. So if you aren't clinically depressed or homeless but just stressed out, your doctor may be at a loss as to how to help you.

That is why I wrote this chapter—to help you learn how to cope with stress better, in preparation for your pregnancy. If you don't have any stress in your life, you can skip ahead to the next chapter. But I suspect most of you will want to read this chapter. First I will explain why stress during pregnancy may be harmful to your baby. I will also talk about the difference between feeling "stressed" and feeling "stressed out"; you might not be able to avoid stress, but it is being stressed out that you really need to avoid. I will then suggest ten steps you can take to reduce your stress levels and build up your stress resilience *before* you get pregnant. Given the important impact of stress on your health and your future baby's development, learning to stay resilient in the face of stress may be one of the best things you can do to get yourself ready for pregnancy and parenting.

warning: stress during pregnancy can harm your baby

And his daughter in law, Phinehas' wife, was with child,
near to be delivered; and when she heard the tidings
that the ark of God was taken, and that her father in law
and her husband were dead, she bowed herself
and travailed; for her pains came upon her.
SAMUEL 4:19

It has been known since biblical times that stress can cause pregnancy complications. In recent years, stress is emerging as one of the most important risk factors in pregnancy. Stress has been linked to a whole host of pregnancy complications, including miscarriages, birth defects, preeclampsia, low birth weight, and preterm birth.

Take preterm birth, for example. Preterm birth is a leading cause of infant mortality and childhood disabilities in the United States; the 12 percent of babies born preterm (more than 3 weeks early) each year accounts for more than two-thirds of all infant deaths, and more than half of all neurological disabilities in children.

Stress can cause preterm birth in several different ways. First, stress can stimulate the placenta to produce more corticotropin-releasing hormone (CRH), a key hormone involved in the initiation of labor. Second, chronic stress can suppress your immune functions and promote infection and inflammation, which are leading causes of preterm birth. Third, stress can decrease blood flow to the placenta, and poor placental blood flow can precipitate preterm labor. Lastly, stress can induce unhealthy behaviors, such as smoking or drug use, in some people as a means of coping; these unhealthy behaviors have been linked to preterm birth. Thus stress can cause preterm birth via several different pathways—hormonal, infectious/inflammatory, vascular, and behavioral.

Of course, not every woman who experiences stress during pregnancy is going to have a premature baby. It has to do with the nature, timing, and duration of stress. Generally speaking, chronic stress is more strongly linked to preterm birth than acute stress, though in some pregnant women a traumatic acute stressful life event such as bereavement (as was the case with Phinehas' wife), earthquake, or 9/11 can precipitate preterm labor. It also has to do with one's stress response. While this stress response may be genetically predetermined, it is also largely modified by one's life experiences. As I discussed in Chapter 1, chronic stress causes wear and tear (allostatic overload) to one's stress response. If a woman enters the pregnancy all "stressed out," she may be at greater risk for preterm delivery. Lastly, what stress does to pregnancy may also have to do with one's stress resilience, a concept I will explain later in this chapter. A positive outlook, loving family, or social support—what are sometimes called "resilience factors"—can help one stay resilient in the face of chronic stress.

maternal stress and fetal programming

Beyond immediate pregnancy outcomes, there are now growing concerns that maternal stress during pregnancy may also have lifelong consequences on children's health and development.

Maternal stress can cross the placenta (see Box 4.1) and cause damage to the fetal brain. Structural damages in learning centers like the hippocampus, amygdala, and the prefrontal cortex, which are particularly vulnerable to the neurotoxic effects of cortisol, can lead to learning disabilities and behavioral problems in children. At least 14 studies have now linked maternal anxiety and stress during pregnancy to cognitive, behavioral, and emotional problems in children, including ADHD. One study found that these children performed poorly on developmental testing and had more behavioral problems during infancy. Another study found that these children showed more attention deficits, had more problems with inhibition, and were more aggressive at nine years of age.

box 4.1: how does maternal stress cross the placenta?

The answer: cortisol. When mom is stressed out, she produces lots of stress hormones, including cortisol. Normally the baby is protected from maternal cortisol by the placenta, which inactivates cortisol before it crosses the placenta. However, under some circumstances (e.g., poor nutrition, placental defects) this protection is incomplete, and maternal cortisol can still pass through.

Mom's stress can also get to her unborn baby by a different route. Cortisol stimulates the placenta to produce more corticotropin-releasing hormone (CRH). In turn, CRH stimulates the baby's own hypothalamic-pituitary-adrenal (HPA) axis to produce more cortisol. So when mom is stressed out during pregnancy, the baby is immersed in both maternal and fetal cortisol.

Maternal stress can also heighten fetal stress response. Maternal stress can turn on the baby's "stress genes" inside the brain (see Box 4.2). In turn, these "stress genes" can rev up the baby's HPA axis. In a way this makes a lot of sense. One of mom's main objectives during pregnancy is to get her baby ready for the outside world. If the outside world is stressful and hostile, mom needs to get her baby ready for fight or flight—by revving up the baby's HPA axis. A hyperactive fight or flight response may confer upon the baby some survival advantage *in the short run*, but can lead to a whole host of health and developmental problems *in the long run*, including attention deficits, leaning disabilities, behavioral problems, hypertension and heart disease, diabetes and obesity, chronic inflammation, depression, and other psychopathologies later in life.

box 4.2: turning on the baby's stress gene

How does mom rev up her baby's stress response? Epigenetics may be the answer. Animal studies have shown that maternal stress can methylate (turn off) a gene that makes cortisol receptors in an area of the brain called the hippocampus. The hippocampus acts like a set of brakes on the HPA axis; turning off the receptor gene is like loosening the brakes. The end result is a hyperactive HPA axis.

I think epigenetics is fascinating because you can have two individuals with identical genetic codes, and they can end up with very different levels of stress reactivity for life, based on whether their stress genes are methylated or de-methylated, which has to do with whether or not their moms were stressed out during pregnancy. These studies demonstrate how maternal stress during pregnancy can have an important and potentially lifelong impact on children's health and development.

the difference between "stressed" and "stressed out"

It's not stress that kills us; it is our reaction to it.
- HANS SELYE

In today's world stress is unavoidable, but being stressed out is not. The difference is in how you react to stress.

To understand this, you need to know how your body's stress response works. Let's go back about 10,000 years: Imagine you are out and about gathering berries when you come face to face with a saber-toothed tiger.

What do you do? You RUN!

And what helps you run faster is your innate fight-or-flight response. Your brain immediately fires a signal via sympathetic nerves to the adrenal glands, which release adrenalin (epinephrine and norepinephrine) into your circulation. The brain also activates the hypothalamic-pituitary-adrenal (HPA) axis to produce cortisol. Adrenalin and cortisol have many functions designed to help you "fight or flight." This stress response is protective; it is the product of strong evolutionary pressure to survive in the face of real threats to our survival—such as running from a saber-toothed tiger.

What happens once you've gotten away from the big cat? Your heart stops racing. Your breathing slows down. You relax.

That's what always amazes me about the human body! It is self-regulating—it automatically shuts off the stress response once you are out of danger (Figure 4.1). In Chapter 1 I introduced the concept of "allostasis," which refers to the body's ability to maintain balance through change.

Most of you are familiar with the concept of homeostasis. Allostasis is a concept akin to homeostasis, but whereas homeostasis describes the body's ability to maintain equilibrium within a narrow range of biological variability (e.g., the ability of the kidneys and other organs to maintain the potassium level in your blood within a certain narrow range), allostasis is a more dynamic concept that involves adaptations to environmental challenges.

Allostasis works largely by negative feedback mechanisms that are common to many biological systems. Peter Nathanielsz, now at the University of Texas in San Antonio, uses an apt analogy of a thermostat to describe a negative feedback loop. When the room temperature falls below a preset point, the thermostat turns on the heat. But once the preset temperature is reached, the heat turns off the thermostat to prevent the room from being overheated. Under stress, your body activates the HPA

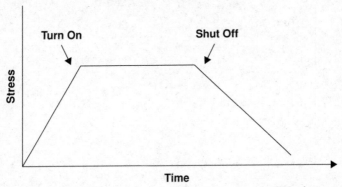

Figure 4.1: Normal stress response. Stress provokes a stress response. Once the stressor is removed, the stress response is shut off through a negative feedback mechanism.

axis to produce cortisol. Cortisol, in turn, feeds back negatively on the HPA axis to keep your stress response in check. That's allostasis at work—maintaining balance through change.

Allostasis works well for stress you can fight off or run from (e.g., a saber-toothed tiger), but it doesn't work as well for stress from which there is no escape (e.g., modern life). In the face of chronic, inescapable stress, your stress response is always turned on. It is not allowed to shut off, and there is no recovery (Figure 4.2).

If your stress response is always turned on and cannot shut off, over time it is going to get worn out. This is when protection gives way to damage, and when you go from feeling "stressed" to feeling "stressed out." There are some major differences.

When you are "stressed," your body activates a sympathetic response that releases adrenalin to make your heart pump harder and faster and constrict your blood vessels. When you are "stressed out," you can't shut off your sympathetic response, and that chronic, uncontrolled sympathetic activation increases your risk for hypertension and cardiovascular diseases in the long run.

When you are "stressed," your body produces cortisol. A main function of cortisol is to convert your body's stored energy into glucose,

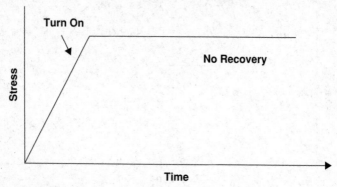

Figure 4.2: Abnormal stress response. Under chronic stress, the stress response is always turned on and does not shut off. Over time the stress response gets worn-out and becomes insensitive to negative feedback controls.

which can be used as readily available fuel for fight or flight. When you are "stressed out," you have too much cortisol. Too much cortisol can cause high blood sugar and insulin resistance, which can lead to obesity and diabetes in the long run.

Under acute stress, cortisol actually enhances your immune functions. But under chronic stress, too much cortisol can suppress your immune system so that you become more susceptible to infections. Moreover, chronic stress can also promote chronic inflammation (see Box 4.3).

box 4.3: how does chronic stress cause inflammation in your body?

Your body has all sorts of built-in checks and balances. A good example is how your HPA axis keeps your immune system in check. Inflammation is the immune system's first line of defense against an infection; it helps the body contain and destroy foreign invaders. But too much inflammation can cause collateral damage to the body. The HPA axis protects the body by putting the brakes on inflammation through the actions of cortisol.

But what happens when someone overuses the brakes? We all hate to drive behind people who drive like that, right? The car isn't going to run very smoothly, just like chronic stress can depress your immune system and increase your susceptibility to infections.

And what happens if you keep on hitting those brakes while driving? Over the long haul those brakes are going to get worn out from overuse. Now you've got a much bigger problem—you can't stop the car, just like chronic stress can cause runaway inflammation in your body.

Acute stress also promotes the growth of neurons in parts of the brain (e.g., the hippocampus, amygdala, pre-frontal cortex) that are involved in learning and memory formation. That's why you can probably still recall vividly exactly what you were doing when 9/11 happened. In contrast, chronic stress does the opposite. Instead of growth of neurons, chronic stress causes atrophy and death of neurons in these learning centers inside the brain. This is why some people who are under chronic stress say that they are becoming more forgetful, that they are losing their memory.

Remember Bruce McEwen's examples of allostasis and allostatic overload in Chapter 1? Allostasis is two 25-lb kids balancing on a seesaw, maintaining balance through change. Allostatic overload occurs when you put two 500-lb sumo wrestlers on the seesaw. You put so much load on that seesaw that sooner or later the seesaw is going to break.

And what would happen if a woman were to enter pregnancy

carrying these two 500-lb sumo wrestlers on her back? She is not going to have a healthy pregnancy and optimal fetal programming, is she?

I've always hated having this conversation with my patients who are already pregnant because it just adds to their stress. They start to get stressed out about how their stress might be ruining their babies' future, and I've often wished that I could've had this conversation with them *before* they got pregnant. The good news is that much as worn-out brakes can be replaced and a broken thermostat repaired, allostasis can be restored. But restoring allostasis takes time—it doesn't just happen overnight. To make a smart and healthy baby, you need to start the repair job now and give yourself enough time to restore allostasis *before* you get pregnant.

ten steps to stress resilience

We've all known people who in the face of stress fall apart, and then there are those who in the face of stress not only survive but thrive. What gives them that edge? What helps them stay resilient so they don't break in the face of stress?

Merriam-Webster's Medical Dictionary defines resilience as "the capability of a strained body to recover its size and shape after deformation caused especially by compressive stress." Stress resilience is what allows you to bounce back in the face of stress. It prevents you from getting broken; it keeps you from getting stressed out.

Let's go back to the image of the two sumo wrestlers on a seesaw. How can you prevent that seesaw from breaking? You can do two things. Either you lighten the load (but good luck moving the sumo wrestlers), or you make the seesaw more resilient so it doesn't break. I might not be able to lighten your load, but I can teach you how to be more resilient so you don't break in the face of stress. Here are ten things you can do to build up your stress resilience, before you get pregnant.

Step 1: Exercise
Step 2: Get a good night's sleep
Step 3: Eat right
Step 4: Learn to relax
Step 5: Learn to prevent stress
Step 6: Work on problem-solving
Step 7: Learn to resolve conflicts
Step 8: Develop positive mental health
Step 9: Get connected
Step 10: Get help

Let me say a word about these ten steps before you get started. You will notice that I am a lot less prescriptive in this chapter than in other chapters. This is because unlike folic acid, for which there is one recommended daily dose (400 micrograms) for everyone, there are different pathways to stress resilience for different people. What works for one person may not work for another. Not all these ten steps are going to work for you; you'll have to pick and choose what's right for you, and find your own path to stress resilience.

1. EXERCISE

The first step you can take to build up your stress resilience is to exercise regularly. Exercise is a great stress reducer probably because it stimulates the production of neuropeptides, including beta-endorphin, that contribute to feelings of happiness. There are numerous reports demonstrating that routine exercise can improve mood. Furthermore, exercise appears to reduce your vulnerability to stress. Animal and clinical studies suggest that exercise may modulate your sympathetic and HPA reactivity to stress, as indicated by findings of lower cortisol and adrenalin levels in response to stressful stimuli in individuals who exercise regularly and are fit. Exercise can also help repair your allostatic overload, as demonstrated by improved insulin sensitivity and actions among individuals with diabetes who exercise regularly.

The National Institutes of Health and the 2005 Dietary Guidelines for Americans recommend that all adults set a long-term goal to exercise at least 30 minutes a day on most, if not all, days of the week. The exercise should be moderate in intensity, and should be something that you enjoy doing so you will sustain it in the long-run and throughout your pregnancy. There are many good forms of exercise, but you should aim for a balanced workout that includes cardiovascular exercise (running, cycling, swimming, aerobics, spinning, elliptical machines, etc.), core conditioning (yoga, Pilates, fitness ball, or such exercises as bridge, sit-up, plank, and quadruped to strengthen your abdominal, back, and pelvic muscles), and strength and flexibility training (which involves primarily lifting or pushing weights and stretching). Many such exercises can be modified once you become pregnant.

One more word about stress and exercise—racing around work or chasing after your kids isn't really good exercise, especially if you are stressed out doing it. While it might give your heart and muscles a good workout, it can also activate your stress response, which adds to rather than reduces your allostatic overload. So even if you run around all day, it doesn't count—make some time for yourself (at least 30 minutes) to exercise every day.

2. GET A GOOD NIGHT'S SLEEP

Stress and sleep are intricately related. Your cortisol level starts to go up in the wee hours of the morning; it tapers off in the evening before you go to bed. Elevated levels of cortisol in the evening are a sign of allostatic overload. Changes in sleep patterns are one of the first things doctors look for in cases of depression.

Sleep allows you to recover from stress; it reduces your allostatic overload. There are a number of websites (e.g., the American Academy of Sleep Medicine, the Food and Drug Administration) that offer tips to help you get a good night's sleep, including the following:

- Avoid caffeine (including caffeine-containing drugs), nicotine, and alcohol for four to six hours before bedtime. The first two are stimulants that can make it difficult to sleep. And while alcohol may have a sedating effect at first, it tends to disturb sleep after several hours.
- Don't exercise within four to six hours of bedtime if it hinders your sleep. Working out earlier in the day, though, not only doesn't hinder sleep but can actually improve it.
- Perform relaxing rituals before bed, such as taking a warm bath, listening to relaxing music, or eating a light snack.
- Before going to bed, try as much as possible to put your worries out of your mind and plan to address them another time.
- Reserve your bed for sleeping. To preserve the association between bed and slumber, don't watch television or do work in bed.
- Go to bed only when sleepy. If you can't fall asleep within 15 to 20 minutes, get out of bed and read a book or do another relaxing activity for a while, rather than trying harder to fall asleep.
- Make sure your bed is comfortable and the bedroom is conducive to restful sleep—quiet and at a comfortable temperature, for example.
- Wake up about the same time every day, even on weekends, to normalize the sleep-wake schedule.
- Don't take naps if they interfere with your sleep. If you nap, nap during the mid-afternoon for no more than 30 minutes.

One more word about sleep: Try as much as you can to avoid staying up late. There are always good reasons that will trap you into staying later and later (e.g., a report due, a project deadline, a big presentation or meeting, or just a good late-night show on TV), but it's a sure way to throw your sleep pattern and circadian rhythm, not to mention your stress response, out of balance, and may be adding another level of allostatic overload to your existing stress levels.

3. EAT RIGHT

When we are stressed out, we tend to reach for foods that are high in fat and high in refined carbohydrates. Cortisol makes us hungry for high-energy carbs and fats, which then get stored in the body in preparation for fight or flight. They also make us fat, especially around the midriff. There is some evidence from animal studies that abdominal fat stores, together with the fats and carbs that we eat, actually send a signal to the brain to blunt our stress response. That is why they are called comfort foods; they actually make us feel better. The problem is, the more carbs and fats we eat, the more cortisol we produce, which make us reach for more carbs and more fats in a vicious cycle. So the chronic, inescapable stress in our lives, I believe, is partly responsible for the growing epidemic of obesity in our nation and in many parts of the world.

To break this vicious cycle, you need to start eating right (see Chapters 2 and 3). Reduce your dietary intake of saturated fats and refined carbs. The average American consumes too much saturated and *trans* fats and refined carbs. Eating right, in the long run, can reduce your stress level and make you feel better.

Besides fats and refined carbs, other things in which we indulge can also increase our stress level. For example, alcohol gives us that initial "rush" that makes us feel revved up and disinhibited by increasing our cortisol level. But with chronic use, alcohol can actually blunt our HPA axis. The blunting of the HPA axis can also leave you more susceptible to infection and inflammation. So part of eating right is avoiding the use of cigarettes, alcohol, and drugs as means of coping with stress.

4. LEARN TO RELAX

A key feature of stress resilience is the ability to relax. Stress resilient people know how to relax. In contrast, stressed-out people don't seem to be able to turn off their stress response. They stay all wound up and tense, ruminating over a heated argument they had with their spouse or co-worker, or feeling overwhelmed by the problems that are piling up. Their stress hormones stay elevated, and that is why they feel stressed out. If you are the type that just don't seem to be able to relax and let go (without turning to smoking, alcohol, or drugs), you need to work on developing some relaxation techniques before you get pregnant.

Here are some techniques that many of my patients have found helpful:

- **Breathing exercises.** You can calm yourself by learning to consciously control your breathing. In *deep breathing*, slowly inhale through your nose while you count to four, expanding your abdomen before allowing air to fill your lungs. Reverse the process as you exhale through your mouth to a count of eight. In *exhalation breathing*, lie on your back with your arms at your side. As you begin to breathe in through your nose, raise your arms toward the ceiling and continue to move them all the way over your head, until they are resting on the floor again. Then exhale slowly and smoothly through your mouth as you return your arms to your sides. The key here is to slow down your breathing to calm yourself down and at the same time to focus your mind on the breath instead of the stress. Pay close attention to the sensations of breathing, expanding, and relaxing.
- **Progressive relaxation.** This is a technique to help relax tense muscles. Lie down on your back and close your eyes. First make tight fists, hold for five seconds, and then relax your hands. Do this three times. Pay attention to the different sensations of tension and relaxation. Then repeat the step with all of your muscle groups: arms, shoulders, chest, abdomen, back, hips, thighs, lower legs, and feet. With practice, you'll be able to do this in about five minutes. For an added benefit, combine this technique with the breathing exercises I described. Some people find they can benefit from using audiotapes available that lead them through these exercises.
- **Meditation.** Meditation involves focusing the mind upon a breath, a sound, or an image in order to increase awareness of

the present moment, promote relaxation, reduce stress, and promote personal or spiritual growth. There are many different forms of meditation, but most involve sitting in silence for 10 to 40 minutes a day to fully experience the present moment with serenity. Dr. Herbert Benson at Harvard Medical School developed a technique of repeating a word, sound, prayer, phrase, or activity (including swimming, jogging, yoga, or even knitting) for 10 to 20 minutes, twice a day, to elicit a *relaxation response*. What is repeated is up to the individual. For example, instead of Sanskrit terms, the person may choose something personally meaningful, such as a phrase from a Christian or Jewish prayer. In *transcendental meditation* (TM), the person sits with closed eyes and concentrates on a single syllable or word (a mantra) for 20 minutes, twice a day. When thoughts or feelings arise, the attention is brought back to the mantra. A growing body of evidence suggests that TM may reduce risks for cardiovascular diseases, largely by restoring allostasis in the neuroendocrine systems (sympathetic and HPA axes) whose functions had been distorted by chronic stress. There is even some preliminary evidence that TM may help remodel your brain.

- **Mindfulness.** A special form of meditation is mindfulness meditation, popularized in the healthcare setting by Jon Kabat-Zinn at the University of Massachusetts. In formal mindfulness practice, the person sits with eyes closed, focusing their attention on the sensations and movement of the breath for approximately 45 to 60 minutes, at least once a day. Informal mindfulness practice involves bringing awareness to every activity in daily life. Wandering thoughts or distracting feelings are simply noticed, without resistance or reaction. The goal of mindfulness is increased awareness of all aspects of self, including body and mind, in the present moment. Studies have shown the efficacy of a mindfulness-based stress reduction (MBSR) program for treating problems as various as chronic pain, anxiety disorders, fibromyalgia, epilepsy, psoriasis, and hypertension.

There are many other relaxation techniques. Try to find at least one technique that works for you—something that you can readily turn to when you are feeling stressed out—before you get pregnant.

5. LEARN TO PREVENT STRESS

In today's world stress may be unavoidable, but some stress is preventable. Learning how to prevent stress is an important skill to acquire before you get pregnant.

- **Plan ahead.** Think back to the last few times when you felt really stressed out. Did they involve deadlines you couldn't meet? Presentations, meetings, or tests for which you felt unprepared? Credit card bills, rent, or mortgage payments you couldn't pay on time? If you are like most of us, some of your stress may be brought on by procrastination, poor time management, and poor planning in general, financial and otherwise.

    We could all do better with planning ahead. Some of the best advice I've ever gotten about life came from my surgery professor at UCSF. He told me that performing surgery is like playing a chess game—the great surgeon doesn't just react; she anticipates several moves ahead. I think the same lesson applies to life; you'd be better off if you can anticipate and stay several moves ahead of the game.

    For many women pregnancy is a time of great change. These changes can be exciting, but they can also be very stressful. If you can anticipate and plan ahead, you might be able to prevent some major stressors during pregnancy. If you are thinking about taking on a new job or a big project, you might want to consider waiting until your life is more settled before you try to get pregnant. If you don't want to wait, then you might want to reconsider the timeline for achieving your career goals so you don't get totally stressed out during pregnancy. If you are thinking about moving, buying a new home, or remodeling your house to build a bigger nest for your baby, you might want to consider doing that now before you get pregnant. Moving is a major stressor you can do without during pregnancy, and remodeling your home can expose you to a number of potential reproductive and developmental toxicants that you should avoid during pregnancy, as I will explain in Chapter 6. Do some financial planning before you get pregnant, whether you are living from paycheck to paycheck or living off of a trust fund. Having a baby and raising a child are expensive; you and your husband/partner need to get yourselves financially prepared for pregnancy. One place to start is by looking into your health insurance coverage; I've had several patients who got stuck with huge hospital bills from deductibles and exclusions they didn't know they had. Plan ahead; don't put yourself in situations where you are going to be stressed out and pregnant. Take care of business before you get pregnant.

- **Avoid stress.** I'm not a big fan of avoidance as a means of coping with stress, but sometimes the best way to deal with a problem is to avoid it. There are some problems you definitely need to confront and not hide from—for example, if you are experiencing abuse at home or harassment at work, these are problems you should not have to put up with. Then there are other problems that just aren't worth stressing about—annoying people you don't need to be around or stressful situations you don't need to put yourself in; you'd be better off staying away from these people or situations and not letting them stress you out.

- **Set limits.** I learned this lesson the hard way. When I first joined the faculty at UCLA straight out of residency training, I was asked to be the medical director of the UCLA ob/gyn clinic. I felt it was a great honor, and so I worked hard to prove myself. For all my hard work, the next year I was rewarded with the added responsibilities of running the ob/gyn residency training program at UCLA. I felt that, too, was a great honor, and so I worked even harder to prove myself. Over the next few years, work kept piling up and the harder I worked the more work I got. It got to a point where I was doing so much that I was completely burnt out and wasn't doing anything very well, and that was stressing me out because I didn't want to disappoint anyone. I finally realized that, for me, one of the ways I get stressed out is by not setting limits. So I am learning to say no, and guess what? No one thought any less of me for saying no! I have become more productive and happier, and now I actually have time to use my brain to think and be creative, which was why I had become a professor in the first place.

  Some of you might have the same problem about setting limits. You might feel that you still have to prove yourself. You don't want to say no because you don't want people to think you can't handle the pressure. So you often take on more than you can handle, and that is a sure formula for getting stressed out. This is especially a problem for some working moms-to-be and moms; you don't want to say no or else you get put on the "mommy track." Many of you take on more than your share not only at work, but also at home. Know your limits and learn to ask for help. While it can be difficult to say no, people might actually respect you more for being able to stand up for yourself. From my experience, I think you will find yourself more productive and creative, or at least much less stressed out, if you learn to set limits for yourself.

Box 4.4 offers a few more suggestions on managing your stress at work.

box 4.4: managing your stress at work

If you are feeling stressed out at work now, it is highly probable that you will be just as (if not more) stressed out during your pregnancy and after your baby is born. Now is a good time to start thinking about how to reduce your stress level, before you get pregnant.

- **Identify where your stress is coming from.** What is stressing you out at work? Is it the work itself? Does your job give you satisfaction and fulfillment, a sense of meaning and purpose, or are you just going through the motions? Does your job allow you much creativity and autonomy, or does it come with high demand but little or no control? Or is it the work overload that is stressing you out? Too much work, not enough time, the long hours, the time pressure, the rat race to make partner, get promoted, or tenured, or the worry that you'll get put on the "mommy track" if you start talking about getting pregnant? Or is it the people you work with? Your boss or supervisor, clients or customers, or some co-worker you just don't seem to be able to get along with? Identifying the source of your stress is the first step to managing stress at work.
- **Find meaning and passion from your work.** The biggest stress comes from doing work in which you find little meaning or passion. If you are really unhappy with your work right now, consider changing your job or career before you get pregnant. Pregnancy and motherhood are extremely challenging times to

make that switch. Be sure to familiarize yourself with the Health Insurance Portability and Accountability Act (HIPPA) and the Consolidated Omnibus Budget Reconciliation Act (COBRA) rules so you don't lose health insurance coverage while making the transition.

- **Manage work overload.** If your stress comes from work overload, learn to manage your workload. Set realistic goals for yourself; avoid unrealistic expectations. Make a to-do list each day that you can check off. Prioritize your tasks; work on things that are important first. Stay focused; avoid distractions—unless you are expected to be on call, select a time of day when you will return phone calls and email. Learn to say no. Learn to delegate. Learn to ask for help.

- **Build better work relationships.** If your stress comes from toxic people at work, avoid them if you can. If you can't, learn to work with them. Surround yourself with optimistic people—people who can lift you up when you are feeling down. Find good mentors who will show you how to be successful not only at work, but in balancing work and family.

- **Don't sweat the small stuff.** Think positive; don't worry so much. Give yourself a break—accept your mistakes, learn from them and move on. Lighten up—use humor to relieve stress at work. Humor is a mark of psychological health; researchers believe we can laugh ourselves to health.

6. WORK ON PROBLEM-SOLVING

Having problems is stressful, but having problems we cannot solve is what stresses us out. Stress-resilient people don't have fewer problems, they are just better at solving problems. Working on improving your problem-solving skills is probably one of the best things you can do to build up your stress resilience.

When you look at people who are good problem-solvers, problem-solving basically boils down to five steps.

1. **Recognize the problem.** To solve a problem, first you need to recognize that there is a problem. Tune in to your emotions and behaviors—often they clue you in on a problem. If you find yourself irritable, tense, moody, overeating, and stressed out around certain people or situations, there is probably a problem. Of course we all tend to blame others, but to problem-solve, you have to look at your reaction to others. That's the part you can tackle.

2. **Define the problem and identify the causes.** It is much easier to solve problems that are well-defined and concrete than those that are vague and global. What is the problem? For problems that seem overwhelming and insurmountable, break them down into smaller, more fixable pieces. Once the problem is defined, you need to identify its cause(s). Is it your job—what about your job that is stressing you out? Is it your relationships—what about the relationships that is stressing you out? Delve in deeper; try to look for the "cause" of the causes until you get to the root of the problem. You might not be able to change the person or the problem, but you can certainly find ways to adapt differently to that problem. Looking clearly at your own responsibility in the problem allows you to make a difference rather than point your finger out there. For instance, if you and your partner tend to fight about communication (or the lack thereof), what can YOU do and say to make a difference? Don't wait for your partner to change; your own actions can cause change to happen.

3. **Propose solutions.** What are you going to do to solve the problem? An effective approach is to "brainstorm" solutions. For the moment, don't worry if they are good or bad ideas—just write them down. I often find talking to my family, friends, colleagues, and mentors helpful at this stage. Ask

them what they would do if they were in your shoes. Generate
a list of as many alternative solutions as possible.

4. **Decide on a solution and plan out action steps.** Go through
your list and weigh the merits of each solution. Consider all
the positive consequences (benefits) and negative consequences (risks, costs) of each solution. Consider the feasibility
and the likelihood of success with each solution. Collect more
information if you need to. Then decide on the best approach.
Once the decision has been made, you need to develop an
action plan—with clearly stated goals, measurable objectives,
and concrete, specific, actionable steps. What are your goals?
What are your objectives? Objectives should be SMART
(specific, measurable, attainable, realistic, and time-bound).
What is your first step? What is the next step? Learn to break
down big problems into little actionable steps.

5. **Evaluate the effectiveness of problem-solving.** Did your
solution work? Did it make a positive change? Is the problem
solved? If yes, what worked? If no, why not? It is important to
learn from both your successes and failures because they will
help strengthen your problem-solving skills in the long-run.

7. LEARN TO RESOLVE CONFLICTS

For many women, interpersonal conflicts lie at the heart of most emotional distress. These conflicts, if unresolved, create wear and tear on your
psyche and your health. Learning to deal with these conflicts is an important tool for building your stress resilience.

Teaching conflict resolution skills is beyond the scope of this book,
but there are three basic things you can work on to improve your capacity for resolving conflicts: emotional intelligence, communication, and
negotiation skills.

1. **Emotional intelligence.** Much of interpersonal conflicts have
to do with emotions, and the capacity to perceive, manage,
and use emotions is called emotional intelligence. Peter

Salovey at Yale and John Mayer at the University of New Hampshire were the first to use the term "emotional intelligence" to describe "a set of skills that contribute to the accurate appraisal and expression of emotion in oneself and in others, the effective regulation of emotion in self and others, and the use of feelings to motivate, plan, and achieve in one's life." Daniel Goleman popularized the idea in his 1995 best-seller, *Emotional Intelligence*, in which he described emotional intelligence as consisting of five competencies: self-awareness, self-regulation, motivation, empathy, and relationship management.

The good news is that unlike IQ, your can improve your EQ (emotional quotient, a measure of your emotional intelligence). There are many self-help books and programs on how to improve your emotional intelligence, such as *The Emotional Intelligence Quick Book* by Travis Bradberry and Jean Greaves. Since it takes two to have an interpersonal conflict, you may want to work with your spouse/partner on improving your collective EQ. My advice is that you start with becoming more aware of your own emotions (self-awareness) as well as each other's emotions (empathy). Working on improving your emotional intelligence together now will help avert a lot of interpersonal conflicts in the future.

2. **Communication skills.** Good communication is key to every successful relationship, and poor communication lies at the heart of many conflicts. An important step to building capacity for conflict resolution is to work on your communication skills.

Much has been written about good communication, most of which starts with good listening. Learning to listen is a lifelong process: Learn to listen actively, ask questions, or paraphrase to make sure you really understand. Listen with empathy and without assumptions or judgment; be willing to look at every angle and understand and respect a different position even if you disagree with it. Learn to express your-self—be clear and to the point. Say what you mean and mean what you say. Be self-aware and aware of other's feelings (see emotional intelligence); pay attention to non-verbal commu-nication (e.g., eye contact, body language). There are a number of useful books and websites that can help you work on improving your communication skills, which I've refer-enced in the appendix. There are also marriage counselors and family therapists who can work with you and your husband/partner on improving your communication styles and conflict resolution skills. If you've been having problems communicating in your marriage/relationship, I'd recommend going to a counselor/therapist, even for brief therapy, just to learn some techniques for conflict resolution before you get pregnant.

3. **Negotiation skills.** Learning to negotiate is another impor-tant skill to have for resolving conflicts. I've long been a big fan of two books by these titles—*Getting to Yes* by Roger Fisher and William Ury at Harvard University, and *Getting past NO* by William Ury. While they are technically business books, they contain such principles as "separate people from the problem" and "focus on interests, not positions" that you can apply for win-win negotiations at home. My goal with this chapter is not to turn you into a skilled negotiator for world peace, but simply to make you aware of the availability of such conflict resolution tools, and the need for practice to make perfect. These skills will help you build your capacity for conflict resolution and stress resilience, and may help make your home, your workplace, and perhaps the world just a little bit better.

8. DEVELOP POSITIVE MENTAL HEALTH

This is probably one of the best things you can do to build up your stress resilience before you get pregnant. Positive mental health is not merely the absence of mental illness or infirmity; it is a state of complete psychological wellbeing. Over the past decade there has been a growing movement in psychology toward positive psychology—psychology that is not only about treating psychopathologies but about promoting that state of complete psychological wellbeing. Positive mental health is defined by the following six characteristics (Box 4.5):

box 4.5: characteristics of positive mental health

A *sense of meaning*—One of the most defining characteristics of positive mental health is having a strong sense of meaning or purpose in life. This sense of meaning defines who we are and what we are all about. It motivates us to set and pursue goals and actualize our potentials. In times of personal crisis, it redefines challenges as opportunities for personal growth.

Self-acceptance—Self acceptance means accepting yourself as who you are, and loving and believing in yourself. Psychologists also call this self-esteem.

Autonomy—Autonomy means "self-governance." It is about being responsibly yourself and not about pleasing others; it is living your life according to your own personal standards and not the opinions and approval of others.

Positive relations with others—Another defining characteristic of positive mental health is the capacity to experience deep connections with others, which I will elaborate on in the next section.

Satisfaction with life—Most people with positive mental health are satisfied with their lives. This doesn't mean that they are rich and powerful, and it certainly does not mean that they always get what they want. Their lives aren't perfect, but they don't sweat the small stuff and live in gratitude for what they have and appreciate all the wonders they find around them.

Optimism—Optimism is what keeps us going in good times and bad. It is a tendency to see the glass half full, a belief that tomorrow will be a better day.

Positive mental health may be one of the best defenses against the wear and tear of chronic stress. A growing body of scientific research now supports the healing power of positive mental health, from warding off common colds to possibly slowing the progression of cancer.

So what can you do to build a positive mental health? Here are some recommendations from several noted psychologists. Remember not everything is going to work for you, and you will have to find your own pathway to positive mental health.

- **Find your purpose.** If you haven't found it yet, this is something you really need to work on before you get pregnant. Your life is about to change, and it is important to be grounded to a purpose through all the changes that pregnancy and parenting will bring. Write a mission statement for yourself. Who are you? What are your mission and goals in life? Remember, don't just talk about your mission and goals at work. What are you all about—your core values? From time to time check in with yourself to make sure you are staying on course, that you are conducting your life according to your mission statement and living true to your core values. And make sure you share this mission statement with your husband or partner, and that you create a joint mission statement based on your own personal mission statements. If you do this, you will also set an example for your children on how to conduct their lives and stay true to themselves.
- **Use your strengths.** What are your top strengths and how are

you using them? Dr. Martin Seligman, a leading expert on positive psychology, has conducted extensive research on what people can do to increase their happiness. He found that one of the most effective ways to increase your happiness is to identify your top strengths and use them in a new way. If you are musically gifted but haven't had much time to play lately, dust off that violin and go teach some underprivileged kid how to play the violin.

- **Count your blessings.** Another effective way to increase your happiness, according to Dr. Sonja Lyubomirsky at University of California, Riverside, is to keep a "gratitude journal" in which you write down three to five things for which you are thankful. Do this once a week and keep it fresh by varying your entries as much as possible.

- **Live in gratitude.** Write a "gratitude letter" and then make a visit to someone who made a big difference in your life whom you never properly thanked.

- **Learn to forgive.** Just as you can learn to live in gratitude, you can also learn to forgive. Some women find it helpful to write a letter of forgiveness to a person who has hurt or wronged them. If you have been abused, maybe you could try a round of counseling to clear your memories before the next generation comes along. You may find more strength and eventually forgiveness. If you can't forgive, you dwell in the past and ruminate on the pain. Rumination has been linked to higher corticotropin-releasing hormone (CRH) levels and lower birth weight in pregnancy. Forgiving may allow you to move on.

- **Savor life's joys.** Dr. Lyubomirsky recommends paying close attention to momentary pleasures and wonders. If your life doesn't give you much of those, learn to find meaning in suffering and see wonders in the mundane. Some psychologists suggest taking "mental photographs" of pleasurable moments to review in less happy times.

- **Spend time with friends and families.** One of the strongest predictors of positive mental health is having strong personal relationships. Make time for your families and friends; make a visit if you haven't seen them for a while.
- **Practice daily acts of kindness.** Offer your seat to an old lady or a pregnant woman on the bus; let that harried mom go ahead of you in the checkout line; offer to babysit your friend's kids so she can go out on a date with her husband; volunteer to be a tutor or big sister for some underprivileged kid. These acts of kindness can help some women build positive mental health by strengthening their self-esteem and self-efficacy, increasing their connectedness to others, and winning them gratitude and reciprocated kindness.
- **Learn to be optimistic.** Optimism can be learned and, according to Drs. Michael Scheier at Carnegie Mellon and Charles Carver at the University of Miami, is associated with better coping and improved health and well-being. One way to increase your optimism is by learning to recognize and dispute catastrophic thoughts. Don't describe situations in the most drastic terms. Another strategy, according to the Dalai Lama, is by "shifting perspective"—learn to look at negative events from a positive angle. But this "supple mind" takes practice. "Generally speaking once you're already in a difficult situation, it isn't possible to change your attitude simply by adopting a particular thought once or twice," the Dalai Lama is quoted as saying in *The Art of Happiness*. "Rather it's through a process of learning, training, and getting used to new viewpoints that enables you to deal with the difficulty."

You can learn more about how to develop positive mental health from Dr. Seligman's book *Learned Optimism: How to Change Your Mind and Your Life,* or at his website on reflective happiness at www.reflective-happiness.com. I'd also recommend reading the Dalai Lama's book *The Art of Happiness*.

9. GET CONNECTED

When I speak of resilience, people generally think of individual resilience such as self-esteem or optimism. But there is another (and perhaps stronger) kind of stress resilience that is relational rather than individual. We draw strength not only from within ourselves but also from our relationships. Having a strong network of positive, supportive relationships is one of the best buffers against the wear and tear of chronic stress. Social support has been shown to be an important protective factor in pregnancy.

So what can you do to build up your relational resilience? As I mentioned, spending time with your friends and families and practicing daily acts of kindness contribute to positive mental health. Here I will focus on four more ways of getting connected:

- **Connect with your spouse/partner.** Your spouse or partner can be a vital source of support and resilience, but he can also be a great source of stress and disappointment. So which will it be? Later in the book I will dedicate a whole chapter to preparing dads-to-be, but you've got to help him get ready. Many guys I know want to be a good husband and a good dad, but often feel clueless (or are made to feel clueless) about how to provide support, emotional and otherwise.

  Here are a few questions you should ask about your relationship before you get pregnant. First, ask yourself honestly: *How strong and resilient is your relationship with your spouse/partner?* If your relationship is on the brink, don't get pregnant now. Pregnancy isn't going to save your relationship; in fact, it might even worsen your relationship with all the added stress. Work on repairing your relationship before you get pregnant, and if you cannot do it on your own, get professional help with couples counseling.

  Second, are there things that both of you need to work on before pregnancy? How well do you communicate with each other? How well do you handle disagreements and resolve conflicts? How well do you deal with problems and manage stress? If communication is a problem (as it commonly is, especially when it comes to communicating needs and expectations), work on improving your communication before you get pregnant. If neither of you handle stress well, find better ways of dealing with stress before you get pregnant (e.g., if you need to share a smoke or have a drink to help you cope with stress, try going for a walk or give a couple's massage to each other instead).

Third, are there things that both of you want to do before you get pregnant? Check in with each other's dreams and goals, read each other's mission statement, write a joint mission statement, and see where having a baby fits in. While there may never be a perfect time to get pregnant, you might want to wait if either of you is not quite ready. Take a trip, go on a vacation, or just go on a date—I still carry with me mental photographs of the wonderful times my wife and I had on our trips before our children were born. Those days of freedom and spontaneity are gone for a while, but I will always have the memories.

Fourth, your relationship with your spouse/partner doesn't have to stop growing after you get pregnant, or even after the baby is born. Keep working at it, and you can keep growing with each other for a lifetime.

- **Connect with a mentor at work.** Do you have a mentor at work? It doesn't need to be someone who is assigned to you, and it certainly doesn't need to be someone who is high and mighty. But it needs to be someone whom you can look up to—perhaps someone who's managed to maintain that elusive balance between work and family, or someone who's managed to keep her personal values and integrity intact in the face of all the pressures and temptations at work. Connecting with a mentor who cares about your professional and personal development is one of the best things you can do to stay resilient at work.

- **Connect with your neighbors and community.** How well do you know your neighbors? How often do you and your neighbors get together? How often do you do favors for each other (e.g., watch over your neighbors' homes when they are away)? How involved are you in the life of your community? The connectedness between you and your neighbors, and among members of a community, is what sociologists and political scientists call social capital. Social capital has been linked to maternal and infant health; the greater the social capital in a community, the lower its infant mortality rate. It is thought that social capital affects health to a large part by ameliorating the wear and tear of chronic stress on health. Thus the more connected you are to your neighbors and the more engaged you are in the civic life of your community, the more you contribute to building a healthy community in which you will raise your children.

- **Connect with your spirituality.** Spirituality is another (and some might consider it a "higher") dimension of feeling connected. Spirituality is the way you find meaning, hope, comfort, and inner peace in your life. Many people find spirituality through religion. Some find it through music, art, or a connection with nature. Others find it in their values and principles. Spirituality has been found to be helpful in the prevention of physical and mental illness, and in coping with or recovery from illness. The mechanisms by which spirituality confers health is unclear, but is thought to be related in part to the resilience it affords against stress.

There are two things you can do to improve your spiritual health. First, identify the things in your life that give you a sense of inner peace, comfort, strength, love, and connection. Second, set aside time every day to do the things that help you

spiritually. These may include doing community service or
volunteer work, praying, meditating, singing devotional songs,
reading inspirational books, taking nature walks, having quiet
time for thinking, doing yoga, playing a sport, or attending
religious services. Remember, though, that everyone is different,
so what works for others may not work for you. Do what is
comfortable for you. Getting connected with your spirituality
may be one of the most important things you can do to prepare
for pregnancy and parenting.

10. GET HELP

You don't have to go it alone. When the stress gets overwhelming, learn to
ask for help. Recognizing that you need help and learning to ask for help is
one of the most important steps toward building your stress resilience.

Three examples of common problems for which you need to seek immediate help before pregnancy are domestic violence, depression, and
substance abuse.

Domestic violence. While the home is often thought of as a safe haven,
it is the site of the most common manifestations of violence in our society today. One in five American women will be physically assaulted by a
partner or ex-partner at some point during her lifetime. Some 4 to 8
percent of pregnant women are beaten up by their intimate partners *during* pregnancy, though in some studies as many as 19 percent of women
report physical abuse during pregnancy. The violence may wax and wane,
and he may genuinely feel remorseful at times, but the cycle of violence
is likely to continue and may even escalate during pregnancy or after
childbirth. It is estimated that child abuse occurs in half of all families
where there is spousal abuse.

If you answer **yes** to *any* of the following questions in Box 4.6, get help
now.

box 4.6: domestic violence

- Have you been hit, kicked, punched, or otherwise hurt by someone in the past year? If so, by whom?
- Do you feel safe in your current relationship? Are you afraid of your partner?
- Is there a partner from a previous relationship who is making you feel unsafe now?
- Has anyone, including your partner, ever forced you to have sex?
- Does your partner physically scream or curse at you? If so, how often?
- Does your partner insult or talk down to you? If so, how often?
- Does your partner threaten you with harm? If so, how often?

If you answered yes to even one of these questions, call the National Domestic Violence Hotline at 1–800–799-SAFE (7233) or at TTY 1–800–787–3224. You can call even if you are not ready to leave your husband or partner, or worry what he might do to you or your kids; they will help you find a way that is safe for you and your children.

Depression. Box 4.7 lists the diagnostic criteria for major depression.

box 4.7: diagnostic criteria for major depression

- Depressed mood (feeling sad, depressed, hopeless, blue) most of the day

- Loss of interest or pleasure in almost all activities
- Recurrent thoughts of death or suicide, or making a suicide attempt
- Significant weight loss or weight gain (as a result of change in appetite)
- Insomnia or sleepiness nearly every day
- Slowed thinking, speech, or body movement, or restlessness and agitation
- Fatigue or loss of energy nearly every day
- Feelings of worthlessness or excessive guilt
- Problems with clear thinking, concentration, and decision-making

If this sounds like you, get professional help now. Ask your doctor for a referral to a psychiatrist or a therapist to start working on restoring your mental health before pregnancy.

Substance Abuse. Approximately one in eight pregnant women in the United States reported drinking alcohol during pregnancy, and nearly 3 percent reported binge drinking. Alcohol and substance use during pregnancy has been associated with birth defects, as well as a number of pregnancy complications and long-term neurodevelopmental problems in children. If you answer yes to any of the following CAGE questions (see Table 4.8), you probably have a drinking problem.

You can use similar questions to evaluate drug dependence (e.g., amphetamine, cocaine, marijuana, etc.). Now is a good time to quit, and having a baby is one of the greatest motivating, life-changing forces to help you kick the habit. You can get help by calling the National Drug and Alcohol Treatment Referral Routing Service at 1–800–662-HELP, or going to the U.S. Substance Abuse and Mental Health Services

table 4.1: cage questions

C = Cut-down:	Have you ever felt you should cut down on your drinking?
A = Annoy:	Have people annoyed you by criticizing your drinking?
G = Guilty:	Have you ever felt bad or guilty about your drinking?
E = Eye-opener:	Have you ever had a drink first thing in the morning (as an "eye-opener") to steady your nerves or get rid of a hangover?

Administration (SAMHSA) website at www.samhsa.gov to find an alcohol treatment program near you.

Let me conclude this chapter with a word of advice: Don't get stressed out if you can't do all ten steps at once. The last thing I want is for you to get more stressed out about being stressed out. I know of no one who has mastered all ten steps; I certainly haven't (not even close—I still get stressed out despite knowing a lot about what to do). Don't try to do all ten steps at once. Start with a small step; even one tiny step counts. The only thing I ask is that you make time for that first step—take five minutes a day to do your breathing exercises or keep a gratitude journal. Stephen Covey, author of *First Things First*, talks about how we are so preoccupied in our daily lives with things that are urgent but not all that important (e.g., emails, phone calls, and other interruptions and distractions) that we have little time left for things that are important but not all that urgent (e.g., taking care of ourselves, finding our purpose, savoring life's joy, spending time with family and friends, and connecting with our inner spirituality). Make time for that first step. Once you've fit that one small step into your daily life, go on to the next step. And you know what? That next step is going to get a lot easier once you've taken that first step.

CHAPTER 5

immune tune-up

Infections and inflammation pose perhaps the biggest threat to a healthy pregnancy and optimal fetal programming. If you want a smart and healthy baby, you need to avoid infections and inflammation at all costs during pregnancy. The best way to do that is to give your immune system a good tune-up before you get pregnant. I will show you how in this chapter.

infections and inflammation: setting the womb on fire

Infection is the invasion and growth of pathogenic organisms inside the body. Infection has been linked to a number of pregnancy complications, including miscarriage, stillbirth, birth defects, fetal growth retardation, and preterm birth. A number of infections in early pregnancy have been shown to cause birth defects, most notably the TORCH infections (toxoplasmosis, rubella, cytomegalovirus, herpes, and other infections such as syphilis and chickenpox; I will discuss each of these infections later in the chapter).

Infection is also a leading cause of preterm birth. As mentioned earlier in the book, preterm birth is a major cause of infant mortality in the United

States. The 12 percent of babies who are born preterm (more than three weeks early) each year in the United States account for more than two-thirds of all infant deaths, and the 2 percent of babies who are born very preterm (more than eight weeks early) account for about half of all infant deaths. Moreover, these 2 percent of babies who are born very preterm account for about half of all neurological disabilities in children. Infections may be responsible for up to 80 percent of these very preterm births. Sexually transmitted infections (STIs) such as gonorrhea and chlamydia, reproductive tract infections (RTIs) such as bacterial vaginosis, and urinary tract infections (UTIs) have all been implicated. More recently, periodontal infections have also been linked to preterm birth.

Inflammation is the immune system's first line of defense against an infection. In response to invading bacteria, viruses, or toxins, specialized immune cells (e.g., mast cells, macrophages, neutrophils, lymphocytes) are called into battle. Armed with a wide array of munitions, these immune cells carry out a search-and-destroy mission, but in so doing can cause considerable collateral damage to the body they were supposed to defend. The ancient Romans likened inflammation to being on fire. Inflammation sets the body on fire wherever the battle is being waged. In the case of a splinter, you'll get the characteristic pain and swelling on the skin around the splinter. In the case of a cold, you'll get a runny nose, swollen glands, and a sore throat. In the case of an infection inside the uterus (as in pelvic inflammatory disease), you'll get pelvic pain, fever, and foul-smelling pus coming out of the vagina (pus is the debris from inflammation, composed of the dead bodies of soldiers and invaders alike).

But what if the womb is already inhabited by a baby? If the skirmish is quickly contained and the enemies eliminated, then the baby is safe. However, if the enemy forces are strong and the fighting intense, the baby may get aborted. Inflammation can precipitate miscarriage or preterm labor. By aborting the pregnancy early, the body is ridding itself of an infected abscess so mom has a better chance of survival. In this way inflammation is protective even though the results may be undesired.

born of fire: inflammation and programming of the fetal brain

During pregnancy, the placenta plays a critical role in defending the fetus. The placenta has its own special forces, such as placental macrophages that can do combat with invaders. At the same time, the placenta produces local suppressor factors and blocking antibodies that suppress and block maternal immune cells from attacking the fetus. The fetus carries genetic materials (from dad) that may be recognized by mom's immune system as trespassers; without the protection of the placenta the fetus may be rejected in the same way a transplant gets rejected. Thus the placenta protects the baby from foreign invaders and armed brigades from mom's immune system alike.

Most of the time, the placenta does a good job in keeping out invaders. However, once this placental barrier is breached, the fortress is sieged. Bacteria, viruses, and toxins now gain access to the baby through the amniotic fluid and umbilical cord. Inside the fetus, these invaders run amok and wreak havoc on the baby's developing organs and systems. They are met by infantries from the fetus' immature immune system, as well as armed brigades from mom's immune system that have been transported across the placenta. Fierce battles ensue for the baby's (and the mom's) survival.

A crucial battleground is inside the developing fetal brain. It is now believed that inflammation, perhaps more than the infections it is designed to protect the fetus from, may be responsible for much of the neurological injuries and psychopathologies resulting from perinatal infections. Inflammation can cause damage directly to the developing brain. It can also cause damage indirectly by interfering with the transfer of oxygen and nutrients across the placenta.

A growing body of studies has linked maternal infections during pregnancy to subsequent development of neurological disorders and psychopathologies in her offspring. Several studies have found that babies born to mothers who had chorioamnionitis (infection inside the amniotic sac) during labor have about a two- to fivefold increased risk for cerebral palsy. Other studies have found that children born to mothers who had an infection during pregnancy are at greater risk for developing epilepsy, autism, and schizophrenia, which might not become manifest until years later. One recent study showed that if you had the flu in the first half of pregnancy, your baby has a threefold increased risk of developing schizophrenia over his lifetime. The mechanisms by which maternal flu can cause schizophrenia in her offspring are not known, but inflammation is thought to play a key role in the fetal origin of schizophrenia.

fetal programming of the immune system

Infection and inflammation can interfere with not only the hardwiring of the fetal brain, but also the development of other fetal organs and systems as well, including the baby's immune system. It is hypothesized that infection and inflammation inside the womb, during critical periods of fetal immune development, can permanently alter the structures and functions of the baby's immune system, making him or her more susceptible to infectious or inflammatory diseases in later life (see Box 5.1).

box 5.1: does asthma begin in the womb?

Have you ever noticed how some kids just seem invincible, while other kids are vulnerable to all sorts of childhood illnesses—ear infections, respiratory tract infections, allergies, eczema, asthma, and so forth? There are a lot of reasons why some kids are healthy and other kids are sick, but one of the most important differences between healthy and sick kids is their immune system. The immune system is what protects the body from attacks by outside invaders such as bacteria, viruses, and toxins. Healthy kids are protected by an immune system that is highly competent and fine-tuned, whereas sick kids have an immune system that is either too weak to protect them from invaders, or so clumsy that in stamping out these invaders it causes serious collateral damage to the body.

It turns out that how well your child's immune system works may have a lot to do with fetal programming inside the womb. For example, children whose mothers smoked during pregnancy are more likely to develop allergies and asthma. Toxins from cigarette smoking can cross the placenta and interfere with normal development of the fetal immune system. Maternal infections can also mess with fetal immune development. As discussed earlier, the baby takes cues from mom about what the outside world is like. If the outside world is stressful and hostile, then being born with a revved-up HPA axis may confer some survival advantages. Similarly, if the outside world is crawling with parasites or filled with toxins, then being born with a revved-up inflammatory response may also confer some survival advantages, at least in the short run. A revved-up inflammatory response, however, could put the child at risk for a whole host of immune- and inflammatory-mediated diseases in the long run.

In sum, a growing body of evidence suggests that infection and inflammation pose perhaps the biggest threat to a healthy pregnancy and fetal programming. Maternal infection and inflammation during pregnancy have been linked to major pregnancy complications, including miscarriage, stillbirth, birth defects, fetal growth retardation, and preterm birth. Perinatal infections have also been linked to neurological disorders and psychopathologies such as cerebral palsy, epilepsy, autism, and schizophrenia, possibly because of the programming effects of infection and inflammation on the fetal brain. Infection and inflammation can also program other fetal organs and systems, including possibly the immune system, resulting in greater susceptibility for immune- and inflammatory-mediated diseases later in life. To make a smart and healthy baby, you need to avoid infections and inflammation at all costs during pregnancy.

why do you need an immune tune-up before pregnancy?

So how can you avoid infections and inflammation during pregnancy? It turns out that the best thing you can do to avoid infections and inflammation during pregnancy is to give your immune system a good tune-up *before* pregnancy.

Pregnancy is an immunological balancing act. If your immune system is too weak, you are susceptible to a host of infections that could put your pregnancy at risk. However, if your immune system is too strong, it can cause excessive inflammation that can damage or even abort your baby. Like using cannons to kill a housefly, your baby may become collateral damage to a runaway immune system.

That's why you need an immune tune-up before you get pregnant. If you go into the pregnancy with your immune system already worn-out from chronic stress, persistent infections, poor nutrition, or toxic exposures, you are going to have a hard time achieving that immune balance. By the time you start prenatal care, it may be too late for your body or your doctor to restore your immune allostasis and repair all the wear and tear you've piled up on your immune system quickly enough to optimize fetal programming. In the rest of the chapter, I will teach you how to tune-up your immune system before you get pregnant.

ten steps to tune-up your immune system before you get pregnant

To restore your immune allostasis before pregnancy, there are two things you must do. First, remove all ongoing sources of infection and inflammation that can cause further wear and tear on your immune system. Second, make lifestyle changes to improve your immune fitness. With these two goals in mind, here are ten steps you can take to tune-up your immune system before you get pregnant.

Step 1: Brush, floss, and see your dentist
Step 2: Get check-ups for STIs, RTIs, and UTIs
Step 3: Don't get burnt by the TORCH
Step 4: Eat safe
Step 5: Quit smoking
Step 6: Avoid environmental triggers
Step 7: Get immunized
Step 8: Eat right
Step 9: Exercise
Step 10: Reduce stress

1. BRUSH, FLOSS, AND SEE YOUR DENTIST

Increasingly, periodontal disease is recognized as an important risk factor in pregnancy. Women with periodontal disease have a sevenfold greater risk of preterm delivery. In the long run, they also have elevated risks of heart disease and stroke. The mechanisms by which periodontal disease might lead to preterm delivery, heart disease, and stroke are not clear, but are thought to involve chronic inflammation. Periodontal disease is usually caused by a bacterial infection inside the gum (gingivitis), bone, and connective tissue (periodontitis) that hold the teeth in place. If left untreated, it can become a breeding ground that seeds bacteria and inflammatory mediators into the bloodstream, whereby they can travel to the heart, blood vessels, uterus, placenta, and even the baby to cause inflammation.

To prevent periodontal disease, you need to floss daily, brush after each meal, and see your dentist twice a year for a dental check-up and professional cleaning. Daily flossing is crucial, perhaps more important than even brushing. Flossing prevents the build-up of plaque—a thin film containing bacteria that can inflame the gum and cause it to become red, swollen, and tender; bleed easily when you brush or floss; and pull away from the teeth. This creates pockets between the teeth and the gum where more bacteria can collect. Plaque can harden into tartar, which cannot be removed by brushing or flossing and requires professional cleaning. In severe cases of periodontal disease, your dentist can clean out deep pockets of infection and abscess with a procedure called scaling and root planing, which has been shown to reduce the rates of preterm low birth weight births among pregnant women with periodontal disease. Of course, this is likely to work better, and is probably safer, if it is done before pregnancy than during it, given that such dental procedures during pregnancy could potentially seed more bacteria and inflammation into the bloodstream. So take care of your teeth and gums before you get pregnant.

2. GET CHECK-UPS FOR STIs, RTIs, AND UTIs

Other sources of chronic infection and inflammation include sexually transmitted infections (STIs), reproductive tract infections (RTIs), and urinary tract infections (UTIs). I will discuss the prepregnancy check-up in more detail in Chapter 7.

- **Sexually transmitted infections**—STIs can cause infertility (with gonorrhea and chlamydia), birth defects (with syphilis), preterm delivery (with gonorrhea, chlamydia, and trichomoniasis), and other pregnancy complications. Some STIs can be transmitted from mom to baby; without treatment, nearly one in three babies born to HIV-positive women will become infected with HIV. STIs are sexually transmitted, and the best way to protect yourself against STIs, other than abstinence, is to use condoms every time you have sex. If, however, you are trying to get pregnant, using condoms every time you have sex is not very practical. This is why I routinely screen all my patients who are planning to get pregnant for five of the most common and preventable/treatable STIs: HIV, syphilis, hepatitis B, gonorrhea, and chlamydia. I do so even if the patient is asymptomatic—many women infected with chlamydia, syphilis, hepatitis B, and HIV have no symptoms early on. I also advise their partners to get routine screening because it doesn't make a whole lot of sense to screen just one partner, even if they are (or think they are) in a monogamous relationship. HIV, syphilis, and hepatitis B can be diagnosed with a blood test, and routine screening is recommended for all pregnant women at their first prenatal visit. Gonorrhea and chlamydia can be detected with a urine test or a cervical swab. These are simple tests that can bring a lot of peace of mind to couples who are planning to get pregnant, and for women who are infected but don't know they are infected, getting tested before pregnancy can make a big difference.

• **Reproductive tract infections (RTIs)**—RTIs include bacterial vaginosis (BV), trichomoniasis, and yeast infections.

BV is an overgrowth of abnormal bacteria in the vagina that is often characterized by a foul, fishy odor; its presence in pregnancy is associated with a twofold increased risk of preterm birth. It is still not clear whether BV causes preterm labor since BV is a relatively weak infection. It could be that the presence of BV is a sign of a weakened immune system that isn't able to clear a relatively weak infection; that weakened immune system may be the underlying cause of the preterm delivery. Douching, smoking, and chronic stress

increase the risk of BV. Douching, routinely used by some
women after intercourse or menses or to clear up odor or
discharge, has been found to alter the vaginal flora and pH
and increase vaginal irritation and inflammation. If you
douche (as do 20 to 40 percent of American women aged
15 to 44 years on a regular basis), give it up before you get
pregnant. BV can be diagnosed by checking vaginal pH and
looking at the vaginal fluid under a microscope (characteristic findings include the presence of something called "clue
cells" and the absence of lactobacilli, bacteria that are part of
normal vaginal flora). It isn't part of a routine gynecologic
exam or pap smear test; if you suspect you might have BV
(e.g., you have grayish vaginal discharge with a foul, fishy
odor) you need to ask your doctor to test you for it.

Trichomoniasis is primarily a sexually transmitted
infection characterized by copious green, watery discharge.
Other symptoms can include painful sexual intercourse, lower
abdominal discomfort, and the urge to urinate. It sets off an
intense inflammatory response that can lead to preterm labor.
Diagnosis is made by collecting vaginal fluid for examination;
under the microscope you can see little trichomonads
swimming in a sea of inflammatory cells. Culturing for the
parasite is the best way to diagnose infection; results may take
three to seven days. No test for RTIs is 100 percent accurate; if
your test is negative but you continue to have symptoms, you
should ask your doctors to repeat the test or order additional
tests.

A yeast infection typically does not pose a threat to
pregnancy, but recurrent yeast infections may be a sign of a
compromised immune system as a result of diabetes, poor
nutrition, chronic stress, and other conditions. If you get
frequent, recurrent yeast infections, you might want to
consider working on fixing the underlying problems and
tune-up your immune system before you get pregnant.

- **Urinary tract infections (UTIs)** include infections of the urethra, bladder, and kidneys. A UTI is associated with increased risk for preterm birth. It is typically characterized by urinary urgency and frequency, pain, and burning upon urination; however, some cases of UTI can be completely asymptomatic. Therefore, routine screening of all pregnant women (with a simple urine test) for asymptomatic bacteriuria (bacteria in the urine) is recommended at their first prenatal visit; I'd recommend getting tested before you get pregnant.

3. DON'T GET BURNT BY THE TORCH

While we are on the topic of infections, let's talk about TORCH infections. TORCH stands primarily for four infections that can cause birth defects and other pregnancy complications if the mother contracts them during pregnancy: **t**oxoplasmosis, **r**ubella, **c**ytomegalovirus (CMV), and **h**erpes. The "O" stands for "other" infections including syphilis, hepatitis B, chickenpox (varicella), and parvovirus. This is one TORCH you don't want to pass on to the next generation.

- **Toxoplasmosis:** Toxoplasmosis is an infection caused by a parasite called *Toxoplasma gondii*. The parasite is commonly found in cat feces and raw meat; you can get toxoplasmosis by accidentally swallowing cat feces (e.g., touching your mouth with unwashed hands after cleaning the litter box or gardening), eating contaminated raw or partly cooked meat, or contaminating food with knives, utensils, and cutting boards that have had contact with raw meat. *Toxoplasma* can be transmitted across the placenta from mother to baby; mothers who become infected for the first time during pregnancy are at risk because they have no immunity to protect their babies against *Toxoplasma*. Infected babies are at risk for severe damage of the brain, eyes, or other vital organs, and possibly schizophrenia as a result of damages to the developing brain caused by the intense inflammation set off by the *Toxoplasma* infection.

To check if you are immune to *Toxoplasma*, your doctor can do a blood test. If you are planning to get pregnant and have no immunity against *Toxoplasma*, you should 1) Wear gloves when you garden or do anything outdoors that involves handling soil, and wash your hands well with soap and water after outdoor activities, especially before you eat or prepare any food; 2) When preparing raw meat, thoroughly wash with soap and hot water any cutting boards, sinks, knives, and other utensils that might have touched the raw meat to avoid cross-contaminating other foods. Wash your hands well with soap and water after handling raw meat; 3) Cook all meat thoroughly; that is, to an internal temperature of 160°F and until it is no longer pink in the center or until the juices become colorless. Do not taste meat before it is fully cooked; and 4) Exercise precautions around cats (see Box 5.2). You can get more information on toxoplasmosis from the CDC website on toxoplasmosis at www.cdc.gov/toxoplasmosis.

---

box 5.2: if you are pregnant or getting ready to get pregnant and own a cat

You should . . .

- Have someone else change the litter box, if possible. If you have to clean it, wear disposable gloves and wash your hands thoroughly with soap and warm water afterward.
- Change the litter box daily. The parasite doesn't become infectious until one to five days after it has been shed in the feces.
- Wear gloves when gardening in a garden or handling sand from

a sandbox because cats may have excreted feces in them. Be sure to wash your hands with soap and warm water afterward.

- Cover outdoor sandboxes to prevent cats from using them as litter boxes.
- Feed your cat commercial dry or canned food. *Never* feed your cat raw meat because it can be a source of *Toxoplasma*.
- Keep indoor cats indoors. Be especially cautious if you bring outdoor cats indoors.
- Avoid stray cats, especially kittens.
- Don't get a new cat while you're pregnant.

http://www.cfsan.fda.gov/~pregnant/beftoxo.html

- **Rubella:** Also known as German measles, rubella is a virus that causes a typical rash and low-grade fever for two to three days in children and adults. However, it can cause congenital deafness, cataracts, heart defects, mental retardation, and liver and spleen damage in a fetus whose mother becomes infected for the first time just before conception or in early pregnancy (there is at least a 20 percent chance of damage to the fetus if a non-immunized woman is infected for the first time right before or in early pregnancy). The timing of infection is critical. For example, rubella infection can cause congenital cataracts during week six of pregnancy, when the lens is forming, deafness during week seven to eight due to impaired cochlear development, but no major structural birth defects when the infection occurs after the first trimester. Along with influenza and toxoplasmosis, maternal rubella infection during pregnancy has also been implicated as a possible cause of schizophrenia in the offspring. The best way to prevent rubella infection in pregnancy is by getting vaccinated before pregnancy. Your doctor can order a rubella blood test to check your immunity. If the test is positive, it means you are immune against rubella already and there is minimal chance that your baby will be harmed by a rubella infection during pregnancy. If the test is negative (which means you don't have immunity against rubella), you should get vaccinated. The vaccine uses actual live virus (albeit greatly attenuated in virulence) and should not be given during pregnancy; you should wait at least **four weeks** after completion of vaccination before attempting to conceive. For more information on rubella, you can go to the CDC website at www.cdc.gov/rubella.

- **Cytomegalovirus (CMV):** CMV is the most common congenital infection in the United States. Each year, about 40,000 children are born with congenital CMV infection, which is transmitted from the mother to the fetus. While most babies with congenital CMV have no health problems, in some babies congenital CMV can cause hearing and vision loss, mental retardation, and damages to the lungs, liver, spleen, and other organs. CMV is spread from person to person through bodily fluids such as saliva and urine; contact with saliva and urine of young children (especially children 1 to 2 ½ years of age in daycare) is a major cause of CMV infection among pregnant women. If you are planning to become pregnant, a CMV blood test can help you know how careful you must be. If you test positive for immunity (which means you have been infected with CMV in the past and have immunity against it), there is little chance that your baby will be harmed by CMV. But if you test negative (which means you don't have immunity) and become infected for the first time just before or during pregnancy, you have about a 33 percent chance of transmitting CMV to your unborn baby. There is no vaccine for CMV; if you test negative you should carefully follow these precautions just before or during pregnancy: 1) Practice good personal hygiene, especially hand washing with soap and water after contact with diapers or saliva (particularly with a child who is in daycare).

Wash well for 15 to 20 seconds; 2) Do not kiss children under the age of six on the mouth or cheek. Instead, kiss them on the head or give them a hug; 3) Do not share food, drinks, or utensils (spoons or forks) with young children. You need to be especially careful if you work in a daycare center; ask your doctor to check your immunity against CMV. If you test negative (which means you don't have immunity), you can reduce your risk of getting CMV during pregnancy by working only with children who are older than 2 ½ years of age. You can get more information on CMV from the CDC website at www.cdc.gov/cmv.

- **Genital herpes:** Genital herpes is a sexually transmitted infection caused by the herpes simplex viruses type 1 (HSV–1) and type 2 (HSV–2). Most genital herpes is caused by HSV–2. It is one of the most common STIs in the United States; more than one in five Americans are infected with genital herpes. Most people (over 90 percent) have no signs or symptoms and are unaware that they are infected. For some people, however, genital herpes can manifest as recurrent painful blisters on or around the genitals or anus. Genital herpes can cause preterm labor and fetal growth retardation. Neonatal HSV infection, usually as a result of mother-to-child transmission at the time of delivery, can cause seizures, blindness, learning disabilities, and even death. If you already have genital herpes, your chance of passing it on to your baby during pregnancy is relatively low (less than 3 percent) because your body has built up some immunity against the virus to keep it in check. If, however, you are unfortunate enough to get an active outbreak at the time of delivery, a cesarean delivery is usually performed to avoid transmission of the virus to the baby. If you get frequent outbreaks during pregnancy, your doctor might recommend antiviral prophylaxis such as acyclovir, famciclovir (Famvir), and valacyclovir (Valtrex) for the last month of pregnancy to prevent an outbreak at delivery. If you have never been infected (you can ask your doctor for a blood test), it is important for you to avoid contracting herpes during pregnancy because a first episode during pregnancy (especially in late pregnancy) causes the greatest risk of transmission to the baby (a 33 percent chance). The surest way to avoid transmission of any sexually transmitted diseases, including genital herpes, is to abstain from sexual contact, or to be in a long-term mutually monogamous relationship with a partner who has been tested and is known to be uninfected. If your partner is infected, correct and consistent use of latex condoms can reduce the risk of genital herpes; however, since a condom may not cover all infected areas, even correct and consistent use of latex condoms cannot guarantee complete protection from genital herpes. You should refrain from having sex with your partner during an active outbreak. Currently there is no vaccine for HSV. For more information on HSV, you can log on to the CDC website at www.cdc.gov/std/Herpes.

- **Syphilis:** Syphilis is a sexually transmitted infection caused by a bacterium called *Treponema pallidum*. There are over 30,000 new cases of syphilis, and over 400 cases of congenital syphilis (with transmission from mother to child inside the womb), reported each year in the United States. You can ask your doctor for a blood test to screen for syphilis infection; the test is recommended for all pregnant women at their first prenatal visit, so you might as well do it now. If you test positive, you should get treated (with penicillin or other antibiotics) before you get pregnant. Untreated syphilis can cross the placenta to cause stillbirth, birth defects, hydrops, and preterm labor. You can get more information on syphilis from the CDC website at www.cdc.gov/std/syphilis.

I will talk more about the other TORCH infections (e.g., hepatitis B, chickenpox) under the section "Get Immunized" in this chapter.

4. EAT SAFE

The food you eat can be an important source of infection. Raw foods of animal origin (e.g., raw meat and poultry, raw eggs, unpasteurized milk, and raw shellfish) are the most likely to be contaminated. Foods that mingle the products of many individual animals, such as bulk raw milk, pooled raw eggs, or ground beef, are particularly hazardous because a pathogen present in any one of the animals may contaminate the whole batch. A single hamburger may contain meat from hundreds of animals. Fruits and vegetables consumed raw are a particular concern if they are not washed well. Toxoplasmosis can be spread by vegetables, fruit, and salad where the soil has not been properly washed off. Alfalfa sprouts and other raw sprouts pose a particular challenge, as the conditions under which they are sprouted are ideal for growing microbes as well as sprouts, and because they are often eaten without further cooking. See Chapter 3 for a list of toxic foods that may be vectors for infections, and see Box 5.3 for the CDC's recommendations on how to avoid foodborne illnesses:

box 5.3: avoiding foodborne illnesses

The CDC recommends taking the following simple precautions to avoid foodborne illnesses before or during pregnancy:

- **Cook** meat, poultry and eggs thoroughly. Using a thermometer to measure the internal temperature of meat is a good way to be sure that it is cooked sufficiently to kill bacteria. For example, ground beef should be cooked to an internal temperature of 160°F. Eggs should be cooked until the yolk is firm.
- **Separate:** Don't cross-contaminate one food with another.

(continued)

Avoid cross-contaminating foods by washing hands, utensils, and cutting boards after they have been in contact with raw meat or poultry and before they touch another food. Put cooked meat on a clean platter, rather back on one that held the raw meat.

- **Chill:** Refrigerate leftovers promptly. Bacteria can grow quickly at room temperature, so refrigerate leftover foods if they are not going to be eaten within four hours. Large volumes of food will cool more quickly if they are divided into several shallow containers for refrigeration.

- **Clean:** Wash produce. Rinse fresh fruits and vegetables in running tap water to remove visible dirt and grime. Remove and discard the outermost leaves of a head of lettuce or cabbage. Because bacteria can grow well on the cut surface of fruit and vegetables, be careful not to contaminate these foods while slicing them up on the cutting board, and avoid leaving cut produce at room temperature for many hours. Don't be a source of foodborne illness yourself. Wash your hands with soap and water before preparing food. Avoid preparing food for others if you yourself have a diarrheal illness. If you have to stop to change a baby's diaper while preparing food, wash your hands with soap and water thoroughly before resuming food preparation.

- **Report:** Report suspected foodborne illnesses to your local health department.

One foodborne illness of particular concern for pregnancy is **listeriosis**, caused by eating food contaminated with the *Listeria monocytogenes*. The bacterium has been found in a variety of raw foods, such as uncooked meats and vegetables, unpasteurized milk, as well as in processed foods that become contaminated after processing, such as soft cheeses and cold cuts at the deli counter. Each year in the United States, an estimated 2,500 people become seriously ill with listeriosis; of these, 500 die. Pregnant women are about 20 times more likely than other healthy adults to get listeriosis; about one-third of listeriosis cases happen during pregnancy. Infected pregnant women may experience only a mild, flu-like illness; however, infections during pregnancy can lead to miscarriage or stillbirth, premature delivery, or infection of the newborn.

The CDC recommends the following general precautions for reducing your risk for listeriosis:

- Thoroughly cook raw food from animal sources, such as beef, pork, or poultry.
- Wash raw vegetables thoroughly before eating.
- Keep uncooked meats separate from vegetables and from cooked foods and ready-to-eat foods.
- Avoid unpasteurized (raw) milk or foods made from unpasteurized milk.
- Wash hands, knives, and cutting boards after handling uncooked foods.
- Consume perishable and ready-to-eat foods as soon as possible.

Additional recommendations have been made specifically for pregnant women and persons with weakened immune systems. If you are planning to get pregnant, these are good habits to get into to avoid listeriosis:

- Do not eat hot dogs, luncheon meats, or deli meats, unless they are reheated until steaming hot.
- Avoid getting fluid from hot dog packages on other foods, utensils, and food preparation surfaces, and wash hands after handling hot dogs, luncheon meats, and deli meats.
- Do not eat soft cheeses, such as feta, Brie, and Camembert; blue-veined cheeses; or Mexican-style cheeses, such as queso

blanco, queso fresco, and Panela, unless they have labels that
clearly state they are made from pasteurized milk.

- Do not eat refrigerated pâtés or meat spreads. Canned or
  shelf-stable pâtés and meat spreads may be eaten.
- Do not eat refrigerated smoked seafood, unless it is contained
  in a cooked dish, such as a casserole. Refrigerated smoked
  seafood, such as salmon, trout, whitefish, cod, tuna, or
  mackerel, is most often labeled as "nova-style," "lox," "kippered," "smoked," or "jerky." They are often found in the
  refrigerator section or sold at the deli counters of grocery
  stores and delicatessens. Canned or shelf-stable smoked
  seafood may be eaten.

You can find more information on foodborne illnesses, including
listeriosis, at the CDC website at www.cdc.gov. You can also get information on food safety during pregnancy from the FDA website at www.cf-
san.fda.gov.

5. QUIT SMOKING

Cigarette smoking is a potent stimulus of chronic inflammation. Smoking can cause inflammation inside the airway and blood vessels, and
possibly other organs and systems as well. Several studies have shown
elevated levels of inflammatory markers among current smokers. The
more you smoke, the greater the inflammation. If you quit smoking, these
inflammatory markers will gradually decline over time (though they may
take a few years to return to normal). So if you smoke, quit now, before
you get pregnant.

Quitting smoking is never easy, but it's doable. Preparing for a baby is
a great motivator to quit smoking, especially now that you know what inflammation can do to the baby's developing organs and systems. Here are
some tips from the American Medical Association on quitting smoking:

- Be committed. Keep in mind why you want to quit and stay
  motivated.

- Get help from your doctor and continue to follow up with your doctor, especially during the first month.
- Choose a firm date to quit and mark your calendar. Choose a time that is not particularly stressful and that does not involve situations associated with smoking.
- Begin to cut back prior to your quit date.
- Consider joining a support group of ex-smokers or other stop-smoking programs such as those offered by the American Lung Association and the American Cancer Society.
- Tell friends, family, and coworkers that you are quitting smoking so that they can offer motivation and support.
- Remove smoking from your environment. Avoid places where people congregate to smoke. Remove cigarettes from your car, home, and work.
- Anticipate that you may experience withdrawal symptoms, such as cigarette cravings, anxiety, irritability, and restlessness, even with nicotine replacement or drug treatment. These symptoms usually peak at one to three weeks after quitting but generally become manageable within a few weeks.
- Eat a healthy diet and stay active in order to help with stress and to minimize weight gain.

The National Institutes of Health also has a website (www.nlm.nih .gov/medlineplus/smokingcessation), which offers links to information and resources to help smokers quit smoking. While you are at it, get your husband or partner to quit smoking, too. His smoking can also be a potent stimulus of chronic inflammation inside your body, and put your health and that of your future baby in jeopardy, even if you yourself don't smoke. Make him quit smoking before you get pregnant.

6. AVOID ENVIRONMENTAL TRIGGERS

Besides cigarette smoking, a large number of environmental toxins are also potent stimuli of chronic inflammation. I have dedicated Chapter 6 to reducing your environmental exposures. Here I will focus on a few common household exposures that are known to cause inflammation: molds and mildew, dust mites, and cockroaches. They can cause allergies and asthma in adults and children. Their particles can also cross the placenta to trigger inflammation. Instead of putting it off until after the baby comes, now is a good time to get your house in order, before you get pregnant. Here are some recommendations from the American Academy of Allergy, Asthma, and Immunology (AAAAI):

- **Molds and mildew.** Indoor molds and mildew thrive in areas of the house with increased humidity, such as damp basements and bathroom windows. Keeping these areas well ventilated, dehumidified (with a dehumidifier), and consistently cleaned is the best way to prevent molds and mildew. If you find molds and mildew, you should get rid of them right away with a cleaning solution containing 5 percent bleach and a small amount of detergent. If you find them on wallpaper and carpeting, remove these items immediately. Also, promptly repair and seal leaking roofs or pipes.

- **Dust mites.** Dust mites also thrive in high humidity and in areas where human dander (dead skin flakes) is located, such as the bedroom. To reduce dust mites, it is important to keep humidity below 50 percent throughout the home by using a dehumidifier or central or window air-conditioning. Wall-to-wall carpeting should be removed as much as possible, especially if it is laid over concrete floors. Hardwood, tile, or linoleum is better for people with allergies. Washable throw rugs may also be used if they are regularly washed in hot water or dry-cleaned. Weekly vacuuming (using a vacuum with a HEPA filter or a double bag) can help remove dust mites. In the bedroom, encase mattresses, box springs, and pillows in airtight, zippered plastic or special allergen-proof fabric covers. Replace foam mattresses with spring mattresses, as foam mattresses are great breeding ground for dust mites. Bedding should also be washed

weekly in hot water (130°F) and dried in a hot drier. For
waterbeds, regularly wash the mattress pad on top of the
bed. Comforters and pillows made of natural materials such
as down feathers or cotton should be covered with allergy-
proof encasings.

- **Cockroaches.** If you've got a cockroach problem in your
house, take care of it now. Droppings from roaches are a major
trigger for childhood allergies and asthma, and could potentially be a source of chronic inflammation for your pregnancy.
Cockroaches feel less welcome in a clean, dry house—so keep
your home dry and clean. Keep food in tight-lidded containers
and put pet food dishes away after pets are done eating. Vacuum
and sweep the floor after meals, and take out garbage and
recyclables frequently. Use lidded garbage containers in the
kitchen. Wash dishes immediately after use in hot, soapy
water, and clean under stoves, refrigerators, or toasters where
loose crumbs can accumulate. Wipe off the stove top and
clean other kitchen surfaces and cupboards regularly. Cockroaches need water to survive and thrive in high humidity, so
make sure to fix and seal all leaky faucets and pipes. Block
areas where roaches could enter the home, including crevices,
wall cracks, windows, woodwork or floor gaps, the cellar, and
outside doors and drains.

For more information on how to avoid household triggers of chronic
inflammation, you can go to the AAAAI's website at www.aaaai.org, or
check out the EPA's website at http://www.epa.gov. See Chapter 6 for
more information on environmental exposures, many of which can also
trigger chronic inflammation.

7. GET IMMUNIZED

You should also update all your immunizations before you get pregnant.
Ask your doctor if you need any of the following six recommended adult
immunizations:

- **Tetanus-diphtheria-pertussis (Tdap) vaccine**—The new CDC guidelines recommend that all women receive a single dose of Tdap before they become pregnant. If you get pertussis (whooping cough) after your baby is born, you can infect your newborn. About 2,500 infants are infected with pertussis each year, mostly among young infants (<six months old) who have not completed their series of vaccinations. While the Tdap vaccine is safe in pregnancy and postpartum, ideally you should try to get immunized before pregnancy.

- **Hepatitis B vaccines**—If you haven't done so already, you should get immunized against hepatitis B. Hepatitis B can cause liver cirrhosis and cancer in the long run, and the virus can be transmitted to your baby. The vaccines consist of a series of three shots completed over a course of six months. If you are not sure whether or not you have been vaccinated against hepatitis B, your doctor can do a blood test (hepatitis B surface antibody) to check your immunity.

- **Influenza vaccine (flu shots)**—If you are going to be pregnant during the influenza season (usually between December and March in the United States), you should get a flu shot before you get pregnant. A growing body of evidence now suggests that maternal flu in the first half of pregnancy puts the baby at risk for schizophrenia in later life, possibly as a result of damages to the developing brain caused by inflammatory mediators. Pregnant women are at greater risk for influenza-related complications and hospitalization because of their compromised immune status. Flu shots are commonly made with a preservative (thimerosol) that contains small amounts of mercury; ask your doctor for the thimerosol-free flu shots if you are planning to get pregnant.

- **Mumps-measles-rubella (MMR) vaccine**—Measles, mumps, and rubella can cause birth defects, mental retardation, and even fetal death. Unless you were born outside the United States, you were probably immunized against MMR when you were a child. For some adults, however, immunity wanes over time, which would necessitate a booster vaccine for one or more components of the MMR. Your doctor can order blood tests to check your immunity and see if you need a booster before pregnancy. The vaccine is contraindicated during pregnancy.

• **Chickenpox (varicella)**—If you never had chickenpox before and contract it for the first time when you are pregnant, you can get very sick from varicella pneumonia. Furthermore, your baby has about a 2 percent chance of being born with one or more birth defects if he or she is exposed during the first half of pregnancy. If you have had chickenpox before, chances are you have immunity against chickenpox. If you are not sure whether or not you've been exposed to chickenpox in the past, your doctor can order a blood test (varicella IgG) to check your immunity against chickenpox. If you are not immune to chickenpox, you should get vaccinated before pregnancy because the vaccine is contraindicated during pregnancy.

• **Human papilloma virus (HPV) vaccine**—At least half of sexually active people will get HPV at some time in their lives. Every year in the United States, about 6.2 million people get HPV, 10,000 women will be diagnosed with cervical cancer, and nearly 4,000 will die from this cancer, which is caused by HPV. An HPV vaccine was approved in 2006; it protects women against the four subtypes of HPV that cause about 70 percent of cervical cancer and 90 percent of genital warts. Because it does not protect you against all subtypes of HPV that can cause cervical cancer, you will still need to get your routine pap smear. The vaccine is recommended for young girls and women ages 9–26; if you are over 26, the vaccine may still offer you some protection so talk to your doctor and health insurance plan about getting the vaccine. The vaccine consists of a series of three shots; the second and third doses are given at two and six months, respectively, following the initial dose. The vaccine is contraindicated during pregnancy.

Getting immunized against **MMR, chickenpox, and HPV** *before* you get pregnant is particularly important because these vaccines are contraindicated during pregnancy! Unlike Tdap, hepatitis B, and the flu vaccines, which use recombinant proteins to make the vaccines, MMR and chickenpox vaccines use the actual virus (albeit greatly attenuated in their virulence) to induce an immune memory. These vaccines can theoretically cause birth defects and are therefore contraindicated during pregnancy; **it is recommended that you avoid pregnancy for at least four weeks after receiving MMR or chickenpox vaccines.** Given its newness, the HPV vaccine is not recommended for pregnant women even though the vaccine uses recombinant proteins with no live virus and has not been found to cause birth defects or other problems during pregnancy.

8. EAT RIGHT

The foods you eat can be important triggers for chronic inflammation, or they can help enhance your immune fitness and modulate inflammation. Certain foods are thought to be pro-inflammatory because they exaggerate inflammation; foods that are high in saturated fats, *trans* fats, partially hydrogenated oils, added sugars, and refined carbohydrates can be quite pro-inflammatory. Other foods are considered anti-inflammatory because they help dampen inflammation; foods high in omega–3 fatty acids (e.g., fish oil, walnuts, flaxseeds) and antioxidants are known to have potent anti-inflammatory properties.

Inflammation can also cause oxidative stress. Oxidative stress occurs when the production of damaging free oxygen radicals and other oxidative molecules exceeds the body's capacity to detoxify them. Oxidative stress has been implicated in a number of pregnancy complications, including preeclampsia, fetal growth retardation, and preterm rupture of fetal membranes. Antioxidants can reduce oxidative stress. Antioxidants are categorized as either free radical scavengers that trap or decompose existing free radicals, or enzymes that inhibit peroxidase reactions involved in the production of free radicals. Free radical scavengers include vitamin C (ascorbate), vitamin E (tocopherols), carotenoids, and glutathione, which are found in great abundance in many fruits and vegetables. Antioxidant enzymes include glutathione peroxidase, superoxide dismutase, and catalase, which are dependent on the presence of cofactors such as selenium, zinc, and iron. Excellent sources of selenium include asparagus, button mushrooms, shiitake mushrooms, cod, shrimp, snapper, tuna, halibut, and salmon. Excellent sources of zinc include beef, lamb, venison, sesame and pumpkin seeds, green peas, and shrimp. Excellent sources of iron include cooked soybeans, lentils, boiled chards, spinach, meat, and venison. This is another reason why it is so important to eat a balanced diet everyday.

By now most of you should have read Chapter 2 on nutritional preparedness. Most of the ten steps to nutritional preparedness are also steps that could enhance your immune fitness and reduce chronic inflammation:

Step 1: Achieve a healthy weight
Step 2: Eat a balanced diet every day
Step 3: Make every calorie count
Step 4: Go low on glycemic load
Step 5: Load up on smart fats
Step 6: Dump the dumb fats
Step 7: Eat high-quality proteins
Step 8: Eat a rainbow of fruits and vegetables
Step 9: Take a daily multivitamin containing folic acid
Step 10: Eat more brain foods and less toxic foods

Also see Chapter 3 for a list of brain foods you should eat more of, and toxic foods you should avoid.

9. EXERCISE

Exercise, in moderation, can boost your immune functions and reduce chronic inflammation. Several randomized studies have shown that women who walk regularly (for 35–45 minutes a day, 5 days a week) for 12–15 weeks had half as many sick days due to colds and sore throats as those who don't exercise. The health benefits of regular exercise in preventing atherosclerosis, diabetes, and other chronic disease may be due primarily to its anti-inflammatory actions, and it is thought that regular exercise may also prevent several pregnancy complications, including gestational diabetes and preeclampsia, largely by reducing oxidative stress and chronic inflammation.

As discussed in Chapter 4, the National Institutes of Health recommends that all adults should set a long-term goal to exercise at least 30 minutes a day on most, if not all, days of the week. See Chapter 4, Step 1 for more information on exercise.

One cautionary note: While moderate exercise can boost your immune functions and reduce chronic inflammation, prolonged, high-intensity exercise may do the opposite. Athletes engaged in high-intensity exercise are particularly susceptible to infections for up to 72 hours after exercise, an effect that has been attributed to the immunosuppressive actions of stress hormones like cortisol. Physical and psychological stress, nutritional imbalance, and lack of rest may all contribute to the immune perturbations. If you engage in high-intensity exercise, make sure you eat a balanced diet, get plenty of rest, and don't get stressed out. There is some evidence that drinking a sports drink containing carbohydrates following exercise may reduce the immune-suppressive effects of prolonged and intense exercise. You may want to consider training every other day or every third day to allow your immune system (and stress response) a chance to recover. Show up healthy on a race day, and avoid training when you are sick. Watch out for overtraining and compulsive exercise. Remember, your goal is to stay fit before and during pregnancy, and not to win the race.

10. REDUCE STRESS

As discussed earlier in the chapter, chronic stress can suppress your immune functions, thereby increasing your susceptibility to infection. This is due in large part to the immune suppressive effects of the stress hormone cortisol. Studies have shown that women who are under chronic stress are more prone to a number of infections, including bacterial vaginosis (BV), which can increase the risk for preterm labor during pregnancy. Chronic stress can also promote chronic inflammation, which may be due to the loss of counter-regulation from a worn-out HPA axis. Thus chronic stress can mess up your immune system in two ways—it suppresses immune functions and flames inflammation.

So you need to learn to cope with stress and build up your stress resilience before you get pregnant. Chapter 4 can help you learn to cope with stress better. Here is a quick review of the ten steps to stress resilience:

1. Exercise
2. Get a good night's sleep
3. Eat right
4. Learn to relax
5. Learn to prevent stress
6. Learn to problem-solve
7. Learn to resolve conflicts
8. Develop positive mental health
9. Get connected
10. Get help

To sum up this chapter, the best way to avoid infection and inflammation during pregnancy is by tuning up your immune system and restoring your immune allostasis before pregnancy. To do so you need to remove all ongoing sources of infection and inflammation (and avoid new infections and inflammation) that can cause further wear and tear on your immune system, such as periodontal disease, STIs, UTIs, RTIs, TORCH, foodborne illness, mildew, molds, and dust mites. You should also make lifestyle changes to improve your immune fitness before pregnancy, such as quitting smoking, getting immunized, eating healthy, exercising regularly, reducing stress, and building your stress resilience.

Environmental toxicants are another important source of chronic inflammation. Let's turn our attention now to what you can do to clean up your environment before pregnancy.

healthy environment

a silent pandemic

Imagine a chemical so toxic that if it is inhaled by a pregnant woman and crosses the placenta, it can cause permanent damage to her baby's developing brain. Now imagine this chemical is so widespread that it put more than 100 million American children at risk. And let's say this chemical can reduce the number of American children with far-above average intelligence (IQ above 130) by half, and similarly increase the number of American children with mental retardation (IQ below 70) by half.

We would never, ever allow this chemical to pollute our air, would we?

Well, we did (actually, our parents did). Lead has been added to gasoline to boost octane levels in the United States since the 1920s, but it was not until the 1970s that we began to phase out lead additives in gasoline (which was completed by the mid–1990s). If you were born between 1960 and 1990, chances are you were exposed to a substantial dose of lead from gasoline combustion inside the womb. Ever wonder how much smarter you might have been?

During the 1950s, there was a mysterious outbreak of cerebral palsy, mental retardation, microcephaly (small head), and other neurological disorders in children born around the Minamata Bay in Japan. It was several years before the cause was discovered. A nearby factory was regularly dumping mercury into Minamata Bay. At first this wasn't thought to be a problem because inorganic mercury is poorly absorbed by fish, animals, and humans, and people thought the amount of mercury dumped into the bay was insignificant and should have been quickly diluted in the ocean. The solution to pollution is dilution, right?

Wrong. Bacteria in the water can convert inorganic mercury into organic mercury, which is then easily absorbed by the intestines of fish. Inside the fish mercury accumulates, and the mercury level can get up to 100,000-fold greater than the level in the water. Because humans are "top predators," the build-up of mercury gets even higher inside our bodies because we eat all the fish and animals that accumulate organic mercury from polluted waters. So even a trace of mercury in the water can get concentrated hundreds- and thousandsfold by entering the food chain. Eventually this kind of mercury build-up damaged the brains of babies born to mothers living near Minamata Bay.

All right. So we've learned from our mistakes. Lead is now being phased out from gasoline. The EPA/FDA is now warning pregnant women, and women who might become pregnant, about mercury in fish and seafood. Your future baby is safe, right?

Think again. Of the greater than 80,000 known chemicals, fewer than half have ever been subjected to even token laboratory testing for toxicity to humans. Over 1,000 chemicals have been shown to be toxic to the brain in animal experiments, and 201 chemicals have been shown to be toxic to the adult human brain, but only 5 (lead, methylmercury, arsenic, PCB, and ethanol) have been established to be toxic to the fetal brain.

Does this mean that the fetal brain is tougher than the adult brain? To the contrary. The fetal brain is much more vulnerable than the adult brain. This vulnerability stems from the fact that in nine months, the fetal brain has to develop from a small collection of cells into a complex organ consisting of billions of precisely located, highly interconnected, and specialized cells. Any agent that interferes with any developmental process in the fetal brain could cause permanent, irreparable damage. The reason that only five chemicals are known to be toxic to the fetal brain is that most of the other chemicals have not been studied for their neurodevelopmental toxicity.

Not very reassuring, is it? This is why as a parent I get mad. If I am paying taxes to the government to protect my children and family, then why isn't the government doing more testing, or requiring more testing, of the thousands of chemicals that are being released into our environment everyday? As a researcher, I understand the challenges of this kind of research, especially when the damage might not manifest for years or even decades. This kind of research is hard to do and costly, but for the sake of our future generation I don't think we can afford not to.

And why isn't our government doing more to protect our children and families from these chemicals? The answer has always been: "We don't have enough proof that they cause harm." But why should the burden of proof be on us to show that they are toxic to our children and families, instead of on industries (as many other developed countries have done) that are profiting from the sale of these chemicals to show that they are safe? I will come back to this point at the end of the book.

Philippe Grandjean at Harvard School of Public Health warns us about a silent pandemic of developmental neurotoxicity that may be spreading across our nation. This pandemic is silent because its profound effects are not readily apparent from available public health statistics. For decades fetal exposure to lead in gasoline may have caused subclinical decreases in IQ and subtle learning disabilities that we never knew about, and there is some evidence that such fetal exposure may have also been responsible for shortened attention span, increased impulsivity, heightened aggressiveness, slowed motor coordination, and impaired memory and language skills. Lead was an important cause of this silent pandemic for decades, but who knows which of the thousands of chemicals that are polluting our environment, including hundreds that are known to be toxic to the human brain, may be robbing our children of their greatest potentials before they are born, or even conceived?

no escape

You are probably now wondering which chemicals are known to be toxic to the human brain. Table 6.1 provides a list of 201 known neurotoxic chemicals that Dr. Grandjean and his colleagues have compiled. You can also get an updated list of chemicals known to cause reproductive and developmental toxicity (at least the ones that have been studied) at California's Proposition 65 website: http://www.oehha.ca.gov/prop65/prop65_list/files/P65single081106.pdf.

table 6.1: chemicals that are known to be toxic to the human brain.

Metals and inorganic compounds

- Aluminum compounds
- Arsenic and arsenic compounds
- Azide compounds
- Barium compounds
- Bismuth compounds
- Carbon monoxide
- Cyanide compounds
- Decaborane
- Diborane
- Ethylmercury
- Fluoride compounds
- Hydrogen sulphide
- Lead and lead compounds
- Lithium compounds
- Manganese and manganese compounds
- Mercury and mercuric compounds
- Methylmercury
- Nickel carbonyl
- Pentaborane

- Phosphine
- Phosphorus
- Selenium compounds
- Tellurium compounds
- Thallium compounds
- Tin compounds

Organic solvents

- Acetone
- Benzene
- Benzyl alcohol
- Carbon disulphide
- Chloroform
- Chloroprene
- Cumene
- Cyclohexane
- Cyclohexanol
- Cyclohexanone
- Dibromochloro-propane
- Dichloroacetic acid
- 1,3-Dichloropropene
- Diethylene glycol
- N,N-Dimethylformamide
- 2-Ethoxyethyl acetate
- Ethyl acetate
- Ethylene dibromide
- Ethylene glycol
- n-Hexane
- Isobutyronitrile
- Isophorone
- Isopropyl alcohol
- Isopropylacetone
- Methanol
- Methyl butyl ketone

- Methyl cellosolve
- Methyl ethyl ketone
- Methylcyclopentane
- Methylene chloride
- Nitrobenzene
- 2-Nitropropane
- 1-Pentanol
- Propyl bromide
- Pyridine
- Styrene
- Tetrachloroethane
- Tetrachloro-ethylene
- Toluene
- 1,1,1-Trichloroethane
- Trichloroethylene
- Vinyl chloride
- Xylene

Other organic substances

- Acetone cyanohydrin
- Acrylamide
- Acrylonitrile
- Allyl chloride
- Aniline
- 1,2-Benzenedicarbonitrile
- Benzonitrile
- Butylated triphenyl phosphate
- Caprolactam
- Cyclonite
- Dibutyl phthalate
- 3-(Dimethylamino)-propanenitrile
- Diethylene glycol diacrylate
- Dimethyl sulphate
- Dimethylhydrazine

- Dinitrobenzene
- Dinitrotoluene
- Ethylbis(2-chloroethyl)amine
- Ethylene
- Ethylene oxide
- Fluoroacetamide
- Fluoroacetic acid
- Hexachlorophene
- Hydrazine
- Hydroquinone
- Methyl chloride
- Methyl formate
- Methyl iodide
- Methyl methacrylate
- p-Nitroaniline
- Phenol
- p-Phenylenediamine
- Phenylhydrazine
- Polybrominated biphenyls
- Polybrominated diphenyl ethers
- Polychlorinated biphenyls
- Propylene oxide
- 2, 3, 7, 8-tetrachlorodibenzo-p-dioxin (TCDD)
- Tributyl phosphate
- Trichlorotriethylamine
- Trimethyl phosphate
- Tri-o-tolyl phosphate
- Triphenyl phosphate

Pesticides

- Aldicarb
- Aldrin
- Bensulide
- Bromophos

- Carbaryl
- Carbofuran
- Carbophenothion
- alpha-Chloralose
- Chlordane
- Chlordecone
- Chlorfenvinphos
- Chlormephos
- Chlorpyrifos
- Chlorthion
- Coumaphos
- Cyhalothrin
- Cypermethrin
- 2,4-D
- DDT
- Deltamethrin
- Demeton
- Dialifor
- Diazinon
- Dichlofenthion
- Dichlorvos
- Dieldrin
- Dimefox
- Dimethoate
- Dinitrocresol
- Dinoseb
- Dioxathion
- Disulphoton
- Edifenphos
- Endosulphan
- Endothion
- Endrin
- EPN
- Ethiofencarb

- Ethion
- Ethoprop
- Fenitrothion
- Fensulphothion
- Fenthion
- Fenvalerate
- Fonofos
- Formothion
- Heptachlor
- Heptenophos
- Hexachlorobenzene
- Isobenzan
- Isolan
- Isoxathion
- Leptophos
- Lindane
- Merphos
- Metaldehyde
- Methamidophos
- Methidathion
- Methomyl
- Methyl bromide
- Methyl demeton
- Methyl parathion
- Mevinphos
- Mexacarbate
- Mipafox
- Mirex
- Monocrotophos
- Naled
- Nicotine
- Oxydemeton-methyl
- Parathion
- Pentachlorophenol

- Phorate
- Phosphamidon
- Phospholan
- Propaphos
- Propoxur
- Pyriminil
- Sarin
- Schradan
- Soman
- Sulprofos
- 2,4,5-T
- Tebupirimfos
- Tefluthrin
- Terbufos
- Thiram
- Toxaphene
- Trichlorfon
- Trichloronat

The problem with lists like these is that unless you are a chemist, they are not very readable. What do you do with lists like these? This is why I wrote this chapter—to teach you how to avoid harmful exposures and create a safe and healthy nest in preparation for your future baby.

Generally speaking, these chemicals fall into four major categories: **metals, solvents, pesticides,** and **endocrine disruptors**. Among **metals,** lead and mercury have been the most extensively studied reproductive and developmental toxicants. Cadmium, arsenic, and manganese are also likely reproductive toxicants. Cadmium is used in metal plating, semiconductors, wire, plastic, batteries, welding, soldering, ceramics, painting, and cigarettes; it can damage the testes and interfere with sperm production; it is also toxic to the placenta and can cause miscarriage and birth defects. Arsenic is used as a wood preservative and in agricultural chemicals; it has been shown to cause miscarriage, birth defects, and abnormal neurological development, including impairment of hearing development. Manganese exposure *in utero* has also been linked to impaired neurobehavioral development in children. Manganese has been added to gasoline in the United States since 1995 as an octane booster (in the form of manganese methylcyclopentadienyl, or MMT), and many scientists are now concerned that we may be repeating a mistake similar to the original addition of lead to gasoline in the 1920s. There is some evidence that other metals and inorganic compounds, such as chromium, nickel, and fluoride, may also damage fetal development. Fluoride is added to water in communities across the United States to fight cavities, but too much fluoride may cause tooth and bone damage, and possibly IQ deficits in children.

Solvents are substances that can dissolve other substances. The most widely used solvents include benzene, toluene, ethanol, formaldehyde, alcohol, and phenol, which are found in many common household products, including paints, strippers, glues, markers, cosmetics, and some cleaning agents. If you work in electronics, health care, dry-cleaning, auto repair, laboratories, or painting, chances are you are exposed to some solvents at work. Pesticides frequently contain solvents as inert ingredients. A number of solvents have been shown to increase the risk of miscarriage and certain birth defects (particularly those of the central nervous system, urinary system, heart, lip, and palate). There is some evidence that babies born to *fathers* exposed to high levels of solvents may be at increased risk for childhood cancers of the brain and urinary tract, and leukemia.

Pesticide use is widespread in the United States, and you don't have to be a migrant farm worker to be exposed. Common household exposures include the pesticides you use to get rid of ants, roaches, fleas, ticks, fungi, weeds, and other unwanted organisms from your house or yard. Pesticides used outdoors can get tracked indoors, where they collect on carpets, dust, furniture, toys, etc. One survey found that 98 percent of households used pesticides at least once annually, and two-thirds used pesticides more than five times a year. More than 80 percent of households surveyed used pesticides during pregnancy and 70 percent used during the first six months of a child's life! Pesticide sprays can get carried by air, water, and soil into your home. Many parks, playgrounds, golf courses, and even school yards get regularly sprayed with pesticides.

Pesticides can also get into the food chain and accumulate in your body; the EPA is currently reviewing standards on the acceptable level of pesticide residues in food for thousands of pesticides. Many pesticides have yet to be tested for their reproductive or developmental toxicities; of the 600 active pesticide ingredients used in over 20,000 pesticide products marketed in the United States, only 100 have complete toxicological data available. A large body of studies has linked pesticide exposure during pregnancy to miscarriage, stillbirth, birth defects, chromosome and sperm damage, fetal growth retardation, and some childhood cancers.

From 1950 to 1971, a synthetic estrogen called DES (diethylstilbestrol) was given to more than five million pregnant women in the United States to prevent miscarriage. Decades later, it was discovered that these women had a greater risk for breast cancer. Furthermore, their daughters had a greater risk for anomalies of their reproductive organs, reduced fertility, ectopic pregnancies, miscarriages, preterm birth, and vaginal and other cancers, while their sons had greater risk for small and undescended testicles, abnormal semen, and hypospadias (a birth defect in which the urethra opens on the underside or below the penis).

DES is an example of an **endocrine disruptor** that can cause reproductive and developmental abnormalities, immune system malfunction, and cancer in babies exposed inside the womb. While DES and PCB are banned in the United States, other endocrine disruptors such as dioxins, alkylphenols, and phthalates are widespread. Dioxins come primarily from the disposal of chlorinated compounds that are used in many consumer products (e.g., polyvinyl chloride, or PVC); leading sources of dioxins in the environment include emissions from municipal, medical, and hazardous waste incinerators. Alkylphenols are used in detergents, paints, pesticides, plastics, food wraps, and many other consumer products. Phthalates, the most abundant man-made chemicals in the environment, are used in construction; automotive, medical, and household products; clothing; toys; plastic wraps; beverage containers; and packaging. Over one billion pounds of 25 different phthalate compounds are produced each year in the United States. In addition to these three endocrine disruptors, many more chemicals with endocrine-disrupting activity remain unidentified and unstudied (their number could be in the thousands).

I can go on and on, but you get the idea. There is no escape. Everywhere you look, you'll find products made with potential reproductive and developmental toxicants—paints, glues, markers, cosmetics, detergents, plastic wraps, baby bottles, toys, and on and on. They are found in fish and seafood, in meat and dairy products. They are in the air we breathe and the water we drink. There is just no escape. The best thing we can do is to clean up the environment and demand higher standards of consumer product safety for our children and families. Short of that, the best thing you can do is to minimize your exposure and build a safe and healthy nest before pregnancy.

why worry now?

You are not pregnant now. So why worry now? I will give you four major reasons why you should start to worry now and not later.

The first has to do with the idea of **persistence**. Many chemicals persist in your body. Some pesticides persist for months or even years inside your body. If you wait until you get pregnant, you won't be able to get rid of all the chemicals that are stored inside your body that quickly. Many chemicals will cross the placenta, and some will show up in the breast milk after the baby is born.

The second has to do with **bioaccumulation**. Bioaccumulation is the build-up of a substance in an organism. For example, substances that are fat-soluble, such as dioxins or PCBs, are stored in body fat rather than excreted in urine. Other substances like methylmercury can bind to a protein and get concentrated in an organ such as the brain, kidneys, or liver. And because we sit on top of the food chain, we take in all the methylmercury that bioaccumulates in the fish and animals we eat. Talk about *karma*.

The third reason has to do with **timing**. Timing is everything when it comes to developmental toxicity, and there is growing evidence that exposures during critical windows of development in early pregnancy may cause the greatest damage. Exposure to excess carbon monoxide in the second month of pregnancy when the heart is rapidly developing (beginning about 22 days after conception) has been linked to fetal heart defects. Studies now show exposures to air pollution in the three months leading up conception may damage sperm DNA, which may increase the risks for miscarriage, birth defects, and even childhood cancers.

Lastly, I come back to the idea of **allostasis** and **allostatic overload**. Recall from Chapter 1, allostasis refers to the body's ability to maintain balance through change, and allostatic overload refers to wear and tear from chronic stress (biological or psychological) which, over time, will wear out your body's ability to maintain allostasis. In response to a foreign invader, be it molds or dust mites or chemicals, your body activates an immune response. Once the invader has been contained, however, the body automatically shuts off the immune response. That's allostasis. But if the body is bombarded day in and day out with environmental toxicants, your immune system is always turned on and does not shut off. You may end up with chronic inflammation, which could put your future pregnancy at risk. If you want a smart and healthy baby, you need to go into pregnancy with a fine-tuned immune system. As I discussed in Chapter 5, an important step in the tune-up of your immune system is to get rid of environmental triggers of chronic inflammation before you get pregnant.

So even if you are not planning on getting pregnant right away, now is a good time to start building your baby a safe and healthy nest.

ten steps to creating a healthy environment

So how do you build a safe and healthy nest amidst all the environmental toxicants from which there appears to be no escape? Here are ten steps you can take to creating a healthy environment for your baby, before you get pregnant.

Step 1: Make your home a lead-free zone
Step 2: Drink clean water
Step 3: Breathe clean air
Step 4: Detoxify your home
Step 5: Avoid using pesticides
Step 6: Start nesting
Step 7: Survey your neighborhood
Step 8: Choose a cleaner commute
Step 9: Avoid harmful exposures at work
Step 10: Know your rights at work

1. MAKE YOUR HOME A LEAD-FREE ZONE

Lead is stored in the body and can stay in the bones for many years. During pregnancy, lead is released from the body stores and crosses the placenta easily; fetal lead levels can be up to 90 percent of maternal blood lead levels. Lead can interfere with fetal brain development, and prenatal exposure has been shown to result in significant cognitive impairment in children. Common sources of exposures at home include lead paint, consumer products, and drinking water.

Here are a few tips on how to make your home a lead-free zone:

- **Remove lead paint.** Was your home built before 1978? Any home built and painted before 1978 probably has interior lead paint. Lead can also contaminate the home's surrounding soil. Before you buy or lease an old house, ask the owner if the home has been tested for lead paint. The seller or landlord is required by law to disclose any known information about lead paint (though they are not required to test the paint themselves). If the paint hasn't been tested, inspect the house carefully for the presence of peeling paint, especially around the window frames and radiators. You can send the paint chips to a certified lab for analysis; don't buy or lease a home based on the results of home test kits.

If you are living in a house with peeling lead paint, move. If you cannot move, have the paint removed by trained personnel (this is not a do-it-yourself job; you can poison yourself and contaminate the home/yard even more). The U.S. Department of Housing and Urban Development (HUD), as well as most state and local governments, have lead abatement programs and can provide some financial support for low-income families. If it is not possible to remove lead paint and the paint is peeling or flaking, you can cover it with wallpaper, tiles, sheetrock, or paneling, but it is not effective to simply paint over lead paint. Contaminated soil can be covered with a layer of loose dirt. Don't plant any root crops such as potatoes or carrots in contaminated soil since lead collects in the roots.

- **Avoid consumer products containing lead.** Lead can be found in a number of consumer products including lipsticks, hair dyes, and mini-blinds. Check product labels for the presence of lead, and avoid the use of any product that may contain lead. Some products don't come with labels, such as lead-glazed housewares, plates, and potteries that you might buy from a garage sale or a discount store. One consumer group found unacceptably high levels of lead in about 10 percent of the children's vinyl lunchboxes they tested—children's lunchboxes of all places! The 2007 recall by Mattel and other toy manufacturers of millions of toys containing lead paint is a further reminder of the need for greater awareness. You can test for lead in consumer products by using home test kits.
- **Test your drinking water for lead.** Lead can also be found in your drinking water (see Box 6.1). How can you protect your family from leaded water? You can start by testing for lead at

the tap. You can test a water sample using a home testing kit, or call the U.S. EPA Drinking Water Hotline (1–800–426–4791) for a convenient certified testing laboratory. Make a habit of running the tap water for a minute or two after any periods of disuse (such as overnight) to flush out of the system any lead from pipes. Avoid drinking hot water (which causes more leaching) straight from the tap; use cold water and heat it up. Many water filters can filter out lead. Lead is not a major concern in the shower because it is not absorbed through the skin and is not volatile.

box 6.1: is your drinking water unleaded?

In January 2004 in our nation's capital, D.C. residents learned from a *Washington Post* story that hazardous levels of lead had been present in their drinking water for several years, largely as a result of corrosion of lead pipelines. This story raised concerns in communities across the United States about the quality of their own drinking water. Under the Safe Drinking Water Act, anyone concerned about the community water supply can request test results and public notices of any violations from the local water department. However, another *Washington Post* story in October 2004 called attention to misrepresentation of water lead levels in cities across the United States, including Boston, Philadelphia, and New York City. Federal, state, and utility records showed that dozens of utilities had obscured the extent of lead contamination, ignored requirements to correct problems, and failed to turn over data to regulators for years.

(continued)

Even if your municipal water supply is okay, your pipes may not be. Additional lead exposure can come from lead leaching from indoor pipes, even if you have so-called "lead-free" pipes. "Lead-free" pipes usually contain some amount of lead because our Congress (in their infinite wisdom) legislated in the 1996 Safe Drinking Water Act Amendments that so-called "lead-free" plumbing pipes and components (including brass faucet bodies and necks, shutoff valves, and water meters) could have up to 8 percent lead.

Lead was taken out of gasoline because of its toxicity. You wouldn't think of filling your car with leaded gasoline today; so why would you fill yourself up on leaded water? You can test your tap water for lead by using a home testing kit, or by sending a water sample to a certified testing laboratory.

2. DRINK CLEAN WATER

Other than lead, there are many reproductive toxicants that can contaminate your drinking water at home, including organic solvents, pesticide residues, and trace amounts of chloroform and other chlorinated and brominated organic compounds. One 1998 study found that pregnant women in their first trimester who drank at least five glasses of tap water a day were nearly twice as likely to have a miscarriage as women who drank less tap water; the study linked the miscarriage risk to chlorination disinfection by-products called trihalomethanes (THMs) found in the municipal water of three California communities (Santa Clara County and Walnut Creek in the Bay Area, and Fontana in San Bernardino County). THMs have also been linked to cleft lip and palate, neural tube defects, cardiac defects, and other birth defects.

Here are some steps you can take to ensure the safety and quality of your drinking water at home.

- **Know your water.** You can request a copy of the Annual Water Quality Report from your municipal water authority (the one that sends your water bills) to see how clean and safe your tap water is, or simply log on to the EPA website at www .epa.gov to access local water information. You can also send a sample of tap water to a certified laboratory for testing.
- **Use a water filter.** You can use a water filter to remove reproductive toxicants from your tap water. The selection of a water filter very much depends on what is in your water that you want to filter out. For example, most pour-through pitchers that use activated carbon filter do an adequate job in removing organic contaminants that cause taste and odor problems, as well as metals such as lead and copper; some are even designed to remove chlorination by-products, cleaning solvents, and pesticides. However, many such devices do not remove nitrate, bacteria, or dissolved minerals. For guidance on how to select a water filter, go to the non-profit National Sanitation Foundation (NSF) International website at www .nsf.org and look for the water safety kit. You can also verify a product's claims to remove a particular substance of concern on the NSF website. The EPA website also provides some advice on tap water safety.
- **Don't overcook water.** For the most part, you don't need to boil your drinking water in the United States unless there is a "boil water notice" issued by your municipal water supplier. Boiling water for one minute is effective in eliminating most microorganisms. However, boiling water does little to remove such contaminants as nitrates and pesticides; in fact, it may concentrate these contaminants in drinking water if you boil it for more than a minute, since boiling reduces the volume of water by 20 percent. Boiling reduces but does not completely eliminate chlorination by-products in your drinking water.

- **Beware of bottled water.** If you choose to drink bottled water, *caveat emptor* (buyer beware) should be the watchword. About 25 percent of bottled water sold is simply reprocessed municipal water. Both Aquafina from the Pepsi-Cola Company and Dasani from the Coca-Cola Company are nothing but purified tap water from municipal water systems.

  Bottled water may not be any safer than tap water. While the Food and Drug Administration (FDA) regulates the safety of bottled water that is imported or sold between states, 60 to 70 percent of bottled water packaged and sold within a given state is not regulated. And while the EPA mandates daily monitoring of public drinking water for many bacterial and chemical contaminants, the FDA requires less comprehensive testing (and in most cases requires it only once a year) for bottled water. For example, bottled water companies are not required to test their water for *Cryptosporidium* or *Giardia*, and do not have to meet standards required of tap water for toxic chemicals such as phthalates. Furthermore, containers that sit for weeks or months at room temperature can serve as breeding grounds for bacteria, and there is no telling how long your bottled water has been sitting on a loading dock or store shelves, since bottlers are not required to put expiration dates on bottles.

  Even if your bottled water is safe, your water bottle may not be (see Box 6.2). You can write to the bottlers of your favorite bottled water to obtain a report showing what contaminants, if any, are present in their bottled water product. You can also look on the NSF International website or contact NSF Consumer Hotline toll-free at 1–877–8-NSF-HELP (1–877–867–3435) or by email at info@nsf.org to see if your favorite brand carries NSF independent certification.

- **Protect your well water.** If you use water from your own household well, as do 15 percent of Americans, it is especially important for you to pay attention to water safety. The EPA recommends several steps you can take to protect your private water drinking supply. You can also get more information on well water safety at the NSF International website.

box 6.2: how safe is your water bottle?

Even if your bottled water is safe, your water bottle may not be. Some plastic bottles may leak toxic chemicals into the water. For example, water bottles made of #7 plastic (polycarbonate) can leach a chemical called bisphenol-A (BPA), an endocrine-disruptor that could disrupt normal fetal development. Granted, the amounts of BPA found in the water are usually very low, but even very low doses of BPA have been shown to cause a variety of health effects in laboratory animals. In animal studies, BPA causes cells to turn genes on or off, which could predispose a fetus or child to a reproductive disorder later in life. Recent evidence from rat studies suggests that fetal exposure to even low levels of BPA is associated with increased susceptibility for breast cancer as adults. One recent human study found higher levels of BPA in women with recurrent miscarriages. Based on a review of over 500 studies, an expert panel convened by the National Institute of Health expressed "some concern" that BPA exposure could have neurological or behavioral effects on pregnant women, fetuses, infants, and children. Therefore, it makes sense to avoid any unnecessary exposure whenever possible.

Here are some tips from National Geographic's *The Green Guide* on how to choose your water bottles:

(continued)

- **Check the recycling number on the bottom of your bottle** (look inside the recycling symbol).

Plastics to Avoid
#3 (polyvinyl chloride, which may contain phthalates)
#6 (polystyrene)
#7 (polycarbonate, which may contain BPA)
    By the way, #7 polycarbonate is the plastic used to make most 5-gallon clear water coolers and most clear plastic baby bottles!
Safer Plastics for Use
#1 (polyethylene terephthalate, or PETE)
#2 (high-density polyethylene)
#4 (low-density polyethylene)
#5 (polypropylene)

- **Sniff and taste.** If there's a hint of plastic in your water, don't drink it.

- **Keep bottled water away from heat,** which promotes leaching of chemicals.

- **Use bottled water quickly,** as chemicals may migrate from plastic during storage. Ask retailers how long water has been on their shelves, and don't buy if it's been there for months.

- **Do not reuse bottles intended for single use.** Reused water bottles also make good breeding grounds for bacteria.

- **Choose rigid, reusable containers** or, for hot/acidic liquids, thermoses with stainless steel or ceramic interiors.

- **Consider using a reusable filtration water bottle, a glass bottle, or a water filter.** It's better for the environment, and may be safer and healthier for you and your baby.

3. BREATHE CLEAN AIR

Your future baby's health can also be affected by a large number of indoor air pollutants, including cigarette and cigar smoking, gases and particles from stoves, heaters, fireplaces and chimneys, chemicals from dry-cleaning (see Box 6.3), and possibly radon and asbestos. Here are some steps you can take to protect your air quality at home.

- **Make your home a smoke-free zone.** If you smoke, quit now. Smoking during pregnancy can cause miscarriage, fetal growth retardation, preterm birth, stillbirth, and placental separation. Babies whose moms smoked during pregnancy are at greater risk for a whole host of health problems, including sudden infant death syndrome (SIDS), attention deficit hyperactivity disorder (ADHD), and asthma. Waiting until you get pregnant to quit may be too late; smoking just before and in early pregnancy can create inflammatory and hypoxic conditions inside the womb that may interfere with early placental growth and development. And anyone who has ever tried to quit during pregnancy will tell you that it is not all that easy. Only about one in three pregnant women are able to quit—and of those who quit, about one-third will relapse during pregnancy—probably because of the addiction and all the added stress of pregnancy for which smoking is a coping mechanism. So quit now before you get pregnant. I gave several suggestions and links on how to quit in Chapter 5.

  And don't let anyone else smoke inside your home. If they have to smoke, make them go outside. Secondhand smoke or passive smoking does nearly as much harm to your baby as if you were smoking yourself. Smoking in a different room within the house will reduce, but will not eliminate, your exposure to secondhand smoke; so make them go outside. Opening your windows or using exhaust fans to increase ventilation helps, but because smoking produces

such large amounts of pollutants, natural or mechanical
ventilation techniques will not remove them from the air in
your home as quickly as they build up. Bottom line: Make
your home a smoke-free zone.

- **Keep your stoves, heaters, and fireplace burning clean.** In
  addition to cigarette smoke, other sources of air pollutants
  inside your home include woodstoves, gas stoves, unvented
  kerosene or gas space heaters, and fireplaces with blocked,
  leaking, or damaged chimneys or flues. The major pollutants
  released are carbon monoxide, nitrogen dioxide, and particles
  that could cause harm to your pregnancy. Here are a few tips
  on how you can protect yourself and your future baby from
  these air pollutants:

  - Install and use exhaust fans over gas cooking stoves and
    ranges; using a stove hood with a fan vented to the
    outdoors greatly reduces exposure to pollutants during
    cooking. Keep the burners properly adjusted. Ask your
    gas company to adjust the burner so that the flame tip is
    blue. Improper adjustment, often indicated by a persis-
    tent yellow-tipped flame, causes increased pollutant
    emissions;
  - Keep woodstove emissions to a minimum. Choose properly
    sized new woodstoves that are certified as meeting EPA
    emission standards;
  - Take special precautions when operating fuel-burning
    unvented space heaters. While a space heater is in use,
    open a door from the room where the heater is located
    to the rest of the house and open a window
    slightly;
  - Have central air handling systems, including furnaces,
    flues, and chimneys, inspected annually and promptly
    repair cracks or damaged parts. Change filters frequently
    during periods of use;

- Carbon monoxide is a highly toxic gas. It can be lethal at very high levels. It is a by-product of incomplete combustion of fossil fuels from faulty devices such as boilers, furnaces, space heaters, and fireplaces with blocked chimneys. Because carbon monoxide is colorless, odorless, tasteless, and non-irritating, the only way to detect it is by using a detector. If you use any fuel-burning appliances inside your home, consider installing carbon monoxide detectors.

box 6.3: dry-cleaning and your reproductive health

On the way home from work, you go pick up your dry-cleaning. You roll up your car windows to keep dust out. As soon as you get home you hang your clothes up in the closet, still inside their plastic bags.

Sounds familiar?

Perchloroethylene (PCE, or "perc") is the chemical most widely used in dry-cleaning. PCE is a solvent that dissolves grease and oil from clothes without damaging the fibers. It has been linked to spontaneous abortion and infertility and is a suspected carcinogen.

Newly dry-cleaned clothes brought home and placed in a closet may result in PCE levels within the closet more than one hundred times the level the federal government considers safe for workers. The bedroom may have levels eight times as great, and even adjoining rooms may be contaminated at levels five times the worker safety standard.

Here are some steps you can take before and during pregnancy

(continued)

to reduce your exposure to PCE and other chemicals from your dry-cleaning:

- Avoid chemical dry-cleaning before and during pregnancy, whenever possible. If your local cleaner offers safer, PCE-free ("perc-free") cleaning methods such as CO_2 or wet cleaning, consider trying them;
- PCE can leave a pungent smell on clothes. If dry-cleaned clothes have a strong chemical odor when you pick them up, do not accept them until they have been properly dried. If they still have a strong chemical odor on subsequent visits, try a different dry-cleaner;
- Avoid picking up from the dry-cleaner if you are pregnant or planning to be pregnant. Have someone else do it for you whenever possible;
- If you have to pick up your dry-cleaning, make sure the car is well ventilated on the way home. Toxic fumes containing PCE and other chemicals can build up in an enclosed car;
- Remove the plastic bags and air out your dry-cleaning in the garage or outdoors before storing them indoors;
- To reduce your need for dry-cleaning, hang up clothes immediately after you've worn them, give them a day off between wearings, and air them out before returning them to the closet. To spiff up a suit, you can simply steam it.

- **Test your home for radon and asbestos.** Have your home tested for radon and, if you live in an old house, for asbestos as well. While there is no conclusive evidence that radon or asbestos causes any reproductive or developmental hazards, they are known to cross the placenta and can be absorbed by the fetus. Radon and asbestos have been linked to

certain types of cancers and lung disease, which
should be enough reason for you to worry about
them.

Radon. Any home may have a radon problem, whether it is new or old,
well-sealed or drafty, and with or without basements. While radon problems may be more common in some areas, excessive radon levels have
been found in homes in all 50 states. The most common source of indoor
radon is uranium in the soil or rock on which homes are built. Radon gas
enters homes through dirt floors, cracks in concrete walls and floors, floor
drains, and sumps. You can protect your family from radon exposure at
home by doing the following:

- Test your home for radon–it's easy and inexpensive.
- Fix your home if your radon level is 4 picocuries per liter (pCi/L)
  or higher.
- Radon levels less than 4 pCi/L still pose a risk, and in many
  cases can be reduced.
- If you want more information on radon, contact your state
  radon office, or call 800-SOS-RADON.

Asbestos. Asbestos is a mineral fiber that has been used commonly in a
variety of building construction materials for insulation and as a fire-
retardant. Several asbestos products are now banned, and manufacturers
have also voluntarily limited uses of asbestos. Today, asbestos is most
commonly found in older homes, in pipe and furnace insulation materials, asbestos shingles, millboard, textured paints and other coating materials, and floor tiles. You can take the following steps to protect your
family from asbestos exposure at home:

- If you suspect that your home (or the house you are about to
  buy or lease) contains asbestos, take a small sample and send it
  to an EPA-certified lab for testing (costs about $30). Make sure

you dampen the area with water before sampling so that you don't spread asbestos fibers around. You can also hire an inspector for about $100 plus lab costs.

- It is best to leave undamaged asbestos material alone if it is not likely to be disturbed.
- This is not a do-it-yourself job! Use trained and qualified contractors for control measures that may disturb asbestos and for cleanup.
- Follow proper procedures in replacing woodstove door gaskets that may contain asbestos.

For more information on what you can do to safeguard indoor air quality in your home, visit the EPA or NSF websites on indoor air quality.

4. DETOXIFY YOUR HOME

Let's do a walkthrough, room by room, and start detoxifying your home before you start nesting.

- **Bathrooms.** Let's start with the bathrooms. It might surprise you how many reproductive hazards are in your bathroom.
  - Antibacterial soap. Get rid of antibacterial soaps, especially ones containing the pesticides **triclocarban** and **triclosan**. Plain, non-fragrant soap and water are just as effective and may be less harmful.
  - Personal care products. Get rid of cosmetics, deodorants, shampoo, hair spray, lotion, and other personal care products with chemical additives such as **phthalates, formaldehyde, glycol ethers**, and **petroleum**. As much as you can, use natural, organic, chemical-free products with the Eco-Cert label as well as the USDA Organic seal. You can also compare the safety of common brands of personal care products at the Environmental Working Group's Skin

Deep Cosmetics Safety Database website at www.cosmetic-sdatabase.com.

- Air fresheners. Avoid using air fresheners, which may contain **benzene, phthalates**, and other **organic volatile compounds**. Just open the window and air out the bathroom. Baking soda, cedar blocks, or sachets of dried flowers and herbs can also freshen up the bathroom without all the toxicants.

- Bathroom cleaners. Avoid using bleach, disinfectants, cleaning solutions, toilet bowl cleaners, and bathroom scouring powders containing any of the following ingredients: **ammonia, alkylphenol ethoxylates, chlorine bleach** (aka sodium hypochlorite), **d-Limonene, diethanolamine** or **monoethanolamine, fragrance** (which may contain phthalates), **glycol ethers** (aka butyl glycol, ethylene glycol monobutyl, butyl cellosolve), **sodium hydroxide**, and **sodium lauryl sulfate**. Instead, to clean, deodorize, and disinfect your toilet bowl, try baking soda and white vinegar. Sprinkle toilet bowl with baking soda, add white vinegar and scrub with a toilet brush. To get soap scum off tub and tile, use plain soap and water, and baking soda. For more information on other ingredients to avoid, and for comparisons of commercially available non-toxic cleaning products, go to The Green Guide website at www.thegreen-guide.com.

- Learn to read product labels. If a product does not list ingredients but there is a telephone number to call for the manufacturer, call the manufacturer and request the Material Safety Data Sheet (MSDS) for the product, which should contain the list of ingredients and some of the major potential health effects. MSDS is also available online. If you need help understanding a MSDS, you can call the Teratogen Information Service in your state.

- Molds and mildew. Get rid of molds and mildew from your bathroom (see Chapter 5).
- **Kitchen and dining room.** Since this is where you cook and eat, you want to work on making sure you are not ingesting or inhaling reproductive toxicants into your body.
  - Non-stick pans. Toss non-stick pans containing **perfluorinated chemicals** (which are suspected carcinogens), and replace them with stainless steel or cast iron cookware.
  - Don't microwave plastic. Avoid defrosting meat in its Styrofoam tray or reheating leftovers in take-out containers in the microwave. Some plastic containers can leach **phthalates, bisphenol-A**, and other toxic chemicals into your food in the microwave. Avoid microwaving containers made from #3 (PVC, which may contain phthalates) and #7 (polycarbonate, which may contain BPA) plastics. If you must, only use plastic wrap and containers labeled "microwave safe." Better yet, use a glass or ceramic lid, wax paper, or cloth napkin to prevent splattering.
  - Glass and window cleaners. Avoid glass and window cleaners that contain **glycol ethers** or **ammonia.** Instead, try adding ¼ cup vinegar or 1 tablespoon lemon juice to a spray bottle of plain water for cleaning glass and windows.
  - Countertop, stovetop, and oven cleaners. Avoid scouring powders that contain **silica** or **chlorine bleach**. Avoid corrosive oven cleaners, many of which contain lye and sodium hydroxide. Try baking soda instead. For cleaning up grease, try a mixture of 1/2 teaspoon of washing soda, 2 tablespoons of distilled white vinegar, 1/4 teaspoon liquid soap, and 2 cups of hot water with a spray bottle. Be sure to wear gloves when working with washing soda.
  - Drain cleaners. Avoid chemical drain cleaners, which are among the most dangerous of all cleaning products. Most contain corrosive ingredients such as **sodium hydroxide** and **sodium hypochlorite**. Try baking soda and vinegar instead.

Add baking soda and vinegar to a pot of boiled water and pour down the drain, then flush with tap water. For more stubborn clogs, use a "snake" plumbing tool to manually remove blockage, or try suction removal with a plunger.

- Toxic foods. Get rid of toxic foods from your refrigerator, pantry, cabinet, and cupboard (see Chapter 3)

- **Living room and bedrooms.** These are the rooms you probably spend most of your time in so be sure to make them a healthy living space.

  - Wallpaper and blinds. If you have vinyl wallpaper, get rid of it. It may contain phthalates. While you are at it, replace vinyl mini-blinds with wood plantation shutters.

  - Furniture. Replace furniture made of pressed wood containing urea-formaldehyde resins with furniture made of solid wood or "exterior grade" pressed wood products. Even though formaldehyde has not been clearly demonstrated to have specific reproductive or developmental effects in humans, some studies have linked formaldehyde exposure to increased risk for miscarriages.

  - Mattress and sofa. Polybrominated diphenyl ethers (PBDEs) are flame retardants found in many foam mattresses and upholstered furniture. In rat studies PBDEs have been shown to cause detriment to fetal neurodevelopment, though the health consequences of prenatal exposure in humans are not clear at present. Replace your old PBDE mattress and sofa; PBDE-free mattresses and sofas that meet the strictest fire-retardancy standards are now commercially available in such mainstream stores as Ikea.

  - Carpet. Get rid of wall-to-wall carpeting; replace with an area rug or hardwood floor. I am not a big fan of carpets. Carpets and their adhesives may contain volatile organic compounds, some of which are reproductive hazards. They can also trap lead, pesticides, and other reproductive toxins that you bring home on your shoes, and become a breeding ground for molds, dust mites, and other allergens if they become wet. Consider replacing your old carpet with hardwood floors or area rugs that are easier to clean and maintain. If you are keeping the carpet, vacuum and clean frequently. Use a good vacuum cleaner, one with an agitator and a HEPA filter.

- Dust mites. Get rid of dust mites from your bedroom (see Chapter 5).

- **Garage/attic/basement and outdoors.** You may or may not spend a lot of time in these places depending on how you use them.
  - Storage area. Chances are you are using the garage, attic, or basement primarily as a storage area. In addition to all those boxes of books from college that you've kept but will probably never, ever read again (and all sorts of other junk that you will probably never, ever need again), this is probably also where you keep paint, solvents, pesticides, and any other toxicants that you don't want to store in the house. Keep them in well-ventilated areas, and get rid of any unused pesticide, paint, and solvents immediately.
  - Washer and dryer. The garage or basement is probably also where you keep your washer and dryer. Avoid using fabric softeners and detergents containing phthalates. Fabric can be softened by adding one-quarter cup of baking soda to the wash cycle. To remove stains from clothing, try soaking fabrics in water mixed with lemon juice, hydrogen peroxide, washing soda, or white vinegar. Less toxic laundry detergents are also commercially available.
  - Hobbies. Another possible use of this space is for your (or your partner's) hobbies. If your hobbies involve painting, pottery, making stained glass windows, or handling, shooting, or cleaning guns, you may be exposed to lead or other metals. If your hobbies involve refinishing furniture, repairing cars, painting, building models, or anything that

requires the use of strippers, degreasers, non-water-based glues, or paints, you may be exposed to organic solvents. Now that you are thinking about getting pregnant, try to find new hobbies that won't put you or your future baby in harm's way. If you cannot give up your hobbies, use proper precautions. Hobbies involving solvents should be practiced only in very well-ventilated areas; use special masks designed to filter out particular chemicals and rated by the National Institute for Occupational Safety and Health (NIOSH) for various use. Avoid skin contact with solvents (they can penetrate the skin and enter the body), wear chemically resistant gloves, and never use solvents to clean paint or glue off the skin.

5. AVOID USING PESTICIDES

If you are like 75 percent of American households, you have used at least one pesticide product indoors during the past year. Household pesticides contain both active ingredients and so-called "inert" ingredients (which are usually organic solvents and not listed on the container), both of which may be reproductive hazards. Even if you only use weed killers, fungicides, and other pesticides outdoors on your lawn or garden, they can still be tracked indoors on shoes and may persist for long periods of time in carpets. Take the following steps to reduce your family's exposure to pesticides:

- **Use non-chemical methods of pest control whenever possible.** There are many alternatives to combat pests, from using simple substances like cayenne pepper to keep ants out of the house, to employing companion planting to discourage garden pests, to using baits and traps.
- **Minimize exposure.** If you must use pesticides, avoid doing it yourself if you are pregnant or planning to get pregnant. Some pesticides stay in your body for a long time. Ask someone else to apply the pesticides whenever possible. If you have to do it

yourself, minimize your exposure by using the least recommended amount possible and only for special problems (e.g., a
major insect infestation). Choose products carefully, and use
strictly according to manufacturer's directions. If you are using
them indoors, mix or dilute outdoors. Take plants or pets
outdoors when applying pesticides to them. Use pesticides in a
well-ventilated area and open all windows, use gloves and
avoid any skin contact, and allow time for the area to air out
before re-entering. If you are using pesticides outdoors, avoid
tracking them indoors onto your carpet. One study found that
dust vacuumed from a living room carpet contained sixteen
different pesticides, some banned for years.

- **Keep pest control under control.** If you decide to use a pest
  control company, choose one carefully. Ask for an inspection
  of your home and get a written control program for evaluation before you sign a contract. The control program should
  list specific names of pests to be controlled and chemicals to
  be used; it should also reflect any of your safety concerns.
  Insist on a proven record of competence and customer
  satisfaction.

- **Do not store pesticides inside your home** (e.g., under the
  kitchen or bathroom sink); they can leak out of the can and
  contaminate the air you breathe. Store them in areas that are
  separately ventilated from the home, such as an attic or
  detached garage. Buy in small quantities, use immediately, and
  dispose of unwanted containers safely. Follow the directions
  on the label when getting rid of unused pesticides.

- **Keep exposure to moth repellents to a minimum.** Moth
  repellents contain paradichlorobenzene, a chemical known to
  cause cancer in animals, though no information is available
  on the reproductive or developmental effects of paradichlorobenzene in humans. Where possible, paradichlorobenzene,
  and items to be protected against moths, should be placed in
  trunks or other containers that can be stored in areas that are

ventilated separately from the home, such as an attic and
detached garage.

- **Keep your house clean, dry, and well ventilated.** This will go
  a long way toward eliminating the need for pesticides. For
  example, most roach problems will go away if you deny roaches
  food, water, shelter, and entry. Cockroaches come out to eat at
  night, so get into the habit of putting food away (in the
  refrigerator or a tightly sealed container) after use; cleaning up
  food scraps from floors, tables, chairs, and counters right after
  you eat; washing dishes before going to bed or leaving them in
  soapy water in the sink overnight; and keeping trash in a
  closed trashcan.

6. START NESTING

Think you might need a bigger or better nest for you baby? Many couples
move or remodel their home during pregnancy, in anticipation of the
baby's arrival. However, pregnancy is *not* the best time to remodel your
home. Toxic fumes and dust containing substances such as lead and
volatile organic compounds are often stirred up during remodeling. In
one study, carpet lead levels increased 30-fold during remodeling. The
bonded wood products (plywood, particle board, chipboard), drywall
compound, insulation, carpeting, draperies, vinyl molding, cabinets, and
even new furniture that come with remodeling may contain formaldehyde and other volatile organic solvents. If you can, avoid remodeling your
home during pregnancy.

If you are planning to remodel your home, do it now before you get
pregnant. Don't wait until pregnancy. Remodeling gives you a chance to
build a healthy home environment for your future baby—so insist on using non-toxic or low-toxic paints, finishes, and building materials. Here
are some suggestions:

- Ask your builder for product specification sheets, and consider
  using alternatives such as solid woods instead of pressed wood
  products bonded with resins.

- If you are going to use pressed wood products, ask for "**exterior grade**" products for floors, cabinetry, and wall surfaces. "Exterior grade" pressed wood products contain phenol resins instead of urea-formaldehyde resins and emit lower levels of formaldehyde and other volatile organic compounds. Pressed wood products made for indoor use include: particleboard (used as subflooring and shelving and in cabinetry and furniture); hardwood plywood paneling (used for decorative wall covering and used in cabinets and furniture); and medium density fiberboard (used for drawer fronts, cabinets, and furniture tops). Medium density fiberboard often contains a higher resin-to-wood ratio than any other pressed wood product and is generally recognized as being the highest formaldehyde-emitting pressed wood product. Check the product label or call the manufacturer to see what the particleboard, plywood panel, and fiberboard on the furniture you are about to purchase are made of; avoid products with a high content of urea-formaldehyde. Some studies suggest that coating pressed wood products with polyurethane may reduce formaldehyde emissions for some period of time. For further information on formaldehyde and consumer products, call the EPA Toxic Substance Control Act (TSCA) assistance line (202–554–1404).

- Increase and improve ventilation during and after construction; use air-conditioning and dehumidifiers to maintain a moderate temperature and reduce humidity inside your home, since heat and humidity can increase emission of formaldehyde and other organic compounds.

- If you are going to install new carpets, do it now before you get pregnant. New carpets and their adhesives can emit large amounts of volatile organic compounds. Talk to your carpet retailer. Ask for information on emissions from carpet. Ask for low-emitting adhesives if adhesives are needed. Be sure the retailer requires the installer to follow the Carpet and Rug Institute's installation guidelines. You can get more informa-

tion on selecting carpets and rugs and care and cleaning at
the Carpet and Rug Institute's website at www.carpet-rug.org.

7. SURVEY YOUR NEIGHBORHOOD

How clean and safe is your neighborhood? Are you living right next door
to a toxic waste dump? A factory, plant, incinerator, or facility that is
pouring out tons of reproductive toxicants each year? A dry-cleaner? A
gas station or auto repair shop? A farm? A golf course, park, or play-
ground? How clean is the air you breathe? How noisy is your neighborhood? How healthy is your community?

In planning a pregnancy, you need to ask yourself: Is this the neighborhood in which I want to raise my child? If you are looking for a new
home before you get pregnant, these are the questions you need to consider before you buy or lease:

- **Hazardous waste sites.** Are you living next to one of the
  nation's worst toxic waste sites (a so-called Superfund site)?
  There are 1,305 Superfund sites scheduled for cleanup on the
  National Priorities List (NPL), and you might be living next to
  an NPL site or a toxic waste dump and know nothing about it.
  About 11 million people in the United States, including 3–4
  million children, live within 1 mile of an NPL site. Those of
  you who live in New Jersey, do you know that there are 116
  Superfund sites in your state? Those of you in Los Angeles
  County, do you know that there are 17 Superfund sites in your
  county alone? If you are planning to get pregnant and looking
  to move, you don't want to move within a few miles of a toxic
  waste dump or a heavy polluter, especially one with high
  emissions of recognized or suspected reproductive toxicants.
  Log on to the website for the Environmental Defense Fund, a
  leading national nonprofit environmental advocacy group, at
  www.edf.org, and you can get the locations of the Superfund
  sites in your area, along with a list of top polluters and an
  environmental justice report for your county.

- **Dry-cleaners.** If you live right above a dry-cleaner, move. A 1995 study found New York City apartments located above dry-cleaners contained average levels of PCE more than 4 times the health-based guideline set by the New York State Department of Health. Almost one-third of the apartments in the study registered levels of the toxic chemical more than 10 times the standard, and at least one apartment was found to have an average PCE level 250 times greater than the Health Department guideline!

- **Gas stations and auto repair shops.** Gas stations and auto repair shops emit significant quantities of volatile organic compounds into the neighborhood. Gas stations can pollute local air by leaking fumes during pumping and from spillage during fuel transfer; the underground fuel storage tanks may leak and contaminate underground water supplies. Auto repair and body shops may also emit volatile organic chemicals and metals into the air, and the wastes stored on site may leak into the ground and get into the groundwater.

- **Agricultural operations.** If you live near a farm, you may be exposed to the pesticides they use. Depending on weather conditions, pesticides sprayed on a field may drift for some distance. Those applied to a field may wash off after rain or irrigation and may end up in groundwater. If you live next to a farm, you can ask to be notified of spraying schedules so you can stay away during those times.

- **Parks, playgrounds, and golf courses.** Farms are not the only places that get sprayed with pesticides. Parks, playgrounds, and golf courses may be heavily sprayed, and the chemicals can also seep into the groundwater. In a study of the San Francisco Recreation and Parks Department between 1994 and 1995, no fewer than 60 different pesticides, including 20 suspected reproductive toxicants, were used. As a result of the study, San Francisco has implemented an innovative

program to eliminate the use of pesticides in parks, playgrounds, and public buildings, and adopted Integrated Pest
Management (IPM) as the official policy of the city. If you
live near parks or playgrounds, talk to the Parks and Recreation Department in your town or city about adopting
policies and practices similar to those in San Francisco, or at
the least ask to be notified prior to spraying so you can avoid
the areas during those times. Some golf courses have almost
continuous spraying programs. If you are planning to get
pregnant, you probably shouldn't buy or lease near a golf
course (unless it has an IPM program or pesticide-free
maintenance), and avoid playing on a course right after the
application of pesticides.

- **Air quality.** To find out more about air quality in your local
area, visit the nonprofit Environmental Defense Fund's
website and type in your zip code. You will see how your
county stacks up against other counties in the United States
in terms of air pollution, how many days a year the air is
healthy, and who the top air polluters in your area are. You
can also look up information about toxic chemicals released
into your neighborhood at the EPA's Toxic Release Inventory
(TRI) website. The EPA also maintains the Environfacts
website, which allows users to identify the facilities (with
street addresses) monitored by the EPA in their area and the
amount of air emissions released by the facilities into the
neighborhood.

    Motor vehicles are a major source of air pollution in urban
areas. Maternal exposure to air pollutants emitted in vehicle
exhaust, including carbon monoxide, nitrogen dioxide, sulfur
dioxide, and ultra-fine particles, has been linked to birth
defects, preterm birth, and other pregnancy complications. If
you live right next to a freeway or major road/intersection, you
may be exposed to a hefty dose of exhaust toxins on a daily

basis. If you can, move before you get pregnant. The concentrations of air pollutants drop off sharply at about 150 yards, or
a one-block distance, from the freeway or major road/intersec-
tion; so even if you move only a block or two away you'd be
much better off.

- **Noise pollution.** How noisy is your neighborhood? How close
do you live to the freeway or major roads/intersections? Flight
paths for airplane takeoff and landing? You may be exposed to
noise levels of 90 decibels (db) or above if you live right next to
a freeway or major roads/intersections, and in excess of 100 db if
you live right under the airport flight paths. Daily exposure to
noise above 85 decibels (db) has been shown to cause hearing
loss, but noise at 75 db has been linked to high blood pressure,
and noise at just 65 db to stress and depression. A growing body
of evidence now suggests that noise pollution from airports and
other sources may reduce birth weight, possibly by activating
maternal stress response. Noise is a stressor, and noise exposure
has been shown to increase stress hormones in both children
and adults. The Census Bureau reports that noise is Americans'
top complaint about their neighborhoods, and the major reason
for wanting to move. So before you buy or lease your next home,
check out the noise level in the neighborhood (including that
of your neighbors). You may also want to check out Noise Free
America's website, which publishes a list of towns and cities
with the worst noise pollution problems, as well as some actions
you can take to reduce noise pollution in your neighborhood.

- **Community health.** How healthy is your community? If you
ask someone to describe a "healthy community," you are likely
to hear the following: good schools; strong families; friendly
neighbors; safe streets; open space and parks; a clean environment; a diverse, vibrant economy; and high-quality affordable
health care. These are neighborhood characteristics that are
known to be important to health. For the last two decades,
there has been a growing Healthy Cities/Healthy Communi-

ties movement, driven by the recognition that health is the result of much more than medical care. People are healthy when they live in nurturing environments and are involved in the life of their community; that is, when they live in Healthy Cities. You can find examples of healthy cities and healthy communities all over the United States on the Healthy Cities/Healthy Communities website and think about where you want to raise your family.

8. CHOOSE A CLEANER COMMUTE

If you are like most Americans, you spend on average 24 minutes commuting to work each day, more if you live in cities like New York (38.3 minutes); Chicago (33.2 minutes); Newark, NJ (31.5 minutes); Riverside, CA (31.2 minutes); Philadelphia (29.4 minutes); and Los Angeles (29.0 minutes). This means you will spend more than 100 hours commuting to and from work this year and, if you are like most American women who continue to work through their pregnancy, you will spend up to 75 hours commuting to and from work during your pregnancy. If you drive, you may be taking in large amounts of potential reproductive toxicants during your commute. Increased exposure to carbon monoxide in the second month of pregnancy, when the baby's heart is developing, is associated with a near threefold increased risk of fetal cardiac defects, including defects of the heart septum, valves, and pulmonary artery. Studies have also linked high carbon monoxide and particulate matter exposures to preterm as well as low birth weight babies.

Here are a few things you can do to minimize your exposure to air pollution during your commute:

- **Reduce your commute.** Ask you employer about telecommuting or alternative work schedules such as flextime or staggered work hours to avoid commuting during peak rush hours when air quality is at its worst.

- **Find healthier routes.** Air pollutant levels peak in proximity to freeways, major roads, and intersections; map out your commute and find the road less traveled to minimize your exposure.

- **Breathe clean air.** Depending on your car model and ventilation, the levels of certain air pollutants inside the car may be 10 to 15 times higher than those outside the car. To reduce your exposure to air pollutants during your commute, you can re-circulate the air to keep outside air out (but this might reduce oxygen levels in a long commute), and use a portable air purifier with a HEPA filter to clean the air inside the car. Avoid car air fresheners, which may contain reproductive toxicants such as benzene, phthalates, and other organic volatile compounds. Try putting a box of odor-eating baking soda or a bag of volcanic rocks called zeolite on the floor under your car seat instead.

- **Use a vapor-lock gas pump.** Get gasoline only at a station with a vapor-lock system—a rubber gasket that fits around the gas tank opening to prevent fumes from escaping. Talk to the station manager if the service station you go to does not have vapor controls on their pumps, or take your business elsewhere. Use full service and ask an attendant to pump gas for you if you can afford it (but who can these days?). Avoid "topping off" your car's gas tank; fumes can escape even if you don't spill gasoline. Make sure your gas cap fits properly.

- **Go green.** Your car may be the polluter. Use clean fuels and energy-conserving (EC) grades of motor oil. Drive at a steady, medium speed; most cars operate most efficiently at 35 to 45 miles per hour. Avoid excessive idling; idling for more than 30 seconds burns more gas than it takes to restart the engine. Travel light; take unnecessary items out of the trunk to improve fuel efficiency. Make sure your tires are properly inflated and your wheels aligned. Get regular engine tune-ups and car maintenance checks. Keep car filters and catalytic converters clean. Watch for signals from your vehicle's tailpipe that your car or truck may be running inefficiently. Black smoke means there is too much gas in the air-fuel mixture and the fuel injection system should be checked. Blue smoke means the engine is burning oil and too many hydrocarbons are being released. And don't mess with your car's pollution controls; they are there to keep the air clean for you and your baby.

Better yet, consider walking, bicycling, or using mass transit (especially one that does not burn fossil fuels) to get to work. If you have to drive, drive a greener car (e.g., a hybrid), and carpool if you can. Do your part to reduce air pollution; do it for your future baby's sake.

9. AVOID HARMFUL EXPOSURES AT WORK

If you are like most American women, you work now and will continue to work through much of your pregnancy. Census data indicate that more than half (55 percent) of all babies born in 2003 were born to working mothers. For many pregnant women, the workplace poses the single greatest environmental threat. If you work in manufacturing, you may be exposed to organic solvents such as glycol ethers or heavy metals like cadmium. If you work in agriculture, you may be exposed to pesticides and herbicides. If you work in printing, you may be exposed to solvents and inks. If you work in healthcare, you may be exposed to antineoplastics and ionizing radiation. Even if you work in an office setting, there may be solvent exposures from cleaning products, deodorizers, or office products such as markers, glues, adhesives, and toners. Particle board and carpets in the office may emit formaldehyde. Pesticide residues from nighttime spraying may linger in the air and on surfaces.

There are now more than 84,000 chemical compounds in the workplace, and 2,000 new chemicals are being added each year. With so many chemicals, how do you know that what you are being exposed to at work is safe for you and your future baby? Here are a few tips:

- **Ask to see the Material Safety Data Sheet (MSDS).** All employers are required by law to have an MSDS for each hazardous chemical you might be exposed to in the workplace. An MSDS contains information about the chemical and common name, physical and chemical properties, physical and health hazards, possible routes of exposure, any established exposure limits, handling precautions, control measures, emergency procedures, how to contact the manufacturer or importer, and whether the chemical is listed as a carcinogen. Ask to see the MSDS listing the chemicals to which you are being exposed at work, and consult your doctor or a Teratology Information services counselor before you get pregnant.

- **Consult Teratology Information Services.** Some MSDSs can be quite confusing to even doctors. In such instances you can consult your local Teratology Information Services (TIS) counselor. Log onto the Organization of Teratology Information Services (OTIS) website at www.otispregnancy.org to find a TIS in your area. TIS counselors can interpret the information on MSDS for you.

- **Survey your workplace.** Find out where chemicals come into the plant and where they go, the adequacy of the ventilation system, how often that system is checked by the employer, and when (or if) air sampling is done. Also try to find out if any coworkers have had any reproductive health problems they believe to be work related. If you work in an office setting, there may be no MSDSs on file. Check with your office building manager and janitorial staff regarding the types of chemicals and pesticides used in the office.

- **Protect yourself.** Follow instructions for proper handling of chemicals. Use protective clothing, masks, respirators or other protective equipment properly. If you work in a healthcare setting, exercise universal precautions around biologic and chemical agents. Ask for job reassignment or modification if you work with known or suspected reproductive toxicants.

Change your clothing or wash up before going home to
minimize your family's exposure to reproductive hazards at
work.

10. KNOW YOUR RIGHTS AT WORK

You should know your rights at work. Under the **Occupation Safety and
Health Act (OSHA) of 1970,** you have a right to a working environment that is safe for you and your baby. OSHA requires employers to
provide a workplace free from recognized hazards that cause, or are likely
to cause, death or serious physical harm to pregnant women or their babies. Under **OSHA's Hazard Communication Standard,** you have a
right to know what you are being exposed to. The law requires all employers to label containers with chemical names or hazard warnings,
provide an MSDS for every chemical handled at the facility, and provide
training on the health and safety hazards of toxic substances to which
workers are exposed. An employer who does not provide MSDSs when
asked or retaliates against an employee for requesting MSDSs is breaking the law. You should have copies of the MSDSs of all chemicals with
which you are directly working. If you feel your rights are being violated,
you can file a formal complaint with the state health or labor agency or
directly with the regional office of OSHA. You can request anonymity if
you fear retaliation from your employer. You (along with two corrobo-
rating colleagues, a union representative, or an office of the company)
can also make a request to the National Institute of Occupational
Safety and Health (NIOSH) to request a workplace health study if you
are concerned about exposure to potential reproductive hazards at the
workplace. You can learn more about the 1970 OSHA Act by logging
onto the OSHA website at www.osha.gov.

One final thought for this chapter. Isn't it just crazy that we've gotten
to the point where we can't eat fish without worrying about mercury and
PCB? Can't consume dairy without worrying about pesticides and dioxins? Can't drink tap water without worrying about lead and THM? Can't
drink bottled water without worrying about phthalate and BPA? Can't
go outside our house without worrying about ozone, carbon monoxide,

nitrogen dioxide, sulfur dioxide, and particulate matter? What have we done to our children's world? What are we doing to their developing brains and bodies?

Most important, what can we do as parents to take back our children's future? I will come back to this question at the end of the book. Let's now turn our attention to getting you ready for preconception care.

preconception care

If you are like most American women, you probably haven't heard much about preconception care, which I believe is just as important as (if not more important than) prenatal care to making a smart and healthy baby. This is why I wrote this chapter. I will first answer the who, what, when, where, and why of preconception care, and then I will help you get ready for preconception care so that your doctor can help you get ready for pregnancy.

the five ws of preconception care

First, I will answer the Five Ws of preconception care.

WHO?

Who needs preconception care? I believe every woman should get preconception care before she gets pregnant. It doesn't matter if this is going to be your first pregnancy or your fifth. And it doesn't matter if you are "high risk" or "low risk"; everyone can benefit from preconception care. And according to the Centers for Disease Control and Prevention (CDC), it doesn't even matter if you are actively trying to get pregnant or not, since half of all pregnancies in the United States happen to women who are not trying to get pregnant.

If you are reading this book, you definitely should get preconception care. Call your doctor's office today to make an appointment for preconception care.

(By the way, your man should get preconception care, too. Tell him to read Chapter 8 and then go see his doctor for a preconception check-up).

WHAT?

What is preconception care? As defined by the CDC, preconception care is a set of prepregnancy interventions that aim to identify and modify biomedical, behavioral, and social risks to a woman's health or pregnancy outcome through prevention and management.

Simply stated, preconception care is the healthcare you get before you get pregnant. The goal of preconception care is to get you ready for pregnancy by optimizing your health and minimizing your risks. It includes risk assessment, health promotion, and clinical and psychosocial interventions. Risk assessment should identify reproductive, medical, genetic, nutritional, social, psychological, and behavioral risk factors that can put your future pregnancy at risk. This would typically include a routine physical and laboratory testing. Health promotion should cover such topics as healthy weight and nutrition, behavioral change, stress reduction, and avoidance of environmental toxicants. Clinical interventions should address any ongoing problems, such as diabetes, depression, or smoking, before you get pregnant.

For some women, preconception care may take one prepregnancy check-up, and they are ready to go. For others, it will require a series of visits, including referrals to specialists. Because every woman is different, the content of preconception care needs to be individualized.

WHEN?

When should I go see my doctor for preconception care?

The sooner, the better.

If you are planning to get pregnant in the next few months, **now** would be a good time for your prepregnancy check-up.

But even if you are planning to wait a year, it is still a good idea to start your preconception care now. This is especially the case if you need to lose some weight, change medication, stop smoking, or get your blood pressure or diabetes under control before you get pregnant. But even if you are in perfect health, your doctor may discover a problem during the check-up that might take some time to resolve. The sooner you start preconception care, the more time you and your doctor will have to minimize your risks and optimize your health before you get pregnant.

What I usually do is ask my patients to come in and see me for a check-up as soon as they start *thinking* about getting pregnant. This way I can start working with them on any problem that I might identify during the visit. If they are planning to wait a while before getting pregnant, I would ask them to come back and see me again a month or two before they actually start *trying*, just to make sure that all systems are still ready to go.

WHERE?

Where should I go for preconception care? Start with your ob/gyn or family physician. Ask your doctor if she offers preconception care. If she doesn't, ask if she could refer you to a doctor who does. Your doctor may also refer you to other specialists, such as an endocrinologist to get your diabetes under optimal control, or a dietician to help you achieve a healthy prepregnancy weight, or a family counselor to get your marriage in order before you get pregnant.

(I use the word "doctor" in a generic sense; some midwives and nurse practitioners are actually more experienced and better trained in providing preconception care than some doctors. The important thing is to find someone who knows what he or she is doing, and is willing to spend the time, give you the attention, and make all the referrals you need to help you get ready for pregnancy.)

WHY?

Why do I need preconception care? Remember Angie's story in the Introduction? Had Angie waited to see me until after she had gotten pregnant, it would've been too late to turn back the clock on implantation and prevent a three-peat of her preeclampsia. As I explained in Chapter 1, even early prenatal care may be too late to prevent some birth defects, reverse implantation errors, and restore your body's allostasis quickly enough to optimize fetal programming. If you want a smart and healthy baby, you need to get ready *before* you get pregnant. Preconception care can help you get ready.

ten topics to discuss with your doctor during your preconception visit

Before you go see your doctor for preconception care, you should make a checklist of things you want to discuss with him or her. Here is a list of the ten most important topics to cover:

Topic 1: Your reproductive life plan
Topic 2: Your past pregnancy history
Topic 3: Chronic medical conditions
Topic 4: Medications you are taking
Topic 5: Family history and genetic risks
Topic 6: Social history
Topic 7: Health behaviors
Topic 8: Depression and anxiety
Topic 9: Preventive and primary care
Topic 10: Preconception laboratory tests

Your doctor probably won't have time to go over all of these topics with you. So read this chapter first. Get organized. Make a checklist of things you want to talk to your doctor about. This will help you get the most out of your preconception care.

1. YOUR REPRODUCTIVE LIFE PLAN

The first thing you should talk to your doctor about is your reproductive life plan. A reproductive life plan is a set of personal goals about having (or not having) children based on your personal values and resources, and a plan and timeline to achieve those goals. This means deciding whether or not you want to have any (more) children, and if yes, when and under what conditions you want to become pregnant.

You should tell your doctor when you want to get pregnant. If you are thinking about it but don't know when, ask your doctor. Your doctor cannot decide for you, but he or she may be able to give you the information you need to help you make a plan. For example, if you are worrying about your biological clock (see Box 7.1), get the facts before you make your plan. Some women in their mid-thirties start to worry a lot about infertility and Down syndrome, when in reality their fertility chances are still pretty good (about 80 percent will get pregnant in one year), their miscarriage rates are still relatively low (less than 20 percent of pregnancies will end up in miscarriage), and their risk for having a baby with Down syndrome or any chromosomal defects is still very small (0.5 percent). Your doctor might be able to help put things in perspective for you in making your plan.

Here are some facts you should consider before making your reproductive life plan.

box 7.1: how fast is your biological clock ticking?

Infertility increases with age
Percent of married women who are infertile by age group

(continued)

Age Group	Percent Infertile*
20–24	7
25–29	9
30–34	15
35–39	22
40–44	29

* Infertility is defined as inability to conceive after one year of unprotected sexual intercourse

Miscarriage increases with age
Percent of pregnancies resulting in miscarriage

Age Group	Percent Miscarried
15–19	10
20–24	10
25–29	10
30–34	12
35–39	18
40–44	34
>45	53

Risk of chromosomal abnormalities increases with age
By maternal age

Maternal Age	Risk for Down Syndrome	Risk for Any Chromosomal Defects
20	1/1,667	1/526
25	1/1,250	1/476

Maternal Age	Risk for Down Syndrome	Risk for Any Chromosomal Defects
30	1/952	1/385
35	1/378	1/192
40	1/106	1/66
41	1/82	1/53
42	1/63	1/42
43	1/49	1/33
44	1/38	1/26
45	1/30	1/21
46	1/23	1/16
47	1/18	1/13
48	1/14	1/10

If you are ready to get pregnant, ask your doctor *when* you can start trying. Although you would've liked to have gotten started *yesterday*, your doctor may ask you to wait. If you've just gotten off the pill, you probably should wait a month or two until your natural cycles are reestablished. If you've just gotten started on a new medication or switched to a new dosage, you should wait until a stable therapeutic level has been achieved. If you've just gotten your MMR, chickenpox, or HPV vaccine, you should wait at least four weeks. If you are trying to shed 30 pounds, your doctor may ask you to wait up to a year (at 1 to 2 pounds weight loss per week plus three to six months of stable weight).

If you had a baby before, how long should you wait before you start trying again? The best scientific evidence suggests that the most optimal birth spacing (from the end of one pregnancy to the beginning of the next pregnancy) is 1½ to 2 years, though this may very well depend on a number of factors such as your age (you don't want to wait two years if you are already 42), your overall health, and prior pregnancy outcome. A short interval between pregnancies has been shown to be an important risk factor for preterm birth, low birth weight, and other pregnancy complications. If your prior pregnancy resulted in a miscarriage or abortion, the best available data suggest that you should wait at least six months before trying to get pregnant again. If you had a cesarean section in your previous pregnancy, you should wait at least six months (but best to wait 1½ to 2 years) before attempting to conceive.

Once you are ready to get pregnant, ask your doctor what you can do to maximize your chances of conceiving. Remember in conception as in everything else in life, *timing is everything.* For fertilization to occur the sperm has to be there in the tube waiting for the egg, and not the other way around. This means you need to have sex before you ovulate, with the 2 to 3 days before ovulation being your most fertile days. If you know when you are going to ovulate, you should have sex 5 days, 3 days, and 1 day before you ovulate (for example, if you ovulate on day 14 of your cycle, you should have sex on days 9, 11, and 13 of your cycle). Some of my patients (the overachievers who want to get pregnant fast) use an ovulation predictor kit to help them time their sexual intercourse.

On average your odds of conceiving in any given cycle are about one in four. Approximately 60 percent of couples who are actively trying to conceive (having intercourse two to three times a week) will conceive within the first 6 months of trying, 75 percent within 9 months, 80 percent within a year, and 90 percent within 18 months. If you haven't gotten pregnant after a year of actively trying, it might be helpful to see your ob/gyn or a fertility specialist to do some basic infertility work-up. If you are over 35, I'd recommend that you do so after 6 months of actively trying.

2. YOUR PAST PREGNANCY HISTORY

History repeats itself, and as George Santayana warns, *"those who fail to learn the lessons of history are doomed to repeat them."* This is true for war and peace, but it holds true for past pregnancy history as well. If you've had a preterm baby (born more than three weeks early) in a previous pregnancy, you have about a 20 to 30 percent chance of having another preterm baby in your next pregnancy. If you've had two prior very preterm babies (born more than eight weeks early), you have a nearly 60 percent chance of having another preterm baby in your next pregnancy. If you had postpartum depression with your last pregnancy, there is a good chance that you will get it again in your next pregnancy and your doctor will need to be watching you closely for symptoms of depression. Certain maternal complications, such as postpartum cardiomyopathy (heart failure), have very high recurrence risks and can be fatal if they recur in a subsequent pregnancy; you'd be well advised to avoid another pregnancy.

If you had a complication in a previous pregnancy, you should be prepared to discuss it with your doctor during the preconception care visit.

- **Bring your old records.** Your old records may provide clues as to what might have happened in your previous pregnancy. The records I find most useful include:
  - Admission note and discharge summary
  - Newborn admission note and discharge summary
  - Delivery note or operative report (e.g., for cesarean section)
  - Placental pathology report, if available
  - Reports of genetic consultation and testing, if done
  - Autopsy and cytogenetic studies for fetal or infant death
  - Reports of laboratory tests and diagnostic procedures (e.g., ultrasound)

  If you are seeing a new doctor, you may want to bring copies of your old records to the appointment (since your old records may not have been faxed to your new doctor's office despite your repeated requests, which, unfortunately, happens all too often).
- **Ask about causes and risk factors.** Ask your doctor what are known causes and risk factors for the pregnancy complication you've experienced, and what tests are available to identify any underlying factor that might put you at risk for recurrence in your next pregnancy. Pay attention to preventable causes and modifiable risk factors.

- **Ask about recurrence risks and what you can do to prevent a repeat.** Ask your doctor what the likelihood of recurrence in your next pregnancy is, and what can be done to avoid a repeat. Box 7.2 gives an example of what I would do for a patient with a history of preterm birth. Your doctor might do things differently, but I just want to give you an example of all the things that can be done to prevent a repeat *before* you get pregnant again.

box 7.2: if you've had a preterm baby

You have about a 20 to 30 percent chance of having another preterm baby in your next pregnancy. Some of the biological and behavioral risks are carried from one pregnancy to the next. The causes of preterm birth are unknown, but in most cases are thought to involve any of four major pathways: infections/inflammation, stress, poor placental blood flow/clotting, or overstretching of the uterus (e.g., twins). Here are some things that can be done to reduce your risk of a repeat, *before* you get pregnant again.

Risk Assessment

- Review past pregnancy history
  Conduct personal interview
  Review old medical records
  Review placental pathology, if available
- Investigate potential causes of preterm delivery

  1. Infections/inflammation
     Refer to a dentist for a good dental check-up;
     Do a urine test to check for chronic, asymptomatic bladder infection;

Screen for gonorrhea, chlamydia, trichomonas, and bacterial vaginosis;

Consider taking a biopsy of the lining inside the uterus to look for presence of chronic infections or inflammation

2. Stress

Screen for intimate partner violence

Screen for maternal depression and other affective disorders

Assess levels of stress and supports at home and work

3. Poor placental blood flow/clotting

Screen for hereditary or acquired clotting disorders, as indicated

Screen for hypertension, diabetes, and other vascular diseases, as indicated

- Review medical history
- Review family history of preterm delivery
- Identify behavioral risk factors (e.g., smoking, drug use, douching)

Health Promotion

- Promote family planning and optimal birth spacing
- Promote healthy weight and nutrition (e.g., folic acid or omega–3 fatty acids)
- Promote stress resilience
- Promote healthy behaviors (e.g., smoking cessation)
- Promote healthy environments (e.g., reduce exposure to toxic stress or air pollution)

Interventions

- Target intervention to identified medical, psychological, or social risks

(continued)

- Give progesterone (*e.g., weekly injections with 17-alpha hydroxy-progesterone caproate*) in a subsequent pregnancy

3. CHRONIC MEDICAL CONDITIONS

If you have a chronic medical condition, it needs to be under optimal control before you get pregnant. Untreated or under-treated medical conditions can put you and your baby at risk. For example, if you have diabetes mellitus, you have, on average, a 10 percent chance of having a baby with a major birth defect (which is three times the risk in the general population). However, if your diabetes is poorly controlled before conception and in early pregnancy, your risk goes up to as high as 20 percent. That is, there is one in five chance that your baby will be born with a major birth defect (most commonly a heart or neural tube defect). This is why you need to get your medical problem under control before you get pregnant.

- **Ask your doctor how your medical condition might affect your future pregnancy.** If you have chronic hypertension (high blood pressure), you are at risk for preeclampsia, preterm delivery, fetal growth retardation, placental abruption, and stillbirth during pregnancy. If you have diabetes, your baby is at risk for stillbirth, birth defects, macrosomia (large baby), birth trauma, and diabetes and obesity when he or she grows up. Ask your doctor how your medical condition might affect your future pregnancy, and what you can do to reduce the risk before you get pregnant.
- **Ask your doctor how your future pregnancy might affect your medical condition.** Pregnancy is a big stress test on your body. For example, your heart has to pump 50 percent more blood during pregnancy, and 80 percent more blood in the immediate postpartum period. While a healthy heart

can handle the extra workload, a diseased heart may get worn out. For other conditions, pregnancy may actually bring a reprieve. Many, but not all, women with rheumatoid arthritis get fewer flares during pregnancy, possibly due to normal immune suppression in pregnancy. Ask your doctor how your future pregnancy might affect your medical condition.

- **Ask your doctor to help you get your medical condition under control before you get pregnant.** Set goals with your doctor. If you have diabetes, what are the target blood sugar levels you want to achieve and maintain before and during pregnancy? If you have high blood pressure, what are the target blood pressures? If you are underweight or overweight, what is your target weight before you get pregnant? Once you've set your goals, ask your doctor to help you develop a feasible plan to achieve those goals. In the boxes below (Box 7.3 and Box 7.4), you will find a couple examples of what I'd do during preconception care for patients with chronic medical conditions.

box 7.3: if you have chronic hypertension (high blood pressure)

If you have chronic hypertension, your future pregnancy is at risk for preeclampsia, preterm delivery, fetal growth restriction, placental abruption, and stillbirth. You can reduce the risk by getting your blood pressure under optimal control before and during pregnancy. At the preconception visit, you need to get

(*continued*)

- A thorough history and physical examination, including a cardiovascular, neurological, and eye exam (if you haven't had one recently);
- Diagnostic and laboratory tests, including an EKG and testing for kidney functions and lipids (if you haven't been tested recently);
- A plan to lose weight (if you are overweight);
- A plan to exercise for an hour a day on most days of the week;
- A healthy eating plan;
- A plan to stop smoking (if you smoke);
- Blood pressure medications if your systolic blood pressure is greater than 140 and diastolic blood pressure is greater than 90, with a goal of keeping the blood pressure below 140/90;
- If you have diabetes or chronic kidney disease; blood pressure medications should be started at 120/80; with the goal of keeping the blood pressure below 130/80;
- A discussion with your doctor about the medications you are taking. Angiotensin-converting enzyme (ACE) inhibitors (e.g., Capoten, Vasotec, Lotensin), angiotension II receptor blockers (e.g., Cozaar), and the beta-blocker atenolol (Tenormin) should never be used during pregnancy because they can cause birth defects. Ask your doctor to switch you to something safer before you get pregnant;
- Alternative medication if you also have high cholesterol and are on a statin medication. Ask your doctor to switch you to something safer before pregnancy since statin medications can cause birth defects and are contraindicated during pregnancy;
- A plan for frequent follow-up—every month until blood pressure is well-controlled. You should maintain a stable, well-controlled blood pressure for at least three months before attempting to conceive.

box 7.4: if you have diabetes (high blood sugar)

If you have diabetes, your future baby is at risk for stillbirth, birth defects, macrosomia (large baby), delivery complications, newborn complications, and diabetes and obesity when he or she grows up; especially if your diabetes is poorly controlled before and during pregnancy. Studies have shown that tight blood sugar control before and in early pregnancy significantly reduces the risk of birth defects. At the preconception visit, you need to get

- A thorough history and physical examination, including a cardiovascular, neurological, and eye exam (if you haven't had one recently);
- Diagnostic and laboratory tests, including an EKG and testing for glycosylated hemoglobin (HbA1c), serum creatinine and 24-hour urinary excretion of total protein, and thyroid stimulating hormone (TSH) (if you haven't been tested recently);
- A plan for self-monitoring of blood sugar at home;
- A plan for self-administration of oral hypoglycemic medication or insulin therapy at home;
- A plan for emergency response to hypoglycemia (low blood sugar) (your family should be taught to recognize the signs and symptoms of hypoglycemia);
- A plan for dietary changes, with reduced intake of foods high in saturated fats, refined carbohydrates, and added sugars;
- A plan to lose weight (if you are overweight);
- A plan to exercise for an hour a day on most days of the week;
- A plan for effective birth control so you don't get pregnant until you are ready to;

(*continued*)

- A plan for frequent follow-up—you should be seen at least every one to two months until your glycosylated hemoglobin is normal;
- Once your glycosylated hemoglobin is normal, you can start to try to get pregnant.

4. MEDICATIONS YOU ARE TAKING

Ask your doctor about the medications that you are taking. Some medications can cause miscarriage or birth defects when taken in the early weeks of pregnancy. The acne drug Accutane (also known as isotretinoin, Amnesteem, and Claravis) is well known for causing birth defects and should be stopped for at least one month before you attempt to conceive. Some medications can cause serious harm to the baby when taken at any stage of pregnancy. ACE inhibitors, a class of medications that includes Capoten (captopril), Vasotec (enalopril), and Lotensin (benazepril), used to treat high blood pressure, can cause birth defects when taken in the first trimester, and kidney damage and even fetal death when taken in the second and third trimesters. Some medications can cause harm to your baby even when taken long *before* pregnancy. The psoriasis drugs Tegison (etretinate) and Soriatane (acitretin) can cause birth defects even when taken up to three years before pregnancy. Some over-the-counter drugs, vitamins, and herbal supplements can also cause harm to your baby. High intake of vitamin A (in excess of 10,000 IU daily from supplements) has been shown to cause certain birth defects, and aspirin or nonsteroidal anti-inflammatory drugs like Motrin (ibuprofen) can cause heart, kidney, and placental problems when taken during pregnancy.

Not all medications are bad. Some medications are needed to treat conditions like asthma, epilepsy, high blood pressure, or depression. Stopping these medications may cause more harm than good to the baby. If you are taking any medications now (as do four out of five U.S. women in their childbearing years; about half of them use a prescription drug), ask your doctor if you need to stop, switch, or continue. Specifically, ask your doctor the following questions:

- **"What FDA category do the medications I'm taking belong to?"** The FDA categorizes drugs as A, B, C, D, or X, based on what is known about their effects during pregnancy (Table 7.1).

Generally speaking, category X medications are a big no-no; they should never be used just before or during pregnancy. Category D medications should also be avoided, unless your doctor believes the benefits outweigh the risks and there are really no safer alternatives. Category A and B medications are generally safe to take. For category C medications, you and your doctor need to weigh carefully risks versus benefits of the medication in deciding whether or not you should stay on the medication before you get pregnant.

In May 2008, the FDA proposed major revisions to prescription drug labeling that would gradually phase out the letter categories. Under the FDA's proposal, the drug label would include three subsections:

- Fetal Risk Summary: What's known about the effects on the fetus
- Clinical Considerations: Dosing, risks of not treating the conditions, and complications
- Data: More details on the data used to write the fetal risk summary and clinical considerations

Once the new rule is fully implemented, your doctor will no longer be able to tell you which FDA category the medications you are taking belong to, but you can still ask her, "what does the drug label say about its use in pregnancy?"

- **"Are there safer alternatives to the medications I'm taking?"** Ask your doctor if there are safer alternatives to the medications you are taking. For example, if you are taking an

table 7.1: food and drug administration current categories for drug use in pregnancy

Category A   Adequate and well-controlled studies have failed to demonstrate a risk to the fetus in the first trimester of pregnancy (and there is no evidence of risk in later trimesters).

Category B   Animal reproduction studies have failed to demonstrate a risk to the fetus and there are no adequate and well-controlled studies in pregnant women OR Animal studies have shown an adverse effect, but adequate and well-controlled studies in pregnant women have failed to demonstrate a risk to the fetus in any trimester.

Category C   Animal reproduction studies have shown an adverse effect on the fetus and there are no adequate and well-controlled studies in humans, but potential benefits may warrant use of the drug in pregnant women despite potential risks.

Category D   There is positive evidence of human fetal risk based on adverse reaction data from investigational or marketing experience or studies in humans, but potential benefits may warrant use of the drug in pregnant women despite potential risks.

Category X   Studies in animals or humans have demonstrated fetal abnormalities and/or there is positive evidence of human fetal risk based on adverse reaction data from investigational or marketing experience, and the risks involved in use of the drug in pregnant women clearly outweigh potential benefits.

anti-epileptic medication, ask your doctor which one is safest
for pregnancy. While most of the older anti-convulsants (e.g.,
Dilantin or *phenytoin*, Tegretol or *carbamazepine*, Depakote or
valproic acid) have been linked to birth defects, some of the
newer anticonvulsants (e.g., Lamictal or *lamotrigine*, Topamax
or *topiramate*) appear to be safer. Similarly, if you are on an
anti-depressant, ask your doctor if there are safer alternatives
for pregnancy.

- **"What is the smallest effective dose to treat my condition?"**
As a rule of thumb, you want to minimize any potential fetal
exposure; so use the smallest effective dose recommended by
your doctor to treat your condition. Any medication, no
matter how safe, can still cause fetal harms when used in
excess. A corollary of this rule is that you want to use the
fewest number of medications for the shortest duration that
are effective for treating your condition.

- **"Do the benefits outweigh the risks?"** Decisions about
medication use during pregnancy, or when you are planning
to get pregnant, should ultimately be based on a careful
risk-benefit calculus. You should ask your doctor these
questions: What are known benefits, what are known risks,
and do the benefits outweigh the risks? For example, if you
haven't had a seizure in two to three years, ask your doctor if
you can stop your anti-epileptic medication. You should stay
seizure-free for six months off the medication before attempting to conceive.

- **"When can we start trying?"** If your doctor is switching or
stopping your medication, ask her how long you have to wait
before you can start trying. If she is switching you to a new
medication or a new dosage, she may ask you to wait until a
stable, therapeutic level has been achieved. Some medications
have a long "half-life" (the time it takes to get rid of half the
quantity of a drug or substance from your body); your doctor

may ask you to wait a while after stopping your medication before attempting to conceive.

- **"What about herbs and supplements?"** Presently little is known about the potential fetal risks of most herbs and supplements. Therefore, the American College of Obstetricians and Gynecologists and the Teratogen Society caution against the use of any herbal preparations in large quantities or for medicinal purposes during pregnancy (see Chapter 3). If you are planning to get pregnant soon, you should discontinue the use of herbs and supplements that are not prescribed by your doctor, or at least let your doctor know what you are using. You can also call up your local Teratogen Information Service and talk to a counselor about the herbs and supplements that you are taking.

5. FAMILY HISTORY AND GENETIC RISKS

You should talk to your doctor about your family history and genetic risks. You can help your doctor out by learning as much as you can about your family history before your preconception visit.

- **Family history.** You should let your doctor know if anyone in your family, or your husband's (or partner's) family (including parents and grandparents, if known), has any genetic disorders (e.g., muscular dystrophy, cystic fibrosis, sickle cell disease, Fragile X syndrome), unexplained mental retardation, birth defects, medical problems (e.g., bleeding or clotting disorders) or pregnancy complications (e.g., multiple miscarriages, gestational diabetes). If possible, be sure to include your grandparents' history because some genetic disorders may skip a generation. Your doctor may refer you to see a genetic counselor to further evaluate your genetic risks.
- **Ethnic background.** Your ethnicity may put your baby at risk for certain genetic disorders. Table 7.2 summarizes the

likelihood that you are a carrier for certain genetic disorders, based on your ethnic origin:

table 7.2: common genetic disorders based on ethnic origin

Ethnic Origin	Genetic Disorder	Carrier Frequency
African	Sickle Cell	1 in 10
	Cystic Fibrosis	1 in 65
	Beta Thalassemia	1 in 75
Ashkenazi Jewish	Gaucher Disease	1 in 15
	Cystic Fibrosis	1 in 26 to 1 in 29
	Tay-Sachs Disease	1 in 30
	Dysautonomia	1 in 32
	Canavan Disease	1 in 40
Asian	Alpha Thalassemia	1 in 20
	Beta Thalassemia	1 in 50
Caucasian	Cystic Fibrosis	1 in 25—1 in 29
French Canadian, Cajun	Tay Sachs Disease	1 in 30
Hispanic	Cystic Fibrosis	1 in 46
	Beta Thalassemia	1 in 30—1 in 50
Mediterranean	Beta Thalassemia	1 in 25
	Cystic Fibrosis	1 in 29
	Sickle Cell	1 in 40

For example, 1 in 10 African Americans is a carrier for sickle cell, and 1 in 25 Caucasians (Northern European Americans) is a carrier for cystic fibrosis. Here is a list of 10 genetic conditions that I routinely screen for women of Ashkenazi Jewish ancestry who are pregnant or planning to get pregnant; these comprise what is often referred to as the "Ashkenazi Jewish panel":

- Bloom syndrome
- Canavan disease
- Cystic fibrosis
- Familial dysautonomia
- Fanconi anemia group C
- Gaucher disease
- Glycogen storage disease Type I
- Mucolipidosis type IV
- Niemann-Pick disease types A and B
- Tay-Sachs disease

If you are of African ancestry, you should be screened for sickle cell disease. If you are of Mediterranean, Middle Eastern, African, Southeast Asian and Southern Chinese, or Hispanic ancestry, you should be screened for beta thalassemia. If you are of northern European descent, you should be screened for cystic fibrosis (although the American College of Obstetricians and Gynecologists now recommends that *all* couples who are pregnant or contemplating pregnancy be offered cystic fibrosis screening if requested, regardless of their ethnic background). Since most these disorders are autosomal recessive, both parents must be carriers for their child to be at risk. If you test positive to be a carrier, then your husband/partner should also be tested. Of course, if you and your husband/partner are a mixed-race couple, genetic screening should begin with the person at the greatest genetic risk based on ethnic background.

- **Age.** If you are 35 or older, you have a greater risk for having a baby with Down syndrome or other chromosomal defects compared to women who are younger. But that risk should not be exaggerated. At age 35 your chance of having a baby with Down's is 1 in 378, and your baby's risk for *any* chromosomal defect is 1 in 192—still far less than a 1 percent risk (see Box 7.1).

If you are 35 or older, your doctor may offer you an amniocentesis or chorionic villus sampling (CVS) during pregnancy to see if your baby has Down syndrome or other chromosomal defects. Amniocentesis and CVS are procedures used to diagnose genetic and other abnormalities of the fetus. Amniocentesis involves taking a sample of the amniotic fluid through a needle inserted in the abdomen, and CVS involves taking a sample of the placenta through a needle inserted through the cervix. Due to the availability of non-invasive screening tests these days, not all of my patients who are 35 or older would go for an amniocentesis or CVS. If their first- and/or second-trimester screening tests and ultrasound are normal, their risk for having a baby with Down's or any other chromosomal defects goes from a pre-test probability of 1 in 192 to a post-test probability of less than 1 in 3,000. One in 3,000 isn't a 100 percent guarantee, but for many couples these odds are good enough that they will forego a procedure that has a 0.5 percent (amniocentesis) to 1 percent (CVS) chance of causing a miscarriage. For other patients, their need for medical certainty, coupled with low procedure-related risk, will compel them to seek reassurance from CVS or amniocentesis.

Your husband's age does not appear to increase the baby's risk for Down syndrome or other chromosomal abnormalities, but he does have a biological clock, too. Older men are more likely to father a child with achondroplasia (the most common form of dwarfism), Marfan syndrome (allegedly what Abraham Lincoln had), and schizophrenia (see Chapter 8).

- **Known genetic disorder.** If you have a known genetic disorder such as sickle cell disease, you may be at greater risk for a number of pregnancy complications. Talk to your doctor about your risks, and what you can do to reduce the risks before and during pregnancy. Some genetic diseases require you to take actions now before you get pregnant. For example, if you have phenylketonuria (PKU), your body cannot metabolize the amnio acid phenylalanine, which is present in nearly all foods, diet soft drinks, and aspartame-containing artificial sweeteners such as Equal. During pregnancy, high blood levels of phenylalanine build up in the mother, which can cross the placenta with devastating consequences to the fetus. In up to 90 percent of such cases, the babies will have mental retardation and/or a small head size (microcephaly). Many will also have heart defects, low birth weight, and characteristic facial features. If you have PKU, you need to get on a special PKU diet for at least three months before you get pregnant, and continue the diet throughout pregnancy. Your doctor will need to do blood tests to check your blood phenylalanine levels on a monthly basis before and during pregnancy.

6. SOCIAL HISTORY

Help your doctor out. Your doctor may be so busy taking care of your medical needs that he or she may overlook social issues that are equally important to your (and your future baby's) health. You can really help your doctor out by bring up social issues of concern to you, including problems at home, exposures at work, and major stressors in your life.

- **Problems at home.** As I mentioned in Chapter 4, one of the most serious problems at home is family violence. Unfortunately, family violence occurs all too often in our society. If you answer yes to any of the questions in Box 4.6, you need to bring it up with your doctor. This is especially important if your partner has threatened to kill you, if there are weapons in the house, or if he abuses alcohol or uses drugs. Get help now before you get pregnant! Tell your doctor, or call the

National Domestic Violence Hotline at 1–800–799-SAFE
(7233) or TTY 1–800–787–3224, 24 hours a day, 365 days a
year from all 50 states.

Even if there is no violence, talk to your doctor if you are
having problems with your partner. She may refer you for
marital counseling or other types of support to help you work
out your problems before pregnancy. By all means don't use
the pregnancy as a way of keeping your man. If he is going to
leave you, having a baby is only going to magnify the problems and may drive him away even sooner. Work out your
problems before you get pregnant, or leave him and find
someone with whom you truly want to have a baby, raise a
family, and spend the rest of your life.

- **Exposures at work.** Bring a copy of MSDS from work to your
  preconception visit (see Chapter 6). If you are exposed to any
  known or suspected reproductive toxicant at work, ask your
  doctor to intervene on your behalf. For example, he or she
  can write a letter to your employer requesting job modifications or setting limits to your occupational exposures before
  you get pregnant.

- **Major stressors.** Let your doctor know if there are any major
  stressors going on in your life. Don't assume there is nothing
  he or she can do to help. Don't forego health care if you lose
  your job or health insurance. He or she may be able to
  continue to see you at a discounted rate, sign you up for
  government health insurance programs, or refer you for
  indigent health care. Your doctor may also be able to connect
  you to resources in the community, such as housing assistance, food banks, and government, community, or faith-
  based programs that can help get you back on your feet.
  Doctors are modern-day priests; people come to us for all
  sorts of problems that often have little to do with medical
  care. We can help.

7. HEALTH BEHAVIORS

Certain behaviors may put your future pregnancy, and your long-term health, in jeopardy. Your doctor can help you change your health behaviors before you get pregnant. While I can offer you advice here, I want you to understand that some of these behaviors are addictions and require more than my suggestions for you to change. There are professionals who deal with addictive behaviors, from eating disorders to smoking and other dependencies. Just use this time to attack those problems today instead of saying, "I'll quit tomorrow." You and your baby will be glad you did.

- **Cigarette smoking.** If you smoke, tell your doctor you want to quit before you get pregnant. Set a quit date with him or her. You might experience a lot of unpleasant withdrawal symptoms in the first few weeks after quitting, such as cigarette cravings, anxiety, irritability, and restlessness. Your doctor can help you (or refer you to programs that can help you) deal with these withdrawal symptoms and prevent a relapse (see Chapter 5).
- **Alcohol and drugs.** If you have problems with alcohol and drug use, be honest with your doctor. Tell him or her you want to stop before you get pregnant. He or she can refer you to alcohol or substance abuse treatment programs to help you quit.
- **Eating disorders.** Box 7.5 lists the diagnostic criteria for eating disorders. If you have an eating disorder, ask your doctor for help. Pregnancy will change your body shape and weight. Given the importance of nutrition in pregnancy, it is best to wait until you have the disorder under control before you get pregnant.

box 7.5: diagnostic criteria for eating disorders

Anorexia Nervosa

- Body weight <85 percent of expected weight (for age and height)
- Intense fear of gaining weight
- Undue emphasis on body shape or weight
- Amenorrhea (in girls and in women after menarche) for three consecutive months

Bulimia Nervosa

- Recurrent binge eating (at least two times per week for three months duration)
- Recurrent, inappropriate, compulsive behavior to prevent weight gain such as self-induced vomiting, abuse of laxatives, diuretics, or other medications, or excessive exercise
- Persistent overconcern with body shape and/or weight
- Absence of anorexia nervosa

Binge Eating Disorder

- Recurrent episodes of binge eating. An episode is characterized by:

  1. Eating a larger amount of food than normal during a short period of time (within any two-hour period)
  2. Lack of control over eating during the binge episode (i.e., the feeling that one cannot stop eating)

(continued)

- Binge eating episodes are associated with three or more of the following:

  1. Eating until feeling uncomfortably full
  2. Eating large amounts of food when not physically hungry
  3. Eating much more rapidly than normal
  4. Eating alone because you are embarrassed by how much you are eating
  5. Feeling disgusted, depressed, or guilty after overeating

- Marked distress regarding binge eating is present
- Binge eating occurs, on average, at least two days a week for six months
- The binge eating is not associated with the regular use of inappropriate compensatory behavior (i.e., purging, excessive exercise, etc.) and does not occur exclusively during the course of bulimia nervosa or anorexia nervosa.

8. DEPRESSION AND ANXIETY

Depression and anxiety can have a significant impact on your long-term health and your future baby's development. If you answer "yes" to any of the questions in Box 4.7, talk to your doctor. If you are having thoughts about hurting yourself or hurting others, you must tell your doctor right away.

Box 7.6 lists the diagnostic criteria for anxiety disorders:

box 7.6: diagnostic criteria for anxiety disorders

- Excessive anxiety or worry
- Difficulty in controlling your worry
- Restlessness or feeling keyed up or on edge
- Being easily fatigued
- Difficulty concentrating or mind going blank
- Irritability
- Muscle tension
- Sleep disturbance (difficulty falling or staying asleep, or restless, unsatisfying sleep)

If you have any of these symptoms, tell your doctor. Maternal anxiety has been linked to a whole host of pregnancy complications including preterm birth, as well as long-term neurodevelopmental problems in children, including ADHD. Your doctor may refer you to a mental health professional for counseling. Don't think that you have to be crazy to see a psychologist or psychiatrist; these are specialists who are trained to help you restore your mental health and psychological well-being. Your doctor may also prescribe a medication for you. As discussed earlier, the decision whether or not to start you on a medication before or during pregnancy should be based on a careful risk-benefit calculus.

9. PREVENTIVE AND PRIMARY CARE

Preconception care is not all about the baby; it is also an opportunity to get a check-up for yourself. For women in their childbearing years, the following preventive and primary health services are recommended (Box 7.7):

box 7.7: recommended preventive and primary health
services for women of childbearing age

- Height and weight measurements (at least every three to five
  years)
- Blood pressure (at least every two years)
- Total skin examination (at least every one to three years) to
  screen for skin cancer
- Clinical breast examination (at least every three years begin-
  ning at age 20) to screen for breast cancer
- Screening mammography (at least every one to two years be-
  ginning at age 40) to screen for breast cancer
- Papanicolau smear and pelvic examination (see Box 7.8)
- Immunizations: Ask your doctor if you need any of the follow-
  ing six recommended adult vaccinations:
  - Tetanus-diphtheria-pertussis (Tdap) vaccine
  - Hepatitis B
  - Influenza (if you are planning to be pregnant between
    December and March)
  - Mumps-measles-rubella (MMR)
  - Varicella (chickenpox)
  - Human papilloma virus (HPV)

See Chapter 5 for a more detailed discussion on each of the six vaccines. Remember **MMR, chickenpox,** and **HPV vaccines** are contraindicated during pregnancy, and you should avoid pregnancy for at least
four weeks after your receive these vaccines.

box 7.8: all women should have an annual pelvic exam but not all women need annual pap tests

This is what is currently recommended:
Pap Test

- First screen: About three years after first sexual intercourse or by age 21, whichever comes first.
- Women up to age 30 should get annual Pap tests
- Women age 30 and older have three options:
  - Women who have had three negative results on annual Pap tests can be rescreened with Pap tests alone every two to three years,
  - Continue to have annual Pap tests, or
  - Pap test with the addition of an HPV-DNA test. If both the Pap test and the DNA test are negative, rescreening should occur no sooner than three years.
- Women of any age who are immunocompromised, are infected with HIV, or were exposed *in utero* to diethylstilbestrol (DES) should be screened annually (some experts recommend every six months).

Pelvic Exam

- All women age 18 or older need annual gynecologic examinations, including a pelvic examination, as do sexually active adolescents younger than age 18.

10. PRECONCEPTION LABORATORY TESTS

I recommend the following laboratory tests for all women who are planning a pregnancy (Box 7.9):

box 7.9: recommended laboratory tests for
preconception care

- Hematocrit or hemoglobin
- Urine test
- Blood type and antibody screen
- Determination of immunity to rubella virus
- Syphilis screen
- Hepatitis B
- HIV
- Pap test
- Thyroid stimulating hormone
- Glycosylated hemoglobin
- Genetic screen for cystic fibrosis

The first eight tests on my list are routine prenatal labs, typically obtained during your first prenatal visit. My feeling is that if they are going to be done in early pregnancy, it is better to do them now so that if anything needs to be corrected, it can be corrected before you get pregnant. I will give my rationale for testing thyroid stimulating hormone, glycosylated hemoglobin, and cystic fibrosis below.

- **Hematocrit or hemoglobin.** This is a blood test to look for anemia. Anemia is the condition of having less than the normal number of red blood cells, or less than the normal quantity of hemoglobin, in the blood. Red blood cells and hemoglobin transport oxygen in your blood; therefore, anemia in pregnancy can cause poor oxygen delivery to the fetus and poor fetal growth and development. The most common type of anemia is iron-deficiency anemia, which can be caused by excessive blood loss (e.g., from heavy menstrual periods or a peptic ulcer), insufficient iron intake, or poor iron absorption. Other causes include vitamin B12 deficiency (often as a result of a strict vegan diet that excludes eggs, dairy products, meat, and fish), folate deficiency, and certain genetic disorders such as sickle cell anemia or thalassemia. If your blood work shows that you are anemic, ask your doctor to investigate the cause and correct the anemia before you get pregnant.

- **Urine testing.** Some women can harbor bacteria inside their bladder and not know it. Asymptomatic bacteriuria is a condition characterized by a significant number of bacteria in the urine that occurs without any of the usual symptoms of a urinary tract infection (burning during urination or increased frequency of urination). If left untreated, up to 40 percent of pregnant women with asymptomatic bacteriuria will develop a kidney infection, which could lead to preterm birth and other pregnancy complications. If you are actively trying to get pregnant, ask your doctor to test your urine for asymptomatic bacteriuria.

- **Blood type and antibody screen.** Do you know what your blood type is? You should. There are three blood types—A, B, and O. Do you know if you are "A positive" or "AB negative," or "O negative"? The positive or negative refer to the presence or absence, respectively, of a protein called Rh factor on the surface of your red blood cell. If you are Rh positive, you have nothing to worry about.

- If you are Rh negative (as are 10–15 percent of women), your doctor will need to screen your blood for any antibodies that may have already been formed against the Rh factor. If you have anti-Rh antibodies, your next pregnancy becomes a high-risk pregnancy because these antibodies can potentially cross the placenta to attack your baby. If you don't have anti-Rh antibodies, your doctor will give you a shot called Rhogam at 28 weeks, immediately after delivery, and anytime bleeding occurs during your pregnancy to prevent your blood from becoming sensitized to Rh and forming anti-Rh antibodies. While these tests are usually done at your first prenatal visit, you can ask your doctor to do your "type and screen" now so there will be no surprises during your pregnancy.

- **Determination of immunity to rubella virus.** As discussed in Chapter 5, rubella can cause congenital deafness, cataracts, heart defects, mental retardation, liver and spleen damage, and possibly schizophrenia if you are infected during pregnancy and have no immunity against rubella. Your doctor can find out whether or not you are immune to rubella with a blood test. If you are not immune, you should get immunized before you get pregnant since the rubella vaccine is contraindicated during pregnancy. To repeat, you need to wait **four weeks** after you receive the rubella vaccination before attempting to conceive.

- **Syphilis screen.** Universal screening for syphilis is recommended for all pregnant women at the first prenatal visit because untreated syphilis can cross the placenta to cause serious problems including stillbirth, birth defects, preterm birth, newborn seizures, and developmental delays. Syphilis screening is done through a simple blood test. If you have syphilis, you should get treated *before* you get pregnant. Treatment is with penicillin and no vaccine is currently available.

  Some experts also recommend screening for gonorrhea and chlamydia, at least in high-risk populations. Gonorrhea and chlamydia are sexually transmitted infections that, if left untreated, can cause a whole host of reproductive problems, including infertility, ectopic pregnancy, and preterm birth. These tests can be done by swabbing the cervix with a Q-tip or testing the urine.

- **Hepatitis B.** Universal screening for hepatitis B surface antigen is recommended for all pregnant women at their first prenatal visit. If you test positive for hepatitis B surface antigen in your blood, that means you have an active or persistent hepatitis infection that can be passed on to your baby. Your baby will need both active and passive immunizations against hepatitis B at birth. You should also have your liver functions checked every year since hepatitis B can cause liver damage (cirrhosis) and cancer in the long run. If you test negative for hepatitis B surface antigen and have never been immunized, consider getting vaccinated against hepatitis B before you get pregnant. Hepatitis B immunization consists of a series of three injections over a period of six months.

- **HIV screen.** Universal screening for human immunodeficiency virus (HIV) infection is recommended for all pregnant women at their first prenatal visit. It's a voluntary program, which means you have the right to refuse the blood test. Antiretroviral therapy has significantly prolonged the lifespan of women with HIV and reduced mother-to-child transmission of HIV during pregnancy (from about 30 percent to nearly 0 percent); so it is important to know what your HIV status is before you get pregnant.

- **Papanicolau test.** Papanicolau (Pap) test is a screening test for cervical precancer and cancer. Advanced cervical precancer is treated with a procedure called conization (removing a cone-shape piece of the cervix), which can be risky to perform during pregnancy. Therefore, you should get your Pap test done according to schedule (see Box 7.8) before you get pregnant.

In addition to these routine prenatal labs, I also recommend the following tests for women who are planning a pregnancy.

- **Thyroid-stimulating hormone (TSH) and free thyroxine (free T4).** TSH is a hormone produced by the brain to stimulate the thyroid gland; thyroxine (T4) is the major

thyroid hormone produced by the thyroid gland. A **high TSH**
(which suggests that the brain has to work extra hard to
stimulate an underperforming thyroid gland) or **low free T4**
are diagnostic of **hypothyroidism**, and have been linked to a
number of pregnancy complications including stillbirth and
preterm birth. Furthermore, maternal thyroid hormones play a
critical role in early brain development, and low maternal
thyroid hormones in early pregnancy have been linked to low
IQ in children. One recent study tested the IQ of children
born to women who were mildly deficient in thyroid hormones
in early pregnancy. Nearly one in five (19 percent) of these
children had an IQ score of less than 85, as compared to 1 in
20 (5 percent) children born to women who had normal
thyroid hormone levels in early pregnancy. Since many
women with low thyroid hormones have no symptoms, I
screen all my patients for hypothyroidism during preconception care, and advise those with low thyroid hormone levels to
wait until their TSH and free T4 become normal with
treatment before attempting to conceive.

- **Diabetes screen.** Women who are overweight or obese, or have
a family or personal history of diabetes (e.g., gestational diabetes
in a previous pregnancy), should be screened for diabetes before
they get pregnant. Screening can be done with a fasting plasma
glucose or a glucose tolerance test, but the test should be done
twice, at different times, to confirm the diagnosis of diabetes.
For women with an established diagnosis of diabetes, glycosylated hemoglobin, also known as hemoglobin A1C (HbA1C),
can be used to monitor their blood sugar control over a period
of time. If you have diabetes, you should try to get your blood
levels of glycosylated hemoglobin normal (or as close to normal
as possible) before attempting to conceive.

- **Genetic screen for cystic fibrosis.** The American College of
Obstetricians and Gynecologists (ACOG) recommends that
the carrier screening test for cystic fibrosis be available to all

couples who are planning pregnancy or are pregnant. You should get tested if you have a family history or other risk factors (e.g., ethnicity such as Caucasian or Ashkenazi Jew) for cystic fibrosis. If you don't have any risk factors, ask your doctor or go to ACOG's website to get more information on carrier testing.

I hope you will make an appointment to see your doctor soon for preconception care. Now you know how to get yourself ready, let's now turn our attention to getting your man ready for pregnancy.

from here to paternity
(give this chapter to your man)

Let's talk, man to man.

We need to talk because you probably aren't getting much good advice from your wife's doctor. Most ob/gyns aren't trained to deal with men's health, and they probably won't talk to you much if you show up for your wife's preconception care appointment. And you probably aren't getting much good advice from your own doctor. Most doctors who don't take care of pregnant women won't be able to tell you much about how to prepare for pregnancy, and the honest truth is that most doctors don't know what preconception care for men is.

We also need to talk because you probably aren't getting much good advice from most self-help books on pregnancy. Most such books are written for women on self-care *during* pregnancy; few deal with the time *before* pregnancy, and even fewer are written for men.

Most important, we need to talk because you and your wife might not be talking. Sure, you might be talking about starting a family and dreaming about where you want to raise your kids and maybe even toying with a few favorite names for boys and girls, but she may not be telling you what you really need to hear. Believe me. Being an obstetrician, I get to hear a lot of things that women say about their husbands.

I get to hear all their praises and complaints, all the things their husbands say right or wrong, all the things they wish their husbands would or wouldn't do.

In this chapter I am talking to you from the vantage point of not only a doctor and researcher, but also a husband and a dad. I will tell you about the latest research on how you can help make a smart and healthy baby, but I will also tell you a few secrets I've learned over the years from my patients and my family on how to be a good husband and a good dad.

what women want?

Sperm and support! That's what women want—they want your sperm, and they want your support. Sure your good looks are a bonus. And your sense of humor—that's how you got her to fall in love with you in the first place, right? But now what they want most of all from you is one good sperm, and lots of good support.

So what's in a sperm? The sperm carries your DNA (deoxyribonucleic acid) that you will pass on to your children. About half of your future baby's genetic materials come from the DNA carried in your sperm (the other half come from the DNA carried in your wife's egg). Since the DNA contains the genetic instructions for how the baby's organs and systems will develop and function, how smart and healthy your future baby will be depends greatly on the quality of the DNA carried in your sperm.

The DNA carried in your sperm can get damaged in a lot of different ways. Tobacco, alcohol, drugs (e.g., anabolic steroids), poor diet, certain medical conditions such as diabetes and varicoceles (varicose veins around the testes), radiation and chemotherapy, sexually transmitted infections, and even testicular hyperthermia (overheating) can cause sperm DNA damage. An increasing number of environmental pollutants, including phthalates (a type of plasticiser used in food-can linings and many household products), acrylamide (produced during frying, baking, and overcooking), pesticides, and dioxins, have also been shown to cause sperm DNA damage. Sperm carrying damaged DNA are not very good at fertilizing eggs, and men carrying lots of damaged sperm are usually infertile or subfertile. However, pregnancy may still be possible despite some degree of DNA damage, and such DNA damage may get passed on to the next generation, which can result in birth defects and even childhood cancers.

Over your lifetime, you will make trillions of sperm (as many as 12 trillion by some accounts). But for most of us, only one or two sperm will ever get chosen to pass on our genetic legacy. That's less than one in a trillion chance of being the chosen one. So make it a good one. You don't want to pass on damaged goods. If you want a smart and healthy baby, you've got to do all you can now to protect your sperm DNA.

Your other great contribution to making a smart and healthy baby is support. Your support is vital because it can act as a buffer against stress. In Chapter 4, I talked about what maternal stress can do to the baby inside the womb. Maternal stress is an important risk factor for pregnancy complications such as miscarriage, preterm birth, and fetal growth retardation. Furthermore, a growing body of research suggests that maternal stress can "program" the fetus' developing brain and other vital organs, which could lead to future neurodevelopmental and other health problems. Your support buffers mom against stress; it gives her the resilience to withstand stress. Studies have found that married women have lower rates of infant mortality, low birth weight, preterm birth, and other adverse pregnancy outcomes compared to single moms, even after controlling for socioeconomic and other differences, suggesting that marriage may offer some protection against pregnancy complications caused by stress. How much protection may well depend on how much support you give her; unfortunately for some women, their men can be a source of stress rather than support.

Your contribution to making a smart and healthy baby doesn't stop at birth. Kids growing up in families with high levels of father involvement have better cognitive and socioemotional development in early childhood, greater academic achievement and fewer behavioral problems in middle childhood, and better educational, behavioral, and emotional outcomes in adolescence compared to kids whose fathers aren't around much. Conversely, kids growing up in father-absent families are at greater risk for various educational or behavioral problems and poorer developmental outcomes, even after controlling for parental education, income, and other factors. Your support makes a big difference in your kids' lives.

So your greatest contributions to making a smart and healthy baby come down to two things: making good sperm and giving good support. I will show you how to do both in this chapter.

making good sperm in 90 days?

So you haven't been taking best care of yourself (like many of us). You've been a little more stressed out lately. You've been traveling a lot for work and so you haven't been eating very healthily. Or perhaps you've been overindulging yourself. Whatever the reason, you are a little worried about the quality of your sperm. And you want to know how long it'd take to repair the damage you've caused.

I've got good news for you. The answer is—90 days! That's all it takes. And that is because the life cycle of sperm lasts about 42 to 76 days—from production to ejaculation. Sperm production begins in one of several hundred microscopic coils inside the testes known as seminiferous tubules. They are housed within specialized cells called Sertoli cells, which protect them from external insults. As sperm mature, they leave their homes and move to the upper portion of the tubules, where they lose the protection of Sertoli cells and become vulnerable to injury. There they also lose their ability to self-destruct in response to injury, or to repair damaged DNA. Once the development of the head and tail is complete, sperm are released into the epididymis, where they spend about a week completing their maturation. They remain in this 20-foot-long coil until ejaculation, and it is within the epididymis that they are most susceptible to damage.

But unlike women, who are born with a limited supply of eggs, men continue to make new sperm throughout much of their adolescence and adulthood. And unlike women, who are stuck with damaged goods once their eggs are damaged, men can get rid of damaged sperm (via ejaculation) and make new ones. So if you think you may have done something to damage your sperm DNA in the past 42 to 76 days, just get rid of the old sperm and start making new ones. If you follow my ten-step program for the next 90 days, you can *probably* replace most if not all of your damaged sperm with good sperm.

I say *probably* because there may be environmental threats out there about which we know little that could damage your sperm DNA. I can warn you about the things we know (e.g., smoking, alcohol, marijuana, cocaine, anabolic steroids, certain medications, stress, infection and inflammation, xenobiotics, testicular hyperthermia (overheating), and radiation), but I can't warn you about the things we don't know. I say *probably* also because some of these environmental threats can be stored inside your body for a long, long time (e.g., dioxins can be stored in your body fat for up to seven years), where they can continue to cause damage to new sperm. Most important, some of these threats can cause direct and permanent damage to your germline from which all future sperm are derived. Fortunately, your germline DNA is very well protected and most damage is repaired right away. But given all these reasons, it may be a good idea to start taking care of yourself now even if you aren't planning to make a baby within the next 90 days.

from here to paternity: ten steps to fatherhood

So here is a ten-step program to getting yourself ready for fatherhood. The first step is to make a plan. Steps 2 through 6 are about making good sperm, and steps 7 through 10 are about giving good support. Give yourself at least 90 days to complete the program.

Step 1: Make a reproductive life plan
Step 2: Go see your doctor
Step 3: Give up your biggest vices
Step 4: Manage your stress
Step 5: Eat right
Step 6: Protect your sperm DNA
Step 7: Learn to give emotional support
Step 8: Bring home the bacon AND cook it, too
Step 9: Reprioritize
Step 10: Stay faithful

1. MAKE A REPRODUCTIVE LIFE PLAN

The first step toward fatherhood is to make a plan—a reproductive life plan.

A reproductive life plan, as defined by the Centers for Disease Control and Prevention (CDC), is a set of personal goals about having (or not having) children based on your personal values and resources, and a plan to achieve those goals. To make a reproductive life plan, you need to ask yourself these three questions: 1) Do you want to have any (more) children? 2) If yes, how many children do you want, and when would you like to become a father? Unfortunately, you are not forever young. Men, too, have a biological clock (see Box 8.1). 3) Under what circumstances would you like to become a father? When you are married? When you can afford to raise a family? When you can buy a home? When you've finished grad school or made partner at work? These are important questions about personal values and resources to which you should give some serious consideration before making your reproductive life plan.

If you and your wife are ready to make a baby, go see your doctor before you start trying (see Step 2).

What if you and your wife cannot agree on a reproductive life plan? If the two of you cannot even agree on the first question, whether or not you want to have children ever, then you've got a big problem. Go get some counseling to work this out; your marriage may be in trouble if you can't agree on this very fundamental question about your reproductive life plan. If it is a timing issue (she wants to get pregnant now but you want to wait, or vice versa), 'talk it over with her. Talk about your values and resources, share your fears and dreams, and see if you can come to some agreement on a joint reproductive life plan that is right for both of you.

box 8.1: do men have a biological clock, too?

The answer is, painfully, yes. Most women in their late thirties and early forties are keenly aware that their biological clock is ticking, but many older men seem oblivious to their own clock. It is now becoming increasingly clear that the biological clock ticks for men as well as for women. The older you get, the more likely you are to pass on genetic defects to your children. This is because the older you get, the more damaged your sperm DNA can get. Each time your germ cells divide to make more sperm, it creates an opportunity for an error to occur. Your germ cells go through 23 rounds of mitotic divisions every year (once every 16 days); by the time your turn 30, they will have passed through 380 rounds of mitotic divisions; by age 40, 610 rounds; and by age 50, 840 rounds! The older you get, the more chances for genetic mutations to accumulate just from cell replications. The older you get, the more chances also for your DNA to accumulate wear and tear from environmental insults; several studies have found more breaks in the DNA of sperm from older men (>35 years) than from younger men. As you get older, your body's ability to repair or get rid of damaged DNA also declines. Studies have found that apoptosis (programmed cell death), which is one mechanism your body uses

(continued)

to get rid of damaged sperm, also decreases with age. This means the older you get, the more likely that your future baby will be made with a damaged sperm.

There are now more than 20 different diseases that are correlated with paternal age. These include achondroplasia (the most common form of dwarfism), Marfan syndrome (allegedly what Abraham Lincoln had), autism, and schizophrenia. While the risk is small (on the order of one in ten thousands) for most diseases, for schizophrenia the risk is nearly 1 percent. That is, the risk of a 40-year-old man having a child who later develops schizophrenia is about 1 in 110—similar to a 40-year-old woman's risk of having a child with Down syndrome. The risk for autism is nearly six times higher for children born to men over 40 than those born to men under 30.

Unfortunately, we are not forever young. In making your reproductive life plan, keep in mind that you, too, have a biological clock.

2. GO SEE YOUR DOCTOR

When was the last time you saw your doctor for a regular check-up? If you are like most men (myself included), you've probably put it off longer than you should. Most of us are nicer to our cars than to ourselves—our cars get regular tune-ups and we don't.

Well, it's time to get a tune-up for yourself. In the next few months, you may be called upon to fulfill what theologians and evolutionary biologists alike consider one of life's greatest purposes—to procreate. And one sperm, among the trillions that you will make over your lifetime, may be chosen to pass on your genetic legacy. So make it a good one. Change the oil and filter, check the battery and charging system, inspect the brakes and the belts, rotate the tires and flush the coolants, and get the ride in tip top shape. Make an appointment to see your doctor today.

Here are some things to talk to your doctor about during your preconception visit:

- **Past reproductive history.** Tell your doctor about your past reproductive history. This is especially important if you and your wife have had problems conceiving, or had a previous pregnancy that resulted in miscarriage or fetal death, or a child affected by birth defects or mental retardation.
- **Current medical conditions.** If you have any medical condition, ask your doctor how it might affect the pregnancy. Certain medical conditions, such as diabetes, varicoceles, or sexually transmitted infections, can cause damage to your sperm DNA. Other conditions for which you may have received treatment in the past (e.g., radiation or chemotherapy for cancer) can reduce your fertility. Of course, this is not just about the baby; it's also about your own health. Men are notorious for not reporting new symptoms to their doctors. Tell your doctor if you've been experiencing any abnormal symptoms, such as chest pain, headaches, a change in bowel habits or blood in the stool, a swelling or lump in the testes, painful urination or urethral discharge, a rash, bumps, or ulcers in the genital area, erectile dysfunction or premature ejaculation, and so on.
- **Medications you are taking.** Bring a list of medications (prescription and over-the-counter) that you are currently taking (or have taken in the past year) and ask your doctor whether you can continue to take them while trying to make a baby. A number of medications can lower your sperm count and quality, including alkylating agents, calcium channel blockers, cimetidine, colchicine, corticosteroids, cyclosporine, erythromycin, gentamicin, methadone, neomycin, nitrofurantoin, phenytoin, spironolactone, sulfasalazine, tetracycline, and thioridazine. Some medications such as leflunomide used

to treat rheumatoid arthritis can stay around in your body for a long time; ask your doctor how long you should wait after discontinuation of a medication before you and your wife can begin trying to conceive.

- **Family history and genetic risk.** Tell your doctor if you or anyone in your family has a known genetic disorder, birth defect, or mental retardation. Your doctor may send you for further genetic counseling and testing. Certain genetic disorders can impair fertility, such as cystic fibrosis, Klinefelter syndrome, Kartagener syndrome, and polycystic kidney disease. Some genetic disorders may skip generations so you should try to get a three-generation (your grandparents', your parents', and your generation) family history if you can. If your wife is a carrier for certain disorder (e.g., cystic fibrosis, sickle cell disease), then you may be asked to get tested to see if you are also a carrier. If you and your wife are a mixed-race couple, your doctor may test you first if you belong to an ethnic group at greater risk for certain genetic disorders (e.g., Ashkanazi Jewish descent).

- **Work and hobbies.** Ongoing exposures to metals, solvents, endocrine disruptors, and pesticides at work can lower your sperm count, damage your sperm DNA, and possibly lead to infertility, miscarriage, and birth defects. Ask your employer for a copy of the Material Safety Data Sheet (MSDS) and bring it with you to your doctor's appointment. Your doctor may refer you to a Teratogen Information Service counselor if there is any concern about your occupational exposures. Tell your doctor if your hobby involves chemical exposures, especially to solvents.

- **Risk behaviors.** If you are engaged in any behavior (e.g., smoking, alcohol, or drug use) that might put your sperm DNA and your future family at risk, talk to your doctor about quitting.

- **Mental health.** If you feel depressed or have other mental health problems, now is not a good time to start a family. Talk to your doctor about getting help for your mental health problems.

- **Weight.** Your doctor will check your weight at the visit. Men who are overweight have reduced fertility; for every 20 lbs overweight you have 10 percent increased chance of infertility. Men who are overweight also have lower testosterone levels and poorer sperm quality. If you are overweight, talk to your doctor about a weight loss plan.
- **Blood pressure.** Your doctor will also check your blood pressure. If you have high blood pressure, keep it under control with diet, exercise, and prescription medications if necessary. If you want to stay around long enough to see your kids (and grandkids) graduate from college, keep your blood pressure under control.
- **Physical exam.** Your doctor will also do an annual skin exam to look for skin cancer, as well as an annual testicular exam to look for testicular cancer. You should be doing a monthly testicular self-exam at home. If you are over 40, your doctor may also screen you for prostate and colon cancers if you have certain risk factors.
- **Laboratory tests.** The only laboratory tests that are routinely recommended for men are a cholesterol panel every three to five years and blood sugar screen every three to five years if you are overweight or over 40.
- **Immunizations.** Ask your doctor what immunizations you need. Immunization recommendations are updated annually by the CDC.
- **Go see your dentist.** While you are at it, you should also make an appointment to see your dentist. Periodontal disease can be a source of chronic infection and inflammation in your body.

3. GIVE UP YOUR BIGGEST VICES

You've put this off long enough, but now you have even more reasons to quit. If you can't do it for yourself, do it for your legacy. Cigarette smoking, excessive drinking, and drug use can reduce your fertility and damage your sperm DNA. They can also cause collateral damage to the loved ones around you. Most important, as a dad you will be modeling behaviors to your kids. So give up your biggest vices before you become a father.

Quit smoking. If you smoke, it's time to quit. Paternal smoking has been linked to fertility problems. Men who smoke have lower sperm count, on average about 22 percent lower. The more cigarettes you smoke, the lower your sperm count. They also have more defective sperm with abnormal morphology (e.g., sperm with two heads or two tails—not exactly the seeds with which to make smart and healthy babies) or motility (i.e., poor swimmers). Recent research has revealed that chronic exposure to nicotine and tobacco smoke can reduce the fertilizing capacity of sperm. Chronic nicotine overloading prevents sperm from penetrating the zona, the shell surrounding an egg. On average, chronic smokers show a 75 percent decline in fertilizing capacity when compared to non-smokers. Cigarette smoking can also induce oxidative damage to the DNA in sperm. Pregnancy is still possible despite some degree of sperm DNA damage, and the damaged DNA can be passed on to your future baby.

If you smoke, you may not be the only one who is affected by your smoking. Your wife's eggs (and her health) can get damaged by secondhand smoke. If both you and your wife smoke, that's a double whammy, and it is a lot harder for her to quit if you continue to smoke.

Once you've decide to quit, you can **START** by taking these five steps:

S = **Set** a quit date.

T = **Tell** family, friends, and co-workers that you plan to quit.

> A = **Anticipate** and plan for the challenges you'll face while quitting.
>
> R = **Remove** cigarettes and other tobacco products from your home, car, and work.
>
> T = **Talk** to your doctor about getting help to quit.

You can get help with quitting by calling 1–800-QUITNOW (1–800–784–8669), or go to http://www.smokefree.gov. After you've quit smoking, you should wait at least three months smoke-free before attempting to conceive.

Alcohol. The effect of alcohol on sperm quality is less clear. Some studies have shown that moderate drinking may be protective against DNA damage, perhaps in part due to the antioxidant effect of some alcoholic beverages. Other studies have shown that alcohol may be damaging to sperm DNA. The data are clearer on heavy drinking (more than two drinks a day). In a study of alcoholics in an addiction treatment center, testosterone level, semen volume, sperm count, and the number of sperm with normal morphology and motility were lower among alcoholic than non-alcoholic men.

If you answer yes to any of the following **CAGE** questions, you probably have a drinking problem:

> C = **Cut-down:** Have you ever felt you should cut down on your drinking?
>
> A = **Annoy:** Have people annoyed you by criticizing your drinking?

(continued)

G = Guilty: Have you ever felt bad or guilty about your drinking?

E = Eye-opener: Have you ever had a drink first thing in the morning (as an "eye-opener") to steady your nerves or get rid of a hangover?

You can get help by calling the National Drug and Alcohol Treatment Referral Routing Service at 1–800–662-HELP, or going to the U.S. Substance Abuse and Mental Health Services Administration (SAMHSA) website at www.samhsa.gov to find an alcohol treatment program near you.

Drugs. Several recreational drugs have also been linked to male infertility, including marijuana, cocaine, and anabolic steroids. Marijuana can lower your testosterone, sperm count, and semen quality. Cocaine can also decrease your sperm count and cause abnormal sperm morphology and motility, and the effects can linger for up to two years from last use. Anabolic steroids can also lower your testosterone level and sperm quality. In a small study of 15 men who were using anabolic steroids, 11 had low testosterone levels and 9 had no sperm production at all. Even after quitting, only 2 men resumed normal sperm production. If you have a drug problem, you can get help by calling the National Drug and Alcohol Treatment Referral Routing Service at 1–800–662-HELP.

Caffeine. Just a word about caffeine (which is not necessarily a vice). The effect of caffeine on sperm quality is unclear. One Brazilian study found that men who drank more than six cups of coffee per day had *higher* sperm motility. While more research is needed, a few cups of coffee a day probably won't hurt your sperm.

4. MANAGE YOUR STRESS

Most women are well aware of the connection between their stress levels and their babies' health, but many men still don't make the connection. What does your stress level now have to do with your baby in the future?

Stress can interfere with the balance of your reproductive hormones, leading to lower testosterone levels and decreased sperm production. Because chronic stress can increase your susceptibility to infections and inflammation, it can indirectly cause oxidative damage to your sperm DNA. Stress can cause you to do things you know are bad for your health, such as overeating, smoking, heavy drinking, or drug use, which can also lower your sperm count and damage your sperm DNA. Most important, stress can impair your ability to support and nurture. So if you want to make a smart and healthy baby, you need to keep your stress level under control.

To learn about managing your stress, I invite you to read Chapter 4 of this book. In it I talk about ten steps to stress resilience:

- Exercise
- Get a good night's sleep
- Eat right
- Learn to relax
- Prevent stress
- Learn to problem-solve
- Learn to resolve conflicts
- Develop positive mental health
- Get connected
- Get help

While the chapter was written for your wife, many of the lessons still apply to you. Exercise, get a good night's sleep, and eat right are time-proven remedies against stress for men and women alike. You may also want to try some of the relaxation techniques I suggested, such as deep breathing, transcendental meditation, and mindfulness exercises. You can strengthen your stress resilience by building capacities for problem-solving and conflict resolution and developing positive mental health. Pay special attention to the sections on developing your emotional intelligence and communication skills, as these are two areas where many women complain most about their spouses. Learn to get connected and, most important, ask for help if you need it. If you've got a problem with addiction, depression, or anything that could interfere with your ability to be a good husband and a good father, get help now!

5. EAT RIGHT

Most of you have heard the expression "you are what you eat." But did you know that your sperm is also what you eat?

Studies indicate that the quality of your diet may well determine the quality of your sperm. Nutritional deficiencies in several micronutrients, especially zinc and folate, have been shown to lower sperm production and impair male fertility. Both zinc and folate also have antioxidant properties that counteract reactive oxygen species (ROS) and protect sperm against oxidative stress and DNA damage. Several randomized, placebo-controlled trials have found daily supplementation with 5 mg of folic acid and 66 mg of zinc sulfate increases sperm count and improves sperm morphology and motility in both subfertile and fertile men.

Other antioxidants have also been used to treat male infertility, including vitamin C, vitamin E, selenium, glutathione, ubiquinol, carnitine, and carotenoids. However, the safety and efficacy of such treatments have not been clearly established. In one study, the combination of vitamin C and E at high doses resulted in sperm DNA damage in vitro, raising concerns about the potential harms of high-dose antioxidant supplementation. This is why I do not recommend any unproven supplementation for men who are planning a pregnancy, other than a healthy diet and a daily multivitamin.

I encourage you to take a look at Chapters 2 and 3, which talk about steps you and your wife can take to get yourselves nutritionally prepared for pregnancy. Given what we know today about the role ROS play in causing sperm damage, you should try to reduce your intake of foods that are pro-inflammatory, and increase your intake of foods that are anti-inflammatory and antioxidant. This means reducing your intake of saturated fatty acids, *trans* fats, partially hydrogenated oils, refined carbohydrates, and added sugars such as high-fructose corn syrup; and increasing your intake of omega–3 polyunsaturated fatty acids such as DHA, and lots of fruits and vegetables in rainbow colors. Take a good look at the lists of ten brain foods and ten toxic foods; if you can follow the same diet that I prescribed for your wife, your sperm and your future baby will thank you.

6. PROTECT YOUR SPERM DNA

There are a lot of things that can damage the DNA of your sperm. Here are a few things to avoid:

- **Xenobiotics.** A xenobiotic is a chemical, such as a drug or pesticide, that is foreign to the body. Exposures to a number of xenobiotics have been shown to reduce male fertility and sperm quality. These include
  - **1,2-dibromo–3-chloropropane** is widely used in pesticides, insecticides, and soil fumigants. It can disrupt sperm production and cause male sterility and miscarriage. You can reduce exposure by avoiding the use of products containing 1,2-dibromo–3-chloropropane (and pesticides, insecticides, and fumigants in general) while planning to make a baby.
  - **Nonylphenol** is used in waste water treatment plants as well as household detergents, pesticides, and even contraceptives (spermicides containing nonoxynol–9). It is toxic to aquatic life and can induce DNA damage in human sperm. You can reduce exposure by avoiding the use of household products containing nonylphenol, including super-strength specialty detergents (keep it simple and use baking soda, borax, and vinegar for household cleaning instead).

- **Polycyclic aromatic hydrocarbons (PAHs),** such as benzocpyrene, are found primarily in cigarette smoke; heavy smoking can cause oxidative stress and DNA damage in human sperm and possibly induce childhood cancer in the offspring. You can reduce exposure by quitting and avoiding secondhand smoke.

- **Polychlorinated biphenyls (PCBs)** are a mixture of chemicals that are no longer produced in the United States but are still found in the environment. PCBs can lower your sperm quality and cause sperm DNA damage. Since the primary source of exposure comes from eating contaminated fish (especially sportfish caught in contaminated lakes and rivers) and fish-eating wildlife, you can reduce your exposure to PCBs by following local advisories about consumption of fish and wildlife. You may also want to avoid working with old appliances, electrical equipment, and transformers (made 30 years ago, many of which contain PCBs) for at least three months before you and your wife start trying to conceive.

- **Dioxins** belong to the same class of chemicals, called endocrine disruptors, as PCBs. Dioxins can induce oxidative stress and DNA damage in sperm. Dioxins are stored in animal fats; the primary source of exposure comes from dietary consumption of animal fat. You can reduce your exposure to dioxins by reducing your dietary fat intake (e.g., switch to non-fat or low-fat milk and cheese made from skim milk, de-skin poultry, and choose the leanest cuts of organic beef from grain-fed cows).

- **Phthalate esters** are a type of plasticizer, or softening agent, used in many products containing vinyl (soft plastic). These include home furnishings (e.g., vinyl flooring, wallpaper), children's items (e.g., infant feeding bottles, squeeze toys, changing mats, teethers) and packaging (e.g., disposable bottles, microwave food wrap). Phthalates are also found in cosmetics and scented products such as soaps, lotions, and shampoos, as well as insecticides, adhesives, sealants, and car-care products. Phthalate is a known reproductive toxicant and can lower your sperm count and semen quality. You can reduce your exposure by avoiding the use of products (as much as you can) containing phthalate. One way to avoid phthalate exposure is to avoid microwaving foods in plastic if you are not sure whether your food wrap or plastic container is made with phthalate.

- **Acrylamides** are used in water treatment, paper making, ore processing, and the manufacture of diverse products. Interestingly, for unknown reason acrylamide also appears in foods cooked or processed at high temperatures (above 120°C or 248°F) for a long time. Acrylamide can disrupt male reproduction by many mechanisms, including impairment of sperm development and motility. One way of reducing exposure is to avoid overcooking your food, that is, for too long or at too high a temperature.

- **Heavy metals,** such as lead and cadmium, have also been shown to cause sperm DNA damage. Household exposure to lead includes lead paint, tap water (from leaching of old pipes), and common household items such as hair and beard dyes, mini-blinds, lead-glazed houseware, plates, and potteries. Please refer to Chapter 6 for steps you can take to avoid household lead exposure. Cadmium is used in metal plating, semiconductors, wires, plastics, batteries, welding, soldering, ceramics, painting, and cigarettes. You can find out what you are being exposed to at work by requesting the Material Safety Data Sheet (MSDS) from your employer.

- **Infections and inflammation.** Infections and inflammation have been shown to cause oxidative stress and sperm DNA damage. Infections of the male reproductive organs (e.g., testis, epididymis, urethra, and accessory glands such as the prostate) are the major culprits. Most such infections are sexually transmitted (though some might not be), with chlamydia being the most common. So don't be fooling around, and not while you are trying to make a baby with your wife. Get screened for STDs (if there is a reason to do so) before you start trying. Remember some STDs are asymptomatic, and you may be silently harboring an STD from a long time ago. Infections and inflammation from other parts of the body can get carried by the bloodstream to your reproductive organs, where they can cause damage to your sperm DNA. So get rid of any ongoing sources of infections and inflammation (e.g., tooth or gum disease), and avoid getting sick (as much as you can) while you and your wife are trying to make a baby.

- **High temperature.** High temperature inside the scrotum (the sac that contains the testes) has been shown to cause sperm DNA damage and lower male fertility. Heat from hot baths, saunas, long hot showers (more than 30 minutes), down-filled or electric blankets, heating pads, and laptop computers can increase scrotal temperatures. Wearing tight clothing, prolonged driving, and cycling (for more than 30 minutes at a time, especially in tight-fitting bicycle shorts) can also increase the temperature of your testes. For at least three months before you start trying, you need to avoid overheating your sperm (e.g., stay away from saunas and long hot showers, put the laptop on the desktop instead of in your lap, take frequent rests while driving or cycling, and avoid tight-fitting underwear). Metal workers and welders also have lower sperm quality. If you work in an occupation that may put you at risk, you may want to ask for some job modifications so you can protect your sperm from overheating.
- **Radiation.** Some forms of radiation can damage sperm DNA. If you are exposed to radiation at work (e.g., X-ray technicians or certain laboratory researchers), strictly adhere to radiation

safety protocols and guidelines and find ways to protect
yourself. If you are about to undergo radiation treatment (e.g.,
for cancer), consider freezing some of your sperm (called
"cryopreservation") before you do. There is no conclusive
evidence that exposure to computers is harmful to sperm.
There are conflicting reports regarding the effects of electromagnetic fields on sperm quality. Exposure to mobile phone
radiation also remains controversial. One recent study found
that men who used mobile phones for four hours or more a day
have a lower sperm count and semen quality compared to men
with lower phone use. Some have argued that people who are
heavy users of mobile phones might be more sedentary, more
stressed out, or eat more junk food. It may be their lifestyles,
rather than mobile phone radiation, that is the real culprit,
since after all, people hold their mobile phones to their head
and not their testicles when they talk.

7. LEARN TO GIVE EMOTIONAL SUPPORT

Remember I said your greatest contributions to making a smart and
healthy baby come down to two things: making good sperm and giving
good support? Now that you've mastered how to make good sperm, I'm
going to coach you on how to give good support.

First and foremost is emotional support. Unfortunately most guys just
aren't very good at giving emotional support; it doesn't come naturally
and we aren't brought up in our society to be nurturing. Emotional support is something you have to work hard at; it takes practice.

So how do you give good emotional support? Here are five proven
"techniques" you can work on:

- **Pay attention.** Learn to pay attention. Be there for her. Be
  present—not only physically, but with mindfulness. "Mindfulness means paying attention in a particular way," according to
  Jon Kabat-Zinn, "on purpose, in the present moment and
  non-judgmentally." It's about being completely *present* and in

the moment. When was the last time you were completely
present and in the moment when she was talking with you?
Practice putting the game and not her on pause—with TiVo
you can always go back to the game, but you can't ever go back
to the moment.

- **Listen.** Listening is one of the best ways to show emotional
support. You don't have to do or say anything. Don't try to
solve her problems. Just listen. Practice actively listening.
Learn to ask her questions or paraphrase what she said so she
can tell you are listening. Listen not only with your ears but
with your heart and your eyes—watch for nonverbal commu-
nications. Many of us men want to be helpful and offer
solutions long before she wants them. Ask her to let you know
if she wants your advice or help. Then go back and listen
again.

- **Empathize.** Empathy is the capacity to identify with and
understand what someone else is feeling. It is about being able
to "get under someone's skin" and "walk in their shoes." Well,
maybe you shouldn't try to get into your wife's shoes, but try to
understand what she is feeling and *why*. Many women get
mood swings during pregnancy, partly because of those crazy
pregnancy hormones, and partly because pregnancy may open
up a Pandora's box of repressed feelings. Some of the feelings
may have to do with her childhood family relationships—her
relationships with her parents, her parents' marital relationships, her mother's role in the family and experience with
pregnancy, childbirth and parenting, issues about trust and
betrayal, commitment and abandonment—there is much she
is afraid of that she may not have opened up to you, or even to
herself. Be patient. Try to understand why she is feeling a
certain way. For starters, acknowledge her feelings and
NEVER discount them.

- **Respect.** Everybody wants a little respect, especially from
someone with whom they are going to make a baby, raise a

family, and spend the rest of their life. Show her some respect. NEVER put her down, in public or in private. Don't roll your eyes when she says something you disagree with. Don't say mean things to her. Don't hurt her, physically, emotionally, or by any means. Don't take her for granted. Do find the good in her. Do tell her how much you appreciate her everyday. Do give her credit for your successes because you know you couldn't have done it without her. And don't get jealous of her successes because behind every great woman is a great man.

- **Touch.** Learn to touch her how she likes to be touched. Learn to give back rubs and foot massages; massages have been shown to reduce stress hormones, elevate moods, and alleviate anxiety and depression. They will score you big points during pregnancy and keep your intimacy alive. Remember that many women do not like to be sexually touched when they are tired or before they feel relaxed, whereas men may use sex as a way to relax. Engaging in non-sexual touching will really make her feel appreciated (especially if you did the dishes also).

Take-home message: Stay **ALERT** (pay *a*ttention, *l*isten, *e*mpathy, *r*espect, *t*ouch) to her need for emotional support. You may also want to read Chapter 4 to learn how you can develop your emotional intelligence and communication skills so you can give better emotional support.

8. BRING HOME THE BACON AND COOK IT, TOO

Another kind of support, in psychologists' jargon, is called instrumental support, which includes such things as financial support or help with household chores. Financial support is about bringing home the bacon (or something healthier). Having a baby is expensive, but I don't think I was fully aware of just how expensive it is until my kids were born. So start your financial planning now; it's never too early. Talk to an advisor, or get started by going to websites that teach you about financial planning for baby, such as the March of Dimes website. The website breaks down financial planning for baby into seven steps:

- Make a budget
- Shop smart
- Check out your health insurance options
- Buy life insurance
- Get long-term disability insurance
- Make a will and update beneficiaries
- Look into maternity and paternity leave policies

Get started now before you make a baby. You can start by reviewing your health insurance policy. Know what your out-of-pocket expenses will be for pregnancy. I've known too many couples who got stuck with big bills for services their health insurance didn't cover. I will add one more point to the list: Start a baby fund now. Put aside a set amount of money from your paycheck each month to cover unexpected expenses (believe me, there will be lots of those) once your baby arrives.

Your job isn't done once you bring home the bacon. You have to cook it, too. And when you are done, make sure you clean and do the dishes and take out the trash and run the bath for the kids and put them in their jammies and read them bedtime stories and pay the bills and run out and pick up some milk and, oh, don't forget to fix that leaky toilet. Okay, you shouldn't have to do all these chores, but neither should your wife. Chores are a major source of conflict in marriage. It's the one thing that women complain most about their husbands—they don't do their share of household chores. The resentment is strongest if both of you work, but even if she is a stay-at-home mom, she can still use your help and support. I know because I've been a stay-at-home dad on numerous weekends when my wife was on-call at the hospital. As soon as she comes home from an overnight call I'd tell her "here, take the kids; I need a break," even though she may have been up for 24 hours straight. Homemaking is not easy. If you grew up in a family where your stay-at-home mom did all the housework and had dinner ready when dad came home and you expect the same from your wife, get over it. Those days are over, and unless you marry your mom it's just not going to happen. Housework should be shared. So make a list now of household chores that need to get done, and you pick the chores that she hates to do (and vice versa). For chores that both of you loath (e.g., house cleaning), hire someone to do them if you can afford it. Do your share of the household chores or, if you really want to give good support, do more than your share.

9. REPRIORITIZE

Over the next few months you are going to start nesting. That's right, I said nesting. Now you probably think of nesting as something pregnant women do, driven by instinct to clean, organize, and decorate their home before the baby arrives. It turns out that men do their own nesting as well, but just in a very different way. Most men nest by getting their financial house in order. You are going to be working extra hard to get that big promotion, land that big account, and win that big bonus. For what? Job security? Higher pay? Down payment for a house (or a bigger house)? Extra money to pay for all the extra expenses that come with a baby? Start a college fund (the way tuition is going up, you'd better get started before the baby is conceived)?

There is one problem. If you are pulling long hours and burning the midnight oil at the office, you are not going to be around very much. That's one of the biggest complaints I hear from my patients about their husbands—*my husband works so much that he's never around.* They don't see their husbands' behaviors as nesting; they see their husbands turning into workaholics. They see their husbands caring more about their work than about them, and you know in the back of their minds they are thinking: *If that's how you are now when I'm pregnant, what kind of father are you going to be when the baby comes?* They are scared that they are going to have to raise the kids on their own because you are never going to be around to help out. And the sad truth is—they are partially right. Once you get that big promotion or land that big account, you are just going to get busier. And as much as you want to be a supportive husband and involved dad, you just might be too tired, grumpy, overworked, and stressed out to be all that you can be.

What makes the matter worse is that your wife probably isn't just sitting around waiting for you to come home (though if she is, she is going to be awfully bored and lonely if you are never around). Most American women work through their pregnancy, and many return to work within a few weeks after giving birth (a national survey found that about a third of women return to work less than six weeks after giving birth, and over 70 percent return to work in less than three months). So she, too, is going to be tired, grumpy, overworked, and stressed out, especially when pregnancy hormones are making her extra tired and moody or when she's been up all night long nursing a crying baby every two hours. So fuses get short, arguments erupt about who is doing more and who is more stressed out, and that lovin' feelin' gets lost. This may be a big part of why 10 percent of couples break up during pregnancy, and another 30 percent end their marriages within two years of having their babies, even though pregnancy is supposed to bring them closer together.

How do you prevent this from happening to your marriage? You start by rethinking your priorities. If you and your wife have decided to start a family, then the family is your priority and everything else has to take a backseat. This might mean that you can't stay as late at work. This might also mean cutting back on your business trips. Go on the "daddy track." If you are not ready, personally or financially, to make fatherhood your top priority, then maybe you should wait on making a baby.

10. STAY FAITHFUL

Of all the advice I give in this chapter, this is probably the most important one: Stay faithful! I've seen so many families get broken up because of infidelity—it is a leading cause of divorce in America. Even if you are able to save your marriage, there will always be that distrust that comes between you and your wife, and that hurt which she can never completely get over. And think about the potential damage your infidelity may inflict upon your children—all the negative influences of the stress hormones inside the womb, growing up in a broken home, and the absence of a father role model. You are about to start a family; don't mess it up.

Cheating on your wife is not a good way to make a smart and healthy baby.

I need to make this point because marital infidelity is all too common in our society. According to a 2002 survey from the University of Chicago's National Opinion Research Center, nearly one in four men (22 percent) said they had sex with someone besides their spouse while married. And that's just the ones who were honest. And while men are more prone to infidelity, women are not impervious to it. The same survey in 2002 also found that 15 percent of women admitted to having had extramarital sex. There have also been reports that about 10 percent of babies are found by DNA testing to be genetically unrelated to their supposed father as stated on the birth certificates. I guess two can play the game.

Pregnancy is a vulnerable time. Your relationship with your wife is about to change. Her body will change. Sex will change. Raging hormones, mood swings, overwhelming fatigue, changing body image, fears, anxiety, and even some medical issues can get in the way of sex during pregnancy. After you have kids, your relationship with her will change even more. There will be many times when she is just too tired to have sex with you. And there will be many times when she has little left in her to pay any attention to you. And all the added stresses of pregnancy and parenting will at times strain the relationship even more. These are times when you might be particularly vulnerable to infidelity. When you stop feeling special in your marital relationship, the affection and attention of another woman can make you feel special again.

This is no excuse for cheating, which is selfish, deceptive, and destructive. But I just want to warn you that there are going to be vulnerable times ahead. How will you stay faithful during those vulnerable times? Here are my suggestions of things you can do to prevent becoming unfaithful:

- **Know thyself.** Infidelity is not all about sex. In fact, it is rarely about sex. It often has to do with some unmet needs other than sex, such as a need for attention, power, control, or love. These needs often arise from past relationships, including family relationships when you were growing up. Get to know yourself well; go see a therapist if you need help. Know what your needs are and understand why it is not a good idea to look for sex outside of marriage to fulfill those needs.

- **Learn to perceive and respond to each other's needs and expectations.** No, I'm not just talking about sex (most of us are pretty good at communicating about *that* need). Sit down with your wife and talk about your fears and worries—how you worry you might not be able to afford having a baby right now, how you worry your life might be slipping away, how you worry your relationship with her will be forever changed. Pay attention to her needs and expectations. Unmet needs go both ways. If you have unmet needs, she probably has unmet needs, too. Find out what her fears and worries are, too. If you can learn to perceive and respond to each other's needs and expectations, you will be less likely to cheat on each other.

- **Learn to stay out of trouble.** Don't put yourself in situations where you might be tempted. Don't go on a business trip alone with an associate to whom you feel an attraction. If you are the President, don't ask the intern to deliver the pizza to your Oval Office at midnight.

- **It's the commitment, stupid.** To paraphrase the slogan (*"It's the economy, stupid"*) that helped Bill Clinton win his first presidential election, we can talk strategies all we want but staying faithful really comes down to one thing—commitment. The strongest defense against infidelity is your commitment to each other. Take your commitment seriously; renew your commitment everyday. Remember your vows—you promised *to be true, to love and to cherish, in good times and in bad, in sickness and in health, for better or for worse, for richer or for poorer, 'til death do you part.* Teach your children to keep their promises and honor their commitments by your personal example, starting now.

To sum up your greatest contributions to making a smart and healthy baby: sperm and support. It will take you 90 days to make a new batch of good sperm, and maybe longer to learn how to give good support. So get started today.

I will leave you with some more food for thought about making a smart and healthy baby.

smart and healthy living

This book is not just about making a smart and healthy baby. Okay, baby may be the hook, but it's really about making a smart and healthy you. It's about getting you started on a smart and healthy way of life. And it's about restoring your allostasis and reducing your allostatic overload—the same allostatic overload that puts your pregnancy at risk can also put your health at risk in the long run.

A growing body of research suggests that pregnancy may reveal a woman's risk for chronic disease in later life. If you had gestational diabetes, you have a 40 percent chance of developing type 2 diabetes over the next ten years. If you had preeclampsia, you have a greater risk of suffering a heart attack in the next 10 to 20 years, compared to women who did not have preeclampsia. My own research showed that women who had a preterm birth have a greater than twofold increased risk of developing high blood pressure by age 40, compared to women whose pregnancies all went to term.

What's the connection? It's thought that gestational diabetes and type 2 diabetes, preeclampsia and heart attack, or preterm birth and hypertension may share common pre-disease pathways. The same allostatic overload that caused problems in your pregnancy can go on, over the next 10 to 20 years, to wreak havoc in your blood vessels and vital organs to cause high blood pressure, diabetes, and heart attack. It's almost as if pregnancy is a test—and if you don't pass the midterm, you are at risk for failing the final, too.

So this is not all about the baby; it's also about you. Start living smart and healthy now so you can make smart and healthy babies, and stay around long enough to watch your kids and grandkids grow up to make smart and healthy babies of their own.

no quick fix

We are a quick fix nation. We want a quick fix for everything.

Prenatal care was supposed to be a quick fix to our nation's infant mortality problem. The United States has one of the highest rates of infant mortality in the developed world, and prenatal care was supposedly our answer. We thought if we could get all women into early prenatal care, then we could really do something about preventing low birth weight and preterm births, which are two of the leading causes of infant mortality in the United States. Over the past two decades, massive public health campaigns have been undertaken to get women into early prenatal care. Yet despite dramatic improvements in access to early prenatal care, the rates of low birth weight and preterm births have continued to rise.

It is perhaps not surprising that prenatal care has not been more effective in preventing low birth weight and preterm births. To expect prenatal care, in less than nine months, to repair all the wear and tear on the body from unhealthy diet, constant stress, chronic inflammation, and environmental toxicants over the years, to undo all the damage from cumulative allostatic overload over a lifetime and restore allostasis over-night, may be expecting too much of prenatal care. It's like cramming for an exam. While cramming might help (somewhat), we've all learned from grade school on that we'd do much better if we prepare ourselves all along; and yet that simple lesson we all learned in grade school seems to have been lost to obstetrics and public health over the past several de-cades. If we want to do something about reducing infant mortality in our nation, we really need to be taking better care of girls and women all along, not just when they become pregnant.

When it comes to making a smart and healthy baby, there is no quick fix. There is no magic pill that you can take that will guarantee a smart and healthy baby. And there is no elixir that can restore your allostasis overnight. I could probably sell more books if I came up with a seven-day get-ready program that would guarantee a smart and healthy baby, but I won't. I don't want to sell you a quick fix that won't work.

For some of you restoring your allostasis will take more than seven days; it may take more than seven weeks or even seven months. If you haven't been eating healthily, it will take you some time to get rid of all the junk from your body's stores and start a nutritional savings account for your future baby. If you've been stressed out, it will take you some time to turn down the dial on your stress response and build up your stress resilience. If you are chronically inflamed, it will take you some time to put out the fire within and tune-up your immune response before you get pregnant. If you haven't paid much attention to all the potential reproductive toxicants in the air you breathe, the water you drink, and the foods you eat, it will take you some time to clean house in your body and your environments.

Making a smart and healthy baby takes a lot of preparation. Give your body enough time to repair all the wear and tear that has piled up and restore its allostasis before you get pregnant.

unless

Isn't it just crazy we've gotten to the point where we can't eat fish without worrying about mercury and PCB? Can't have dairy without worrying about pesticides and dioxins? Can't drink tap water without worrying about lead and THM? Can't drink bottled water without worrying about phthalate and BPA? Can't go outside our house without worrying about ozone, carbon monoxide, nitrogen dioxide, sulfur dioxide, and particulate matter? What have we done to our children's world? What are we doing to their developing brains and bodies?

One of my favorite bedtime stories to read to my daughters is *The Lorax* by Dr. Seuss. *The Lorax* is a story about the tree-loving Lorax and the greedy Once-ler. The story begins with the Once-ler arriving at a beautiful, sunny forest of Truffula trees where the Swomee-Swans sing, the Humming-Fish hum, and the Brown Bar-ba-loots play in the shade while eating the fruit of the Truffula Trees. Enchanted by these gorgeous trees, the Once-ler builds a small shop, where he chops down a tree and knits a Thneed. Out of the stump pops a strange little man called the Lorax, who claims to "speak for the trees, for the trees have no tongues." Someone comes along and buys a Sneed. Spurred by greed, the Once-ler invites all his relatives to town, where they start a huge Thneed-making factory, chopping down Truffula Trees left and right to make more Thneeds, much to the Lorax's distress. The Once-ler keeps chopping until the last tree is cut. The land is left gray and desolate. The Bar-ba-loots are forced to move because without the trees they do not have food. The Swomee-Swans have to fly south because of the smog. The water pollution causes all of the fish to leave. At last the Lorax drifts away from the polluted mess, leaving a pile of rocks where he stood, with one word . . . **"Unless."**

Unless we start to clean up the mess we've made. Unless we start to think twice about all the Thneeds we buy, all the Truffula trees that get chopped down, and all the natural resources we use up. Mohandas Gandhi says that "there is a sufficiency in the world for man's need but not for man's greed." I don't know who is making all the profits, but our children are paying a high price for their profits. We all want our children to be smart and healthy, and we all want them to grow up in a safe and healthy environment. But "**UNLESS** someone like you cares a whole awful lot, nothing is going to get better. It's not."

What can we do as parents to take back our nation? One way is to vote with our wallets. Reward businesses that are protecting the earth, and punish businesses that are stealing our children's future. That was what happened to Ikea. Under pressure from consumer groups in the 1990s for their lines of bookshelves that emitted high levels of formaldehyde (hyped as "Deadly Poisoned Bookshelves" by the European media) and for their wastage of paper and other natural resources, Ikea knew it had to change. It adopted a new set of corporate strategies that are ecologically responsive, including the use of environmentally friendly and safe materials in making its products. Consumers in over 30 countries now reward Ikea for its bold transformation with over $7 billion of business annually. So vote with your wallets; send businesses a clear signal about what you truly value.

Another way to take back our nation is to vote with our votes. Don't let politicians steal your vote with sound bites about family values; tell them what truly matters to you and your family. Tell them you want tougher standards and more testing of chemicals that are released into our environments. The burden of proof should be on industries that are profiting from these chemicals to show that they are safe for our children and families, and not on consumers to prove that they are toxic. Tell them you want public policies that will clean up the environment and support the use of cleaner, greener, and safer alternative energy sources. Tell them you want more research on environmental influences of children's health and development.

One such study is the National Children's Study, which will follow a cross-section of 100,000 American children from before conception to 21 years of age. Information from this study will help advance our understanding of the causes and prevention of major childhood diseases including asthma, obesity, diabetes, autism, and developmental delay, and elucidate pathways to optimizing children's health and development. This study needs your support; tell your elected representatives in Congress this is one of the best investments they can make with your tax dollars—an investment on our children's health, which is really our nation's future wealth.

It takes smart and healthy children to make a smart and healthy nation. How smart and healthy our kids' nation will be tomorrow will very much depend on how smart and healthy the choices are that their parents make today.

are you ready?

What Is Your Pregnancy Readiness Quotient (PRQ)?

For each question below, circle the number in the "yes" column if your answer is yes, and circle the number in the "no" column if your answer is no. If your answer is "not sure," "maybe yes, maybe no," "sometimes yes, sometimes no," or "not applicable," then circle the number in the "don't know" column. At the end of the self-test, add up your total score to see how ready you are for pregnancy.

	Yes	No	Don't Know
1. Are you more than 10 pounds over or under your ideal weight? (see Table 2.1 for your ideal weight)	−1	+1	0
2. Do you eat three meals and two snacks a day on most days of the week?	+1	−1	0
3. Do you snack on healthy foods (e.g., nuts, seeds, fruits, vegetables, yogurt) most of the time?	+1	−1	0
4. Do you eat fast food more than once a week?	−1	+1	0

(continued)

	Yes	No	Don't Know
5. Do you skip breakfast more than once a week?	−1	+1	0
6. Do you eat five to seven servings of whole grains a day on most days of the week?	+1	−1	0
7. Do you eat breakfast cereal made with whole grains on most days of the week?	+1	−1	0
8. Do you eat bread, tortillas, or other grain products made from refined flour more often than those made with whole grains?	−1	+1	0
9. Do you eat baked potatoes, mashed potatoes, or French fries more than once a week?	−1	+1	0
10. Do you get at least 220 mg of docosahexaenoic acid (DHA) a day?	+1	−1	0
11. Do you get more than 5 percent of your total daily calories from saturated fats?	−1	+1	0
12. Do you drink organic low-fat or non-fat milk or eat cheese made from skim milk?	+1	−1	0
13. Do you use a polyunsaturated vegetable oil (safflower, sunflower, sesame, corn, or "vegetable" oils) for cooking?	−1	+1	0
14. Do you use olive oil as your principal dietary oil?	+1	−1	0
15. Do you use margarine and vegetable shortening for cooking?	−1	+1	0
16. Do you avoid most processed foods made with partially hydrogenated oils?	+1	−1	0
17. Do you get more than 25 percent of your total daily calories from protein?	−1	+1	0
18. Do you eat shark, swordfish, king mackerel, or tilefish?	−1	+1	0

	Yes	No	Don't Know
19. Do you eat wild ocean fish (e.g., Alaskan wild salmon) at least once a week?	+1	−1	0
20. Do you eat at least five servings of fruits and vegetables a day on most days of the week?	+1	−1	0
21. Do you take a multivitamin containing at least 400 micrograms of folic acid everyday?	+1	−1	0
22. Do you eat yogurt with live active cultures at least once a day on most days of the week?	+1	−1	0
23. Do you eat any of the following at least once a week: spinach, collards, kale, or broccoli?	+1	−1	0
24. Do you eat any of the following at least once a week: prunes, raisins, or blueberries?	+1	−1	0
25. Do you eat any of the following at least once a week: oranges, red bell peppers, or tomatoes?	+1	−1	0
26. Do you know what kinds of cheese you should avoid during pregnancy?	+1	−1	0
27. Do you drink unpasteurized milk or juices?	−1	+1	0
28. Do you always wash vegetables thoroughly before serving raw, even if they come pre-washed?	+1	−1	0
29. Do you know why you should avoid eating liver just before or during pregnancy?	+1	−1	0
30. Do you order deep-fried foods (e.g., French fries, onion rings, fried chicken) in a restaurant?	−1	+1	0
31. Do you avoid eating desserts or snacks high in added sugar on most days of the week?	+1	−1	0
32. Do you use any herbal preparation in large quantities or for medicinal purposes?	−1	+1	0
33. Do you feel stressed out on most days of the week?	−1	+1	0

(continued)

	Yes	No	Don't Know
34. Are you a nervous or anxious person by nature?	−1	+1	0
35. Do you often feel that your problems are piling up so high that you cannot overcome them?	−1	+1	0
36. Do you exercise at least 30 minutes a day on most days of the week?	+1	−1	0
37. Do you include a mixture of cardiovascular exercise, core conditioning, and strength and flexibility training in your exercise routines?	+1	−1	0
38. Do you sleep at least seven to eight hours a night on most nights of the week?	+1	−1	0
39. Do you stay up past midnight at least once a week?	−1	+1	0
40. Do you have trouble falling asleep or waking up early?	−1	+1	0
41. Do you practice any relaxation techniques such as breathing exercises, progressive relaxation, mindfulness practice, or transcendental meditation on a regular basis?	+1	−1	0
42. Do you have difficulties setting limits for yourself or taking on more than you can handle?	−1	+1	0
43. Are you good at solving problems most of the time?	+1	−1	0
44. Are you good at resolving interpersonal conflicts most of the time?	+1	−1	0
45. Do you and your husband/partner communicate well with each other most of the time?	+1	−1	0
46. Are you making good use of your top strengths on most days of the week?	+1	−1	0

		Don't
	Yes	**No**	**Know**

47. Do you try to see the glass half full most of the time? +1 −1 0

48. Do you count your blessings on most days of the week? +1 −1 0

49. Do you try to practice daily acts of kindness? +1 −1 0

50. Is there someone in your life whom you can always count on when you need help? +1 −1 0

51. Has your husband/partner ever shoved, slapped, choked, hit, kicked, punched, or hurt you in any way? −1 +1 0

52. Does your husband/partner embarrass you with put-downs? −1 +1 0

53. Do you feel depressed most or all of the time? −1 +1 0

54. Do you feel bad or guilty about your drinking or feel that you should cut down on your drinking? −1 +1 0

55. Do you get infections (e.g., colds, bladder, or yeast infections) often? −1 +1 0

56. Do you floss every day? +1 −1 0

57. Have you received a dental check-up or cleaning in the past 12 months? +1 −1 0

58. Have you smoked cigarettes in the past three months? −1 +1 0

59. Have you douched in the past three months? −1 +1 0

60. Do you know how to avoid toxoplasmosis? +1 −1 0

61. Do you know how to avoid cytomegalovirus (CMV) infection? +1 −1 0

62. Do you know how to avoid foodborne illnesses? +1 −1 0

(continued)

	Yes	No	Don't Know
63. Does your house have any of these problems: molds, mildew, dust mites, or cockroaches?	−1	+1	0
64. Have you been immunized against or are you immune to chickenpox, rubella, hepatitis B, tetanus and pertussis?	+1	−1	0
65. Is your home completely free of lead?	+1	−1	0
66. Do you drink bottled water made with #3 (polyvinyl chloride), #6 (polystyrene), or #7 (polycarbonate) plastics?	−1	+1	0
67. Are you exposed to secondhand smoking?	−1	+1	0
68. Do you use non-chemical dry-cleaning?	+1	−1	0
69. Do you air out your dry-cleaning first before hanging it up in your closet?	+1	−1	0
70. Do you change the air filters in your home every three months, and have the furnace, flue, or chimney inspected once a year?	+1	−1	0
71. Is your home free of radon and asbestos?	+1	−1	0
72. Do you ever use pesticides (e.g., bug spray) in your home or yard/garden?	−1	+1	0
73. Do you have any furniture made of pressed wood bonded with urea-formaldehyde resins?	−1	+1	0
74. Do you have mattress or furniture made with materials containing polybrominated diphenyl ethers (PBDE)?	−1	+1	0
75. Do you have vinyl wallpaper or mini-blinds containing phthalates?	−1	+1	0
76. Do you use any antibacterial soap containing the pesticides triclocarban and triclosan?	−1	+1	0
77. Do you use any cosmetics or other personal care products containing phthalates,			

	Yes	No	Don't Know
formaldehyde, glycol ethers, and petroleum?	−1	+1	0
78. Do you use any air freshener containing benzene, phthalates, and other organic volatile compounds?	−1	+1	0
79. Do you use any bathroom or kitchen cleaning products containing chlorine, solvents, alkylphenols, or pesticides?	−1	+1	0
80. Do you use non-stick pans containing perfluorinated chemicals?	−1	+1	0
81. Do you defrost meat in its Styrofoam tray or reheat left-overs in the take-out container in the microwave?	−1	+1	0
82. Do you microwave foods in plastic wrap and containers that are not labeled "microwave safe"?	−1	+1	0
83. Do you ever use fabric softeners or washing detergents containing phthalates?	−1	+1	0
84. Do you have any hobbies that may expose you to solvents or other reproductive toxicants?	−1	+1	0
85. Are you planning to remodel your home in the next year?	−1	+1	0
86. Do you live near a hazardous waste site, gas station, auto repair shop, farm, or major freeways or intersections?	−1	+1	0
87. Do you live in a noisy neighborhood?	−1	+1	0
88. Do you get gas only at pumps with the vapor-lock system?	+1	−1	0
89. Have you seen the Material Safety Data Sheets (MSDSs) or know what chemicals you are exposed to at work?	+1	−1	0

(continued)

		Yes	No	Don't Know
90.	Do you know your rights under the Occupational Safety and Health Act?	+1	−1	0
91.	Do you feel overloaded at work?	−1	+1	0
92.	Do you know what your health insurance coverage, co-pays, and deductibles are for pregnancy?	+1	−1	0
93.	Do you know when you want to get pregnant?	+1	−1	0
94.	Have you seen a doctor or healthcare provider for a prepregnancy check-up?	+1	−1	0
95.	Are you taking any FDA category D or X medications?	−1	+1	0
96.	Do you know what genetic screening you need before or during pregnancy?	+1	−1	0
97.	Have you had a clinical breast exam, a Pap test, and a total skin exam in the past three years?	+1	−1	0
98.	Have you ever had your thyroid functions (including a TSH) checked?	+1	−1	0
99.	Do you have any medical condition that is not well-controlled?	−1	+1	0
100.	Do you plan to breastfeed your babies in the future?	+1	−1	0

How Ready Are You?

If your total score is:

80 to 100 = Ready

50 to 79 = Almost ready; need some fine-tuning

0 to 49 = Almost half way there; keep working at it

Any negative score = Not ready; it's time to get started

Notes

chapter 1: get ready

16 **Fetal programming refers to the process** Barker DJP. Mothers, babies and health in later life. Edinburgh: Churchill Livingstone. 1998. Also see Nathanielsz PW. Life in the womb: The origin of health and disease. Ithaca NY: Promethean Press. 1999.

17 **Maternal nutrition linked to childhood obesity** Symonds ME, Stephenson T, Gardner DS, Budge H. Long-term effects of nutritional programming of the embryo and fetus: mechanisms and critical windows. Reprod Fertil Dev. 2007;19(1):53–63.

17 **Animal studies have shown that fetal over-exposure to cortisol** Seckl JR, Meaney MJ. Glucocorticoid programming. Ann N Y Acad Sci. 2004 Dec;1032:63–84. Also see Welberg LA, Seckl JR. Prenatal stress, glucocorticoids and the programming of the brain. J Neuroendocrinol. 2001 Feb;13(2):113–28.

17 **A growing body of research in humans now links maternal anxiety or stress during pregnancy to neurological disorders in children** Van den Bergh BR, Mulder EJ, Mennes M, Glover V. Antenatal maternal anxiety and stress and the neurobehavioural development of the fetus and child: links and possible mechanisms. A review. Neurosci Biobehav Rev. 2005 Apr;29(2):237–58. Also see Talge NM, Neal C, Glover V. Early Stress, Translational Research and Prevention Science Network: Fetal and Neonatal Experience on Child and Adolescent Mental Health. Antenatal maternal stress and long-term effects on child neurodevelopment: how and why? J Child Psychol Psychiatry. 2007 Mar-Apr;48(3–4):245–61.

18 **One recent study showed that if you get the flu** Brown AS. Prenatal infection as a risk factor for schizophrenia. Schizophr Bull. 2006 Apr;32(2):200–2.

18   **Maternal flu linked to autism and schizophrenia in child** Meyer U, Yee
        BK, Feldon J. The neurodevelopmental impact of prenatal infections at
        different times of pregnancy: the earlier the worse? Neuroscientist. 2007
        Jun;13(3): 241–56.

19   **Fetal programming probably works by turning on or off genes** Sinclair
        SK, Lea RG, Rees WD, Young LE. The developmental origins of health
        and disease: current theories and epigenetic mechanisms. Soc Reprod
        Fertil Suppl. 2007;64:425–43. Meaney MJ, Szyf M, Seckl JR. Epigenetic
        mechanisms of perinatal programming of hypothalamic-pituitary-adrenal
        function and health. Trends Mol Med. 2007 Jul;13(7):269–77.

19   **In a classic study, researchers were able to turn off a gene that can cause
        obesity in rat pups** Dolinoy DC, Wiedman J, Waterland R, Jirtle RL. Ma-
        ternal genistein alters coat color and protects Avy mouse offspring from
        obesity by modifying the fetal epigenome. Environ Health Perspect
        2006;114:567–572. Also see Dolinoy DC, Das R, Weidman JR, Jirtle RL.
        Metastable epialleles, imprinting, and the fetal origins of adult diseases.
        Pediatr Res. 2007 May;61(5 Pt 2):30R–37R.

21   **The placenta plays a critical role in fetal programming** Myatt L. Placen-
        tal adaptive responses and fetal programming. J Physiol. 2006 Apr 1;572(Pt
        1):25–30.

22   **an increasing number of environmental pollutants (e.g., phthalates,
        acrylamide, pesticides and dioxins) can cause sperm DNA damage** Ait-
        ken RJ, Koopman P, Lewis SE. Seeds of concern. Nature. 2004 Nov
        4;432(7013):48–52.

24   **There are many more dangers** Schettler T, Solomon G, Valenti M, Hud-
        dle A. Generations at risk: Reproductive health and the environment.
        Cambridge, MA: MIT Press. 2000.

25   **One of the most consistent pathological findings of preeclampsia is poor,
        shallow implantation** Burton GJ, Jauniaux E. Placental oxidative stress: from
        miscarriage to preeclampsia. J Soc Gynecol Investig. 2004 Sep;11(6):342–52.

25–26   **Allostasis describes the body's ability to maintain balance through
        change** McEwen B, Lasley EN. The end of stress as we know it. Washing-
        ton DC: John Henry Press. 2002.

chapter 2: nutritional preparedness

30   **Your body becomes somewhat insensitive or resistant to the actions of
        insulin** Salmeron J, Manson JE, Stampfer MJ, Colditz GA, Wing AL, Willett
        WC. Dietary fiber, glycemic load, and risk of non-insulin-dependent diabetes
        mellitus in women. JAMA. 1997 Feb 12;277(6):472–7. Also see Zhang C, Liu
        S, Solomon CG, Hu FB. Dietary fiber intake, dietary glycemic load, and the
        risk for gestational diabetes mellitus. Diabetes Care. 2006 Oct;29(10):2223–30,
        which found a prepregnancy diet with low fiber and high glycemic load was
        associated with an increased risk for gestational diabetes.

31   **Studies have shown that women who are underweight before pregnancy are at greater risk for having a low birth weight baby** Institute of Medicine. Nutrition during pregnancy. Washington DC: National Academies Press. 1990.

31   **Similarly, short birth spacing is associated with greater risk for low birth weight** King JC. The risk of maternal nutritional depletion and poor outcomes increases in early or closely spaced pregnancies. J Nutr. 2003 May;133(5 Suppl 2):1732S–1736S.

32   **Remember, dioxins are stored in your body fat, and the half-life of some dioxins can be as long as seven years** Institute of Medicine. Dioxins and Dioxin-like Compounds in the Food Supply: Strategies to Decrease Exposure. Washington DC: National Academies Press. 2003.

33   **abdominal fat stores, together with fats and carbs, actually send a signal to the brain to blunt our stress response** Dallman MF, Pecoraro N, Akana SF, La Fleur SE, Gomez F, Houshyar H, et al. Chronic stress and obesity: a new view of "comfort food." Proc Natl Acad Sci U S A. 2003 Sep 30;100(20):11696–701.

33   **folate supplementation that begins more than 4 weeks after conception has shown no benefit** Lumley J, Watson L, Watson M, Bower C. Periconceptional supplementation with folate and/or multivitamins for preventing neural tube defects. Cochrane Database Syst Rev. 2001;(3):CD001056.

34   **log onto the website for the National Heart, Lung, and Blood Institute** http://nhlbisupport.com/bmi/bmi-m.htm. Last accessed September 25, 2008.

36   **Sample menus with reduced calories (1,200 to 1,600 calories) can be found on the National Heart, Lung, and Blood Institute website** http://www.nhlbi.nih.gov/health/public/heart/obesity/lose_wt/sampmenu.htm. Last accessed September 25, 2008.

38   **Regular supplements such as Ensure, Instant Breakfast, Sweet Success, Boost, Sustacal, ReSource, Deliver 2.0, and TwoCal HN** Luke B, Eberlein T. Program your baby's health: The pregnancy diet for your child's lifelong well-being. New York: Ballantine Books. 2001.

41   **Skipping meals when you are pregnant causes a placental stress hormone called corticotropin-releasing hormone** Herrmann TS, Siega-Riz AM, Hobel CJ, Aurora C, Dunkel-Schetter C. Prolonged periods without food intake during pregnancy increase risk for elevated maternal corticotropin-releasing hormone concentrations. Am J Obstet Gynecol. 2001 Aug;185(2):403–12.

43   **You can also find the caloric content of most common foods by going to the USDA National Nutrient Database website** Log on to http://www.ars.usda.gov/Ser<#U00AD>vices/docs.htm?docid=9673. Click on the buttons next to Energy (Calories) to sort the list of foods alphabetically or by caloric content. You can also use the USDA's search tool *What's in the Foods You Eat:* http://199.133.10.140/codesearchwebapp/(x4ixysjpgaw0fe45x2w3vd55)/codesearch.aspx, to look up the caloric and nutritional content of a particular food. Last accessed September 25, 2008.

46   **In excess of 25 percent of total calories, high protein intake has been**

shown to be associated with increased risk of very early premature
births and neonatal deaths Rush D, Stein Z, Susser M. A randomized
controlled trial of prenatal nutritional supplementation in New York City.
Pediatrics 1980;65:683–97.

47   During critical periods of fetal development, all this excess insulin can
do three things to the baby Huang JS, Lee TA, Lu MC. Prenatal programming of childhood overweight and obesity. Matern Child Health J. 2007
Sep;11(5):461–73.

48   There are a number of factors that influence how quickly carbohydrates in
food raise your blood sugar, including Source: http://www.hsph.harvard.
edu/nutritionsource/carbohydrates.html. Last accessed September 25, 2008.

49   you can also just follow these few simple guidelines to choosing carbohydrates Adapted from http://www.hsph.harvard.edu/nutritionsource/
carbohydrates.html. Last accessed September 25, 2008.

51   In one study, researchers randomly assigned pregnant women to receive
a daily supplement consisting of 10cc of cod liver oil Helland IB. Maternal supplementation with very long chain n–3 fatty acids during pregnancy and lactation augments children's IQ at 4 years of age. Pediatrics
2003;111:e39-e44.

51   Omega–3 fatty acids are anti-inflammatory McGregor JA, Allen KG,
Harris MA, Reece M, Wheeler M, French JI, Morrison J. The omega–3
story: nutritional prevention of preterm birth and other adverse pregnancy
outcomes. Obstet Gynecol Surv. 2001 May;56(5 Suppl 1):S1–13.

51   In a large European study, maternal supplementation with fish oil beginning at 20 weeks' gestation Olsen SF, Secher NJ, Tabor A, Weber T,
Walker JJ, Gluud C. Randomised clinical trials of fish oil supplementation
in high risk pregnancies. Fish Oil Trials In Pregnancy (FOTIP) Team.
BJOG. 2000 Mar;107(3):382–95.

52   Another study found that maternal cod liver oil supplementation during
pregnancy was associated with reduced risks of childhood diabetes
Stene LC, Ulriksen J, Magnus P, Joner G. Use of cod liver oil during pregnancy associated with lower risk of Type I diabetes in the offspring. Diabe-
tologia. 2000 Sep;43(9):1093–8.

52   You can get DHA and EPA two ways Weil A. Eating well for optimum
health. New York: Quill. 2001:73–102.

53   You should consume 220mg of DHA a day before pregnancy, and
300mg of DHA per day during pregnancy. Institute of Medicine. Dietary Reference Intakes for Energy, Carbohydrate, Fiber, Fat, Fatty Acids,
Cholesterol, Protein, and Amino Acids (Macronutrients). Washington DC:
National Academies Press. 2005.

54   One 4-oz fillet of steamed or poached wild Alaskan salmon contains
830mg of DHA and 136mg of EPA Source: http://199.133.10.140/
codesearchwebapp/(x4ixysjpgaw0fe45x2w3vd55)/codesearch.aspx. Last accessed September 25, 2008.

54   you can go to the website for Environmental Defense Fund at www.edf

.org to see which brands are purifying their fish oil See http://www.edf.org/ page.cfm?tagID=16536. Last accessed September 25, 2008.

55   **Saturated fats come mostly from animal fats found in red meat** See Weil A. Eating well for optimum health. New York: Quill 2001:82–102 for a review of saturated fatty acids, trans-fats, and partially hydrogenated oils.

55   **LDL cholesterol can cross the placenta and get deposited in fetal blood vessels as fatty streaks** Napoli C, Glass CK, Witztum JL, Deutsch R, D'Armiento FP, Palinski W. Influence of maternal hypercholesterolaemia during pregnancy on progression of early atherosclerotic lesions in childhood: Fate of Early Lesions in Children (FELIC) study. Lancet 1999;354:1234–41.

55   **LDL cholesterol oxidation can cause inflammation in the placenta and in fetal blood vessels and organs** Bonet B, Hauge-Gillenwater H, Zhu XD, Knopp RH. LDL oxidation and human placental trophoblast and macrophage cytotoxicity. Proc Soc Exp Biol Med 1998;217:203–11.

58   **Protein comes from two sources—animals and plants** See Weil A. Eating well for optimum health. New York: Quill 2001:102–124 for a review of animal and plant proteins.

59   **In 2003, a panel of scientists convened by the Institute of Medicine concluded that the only practical way to reduce dioxins exposure in fetuses** Institute of Medicine. Dioxins and Dioxin-like Compounds in the Food Supply: Strategies to Decrease Exposure. Washington DC: National Academies Press. 2003.

60   **Box 2.2: What You Need to Know about Mercury in Fish and Shellfish** Source: 2004 Environmental Protection Agency/Food and Drug Administration Fish Advisory http://www.epa.gov/waterscience/fishadvice/advice .html#notp. Last accessed September 25, 2008.

63   **Pay attention to quality because the quality of plant proteins varies** American Dietetic Association; Dietitians of Canada. Position of the American Dietetic Association and Dietitians of Canada: Vegetarian diets. J Am Diet Assoc. 2003 Jun;103(6):748–65.

67   **The Environmental Working Group (EWG) has come up with the "dirty dozen" of fruits and vegetables with the highest pesticide load** Go to: http://www.foodnews.org/walletguide.php for a complete list. Last accessed September 25, 2008.

68   **In four studies involving over 6,000 women who were randomized to receive folic acid supplements versus a placebo** Lumley J, Watson L, Watson M, Bower C. Periconceptional supplementation with folate and/or multivitamins for preventing neural tube defects. Cochrane Database Syst Rev. 2001;(3):CD001056.

69   **One recent study found that women who took a multivitamin *before* pregnancy were half as likely to deliver preterm as women who did not** Vahratian A, Siega-Riz AM, Savitz DA, Thorp JM Jr. Multivitamin use and the risk of preterm birth. Am J Epidemiol. 2004 Nov 1;160(9):886–92.

70   **Table 2.2 Recommended daily intake of micronutrients before & during pregnancy.** Institute of Medicine. Dietary Reference Intakes for Vitamin

A, Vitamin K, Arsenic, Boron, Chromium, Copper, Iodine, Iron, Manganese, Molybdenum, Nickel, Silicon, Vanadium, and Zinc (2000). Dietary Reference Intakes for Vitamin C, Vitamin E, Selenium, and Carotenoids (2000). Dietary Reference Intakes for Calcium, Phosphorus, Magnesium, Vitamin D, and Fluoride (1997). Dietary Reference Intakes for Thiamin, Riboflavin, Niacin, Vitamin B6, Folate, Vitamin B12, Pantothenic Acid, Biotin, and Choline (1998). Washington DC: National Academies Press.

71 **Large doses of vitamin A (in excess of 10,000 IU) and vitamin D (in excess of 4,000 IU) can cause birth defects** Rothman KJ, Moore LL, Singer MR, Nguyen US, Mannino S, Milunsky A. Teratogenicity of high vitamin A intake. N Engl J Med. 1995 Nov 23;333(21):1369–73.

72 **You can go to the March of Dimes website at www.marchofdimes.org or the Harvard School of Public Health website at www.hsph.harvard.edu** http://www.marchofdimes.com/pnhec/173_15354.asp or http://www.hsph.harvard.edu/nutritionsource/vitamins.html. Last accessed September 25, 2008.

72 *Superfoods Rx* **by ophthalmologist Dr. Steven Pratt and his co-writer Kathy Matthews, and the** *Perricone Promise* **by dermatologist Dr. Nicholas Perricone** Pratt S, Matthews K. Superfoods Rx. New York: HarperCollins 2004, and Perricone N. The Perricone Promise. New York: Warner Books. 2004.

chapter 3: brain foods and toxic foods

75 **In this chapter I will feature ten brain foods** Also see Weil A. Eating well for optimum health. New York: Quill 2001:73–102; Perricone N. The Perricone Promise. New York: Warner Books. 2004; Willett WC. Eat, drink and be healthy. New York: Simon and Schuster 2001; and Luke B, Eberlein T. Program your baby's health: The pregnancy diet for your child's lifelong well-being. New York: Ballantine Books. 2001.

78 **Soy isoflavones can potentially cause fetal goiter in women who are iodine deficient . . . genistein, which can act like an endocrine disruptor** Doerge DR, Sheehan DM. Goitrogenic and estrogenic activity of soy isoflavones. Environ Health Perspect 2002;110:349–53.

79 **Eggs have gotten a bum rap** Greene CM, Waters D, Clark RM, Contois JH, Fernandez ML. Plasma LDL and HDL characteristics and carotenoid content are positively influenced by egg consumption in an elderly population. Nutr Metab (Lond). 2006 Jan 6;3:6.

80 **You can find more information about food safety for eggs** at www.cfsan.fda.gov/~dms/fs-eggs.html. Last accessed September 25, 2008.

82 **There is growing concern that if a woman consumes peanuts (or peanut butter) during pregnancy** Frank L, Marian A, Visser M, Weinberg E, Potter PC. Exposure to peanuts in utero and in infancy and the development of sensitization to peanut allergens in young children. Pediatr Allergy Immunol. 1999;10:27–32.

83 **Several intriguing animal studies have shown that feeding the mother a**

diet high in olive oil Stark AH, Kossoy G, Zusman I, Yarden G, Madar Z. Olive oil consumption during pregnancy and lactation in rats influences mammary cancer development in female offspring. Nutr Cancer. 2003;46(1):59–65 and Kossoy G, Madar Z, Ben-Hur H, Gal R, Stark A, Cohen O, Zusman I. Transplacental effect of a 15 percent olive-oil diet on functional activity of immune components in the spleen and colon tumors of rat offspring. Oncol Rep. 2001 Sep-Oct;8(5):1045–9.

85   **Wild salmon is a lot healthier than farm-raised salmon** Shaw SD, Brenner D, Berger ML, Carpenter DO, Hong CS, Kannan K. PCBs, PCDD/Fs, and organochlorine pesticides in farmed Atlantic salmon from Maine, eastern Canada, and Norway, and wild salmon from Alaska. Environ Sci Technol. 2006 Sep 1;40(17):5347–54. Erratum in: Environ Sci Technol. 2007 Jun 1;41(11):4180.

85–86   **A 2001 *Lancet* article showed that this strain could be used safely in pregnant women and reduced in half the episodes of atopic dermatitis in their babies** Kalliomäki M, Salminen S, Arvilommi H, Kero P, Koskinen P, Isolauri E. Probiotics in primary prevention of atopic disease: a randomised placebo-controlled trial. Lancet. 2001 Apr 7;357(9262):1076–9.

86   **many brands of yogurt and kefir, as well as so-called probiotic preparations that are commercially available, have dead or unreliable contents** Reid G, Bocking A. The potential for probiotics to prevent bacterial vaginosis and preterm labor. Am J Obstet Gynecol. 2003 Oct;189(4):1202–8.

87   **Some examples of whole grain and refined grain products are** Source: http://www.mypyramid.gov/pyramid/grains.html#. Last accessed September 25, 2008.

90   **Here are some recommendations on how to increase your daily intake of barley** Source: www.healthcastle.com/index.shtml. Last accessed September 25, 2008.

90   **The 2005 Dietary Guidelines for Americans, issued by the Department of Health and Human Services and the USDA** www.health.gov/dietaryguidelines/. Last accessed September 25, 2008.

96   **Here is my top-ten list of "toxic foods" you should try to avoid, before and during pregnancy** Go to the March of Dimes website at http://www.marchofdimes.com/pnhec/159_826.asp or the FDA website at http://www.cfsan.fda.gov/~pregnant/pregnant.html for more information on foods to avoid before and during pregnancy. Last accessed September 25, 2008.

103   **Table 3.2. Nutritional Contents of Whole-Wheat vs. Refined Wheat Flour** Source: Nutrition Today, 2001; 36:115

104   **One recent animal study tested the effects of five plant essential oils (sage, oregano, thyme, clove, and cinnamon) on growth and development of mouse embryo** Domaracky M, Rehak P, Juhas S, Koppel J. Effects of selected plant essential oils on the growth and development of mouse preimplantation embryos in vivo. Physiol Res. 2007;56(1):97–104.

104   **serious concerns have been raised regarding poor quality control in the production of many herbal preparations** Marcus DM, Snodgrass WR. Do

no harm: avoidance of herbal medicines during pregnancy. Obstet Gynecol. 2005 May;105(5 Pt 1):1119–22.

chapter 4: stress resilience

106   **Stress has been linked to a whole host of pregnancy complications includ-
           ing miscarriages, birth defects, preeclampsia, low birth weight, and pre-
           term birth** Mulder EJ, Robles de Medina PG, Huizink AC, Van den Bergh
           BR, Buitelaar JK, Visser GH. Prenatal maternal stress: effects on pregnancy
           and the (unborn) child. Early Hum Dev. 2002 Dec;70(1–2):3–14.

107   **Thus stress can cause preterm birth via several different pathways—
           hormonal, infectious/inflammatory, vascular, and behavioral** Wadhwa
           PD, Culhane JF, Rauh V, Barve SS. Stress and preterm birth: neuroendo-
           crine, immune/inflammatory, and vascular mechanisms. Matern Child
           Health J. 2001 Jun;5(2):119–25.

107   **At least 14 studies have now linked maternal anxiety and stress during
           pregnancy to cognitive, behavioral, and emotional problems in children,
           including ADHD** Van den Bergh BR, Mulder EJ, Mennes M, Glover V.
           Antenatal maternal anxiety and stress and the neurobehavioural develop-
           ment of the fetus and child: links and possible mechanisms. A review.
           Neurosci Biobehav Rev. 2005 Apr;29(2):237–58.

107–8   **One study found that these children performed poorly on developmen-
           tal testing** Huizink AC, Robles de Medina PG, Mulder EJH, Visser GHA,
           Buitelaar JK, Stress during pregnancy is associated with developmental
           outcome in infancy, J Child Psychol Psychiatry 2003;44:1025–36.

108   **Another study found that these children showed more attention deficits**
           Van den Bergh RH, Marcoen A. High antenatal maternal anxiety is related
           to ADHD symptoms, externalizing problems and anxiety in 8/9-year-olds,
           Child Dev 2004;75:1085–97.

108   **Maternal stress can turn on the baby's "stress genes" inside the brain**
           See Welberg LA, Seckl JR, Holmes MC. Prenatal glucocorticoid program-
           ming of brain corticosteroid receptors and corticotrophin-releasing hor-
           mone: possible implications for behaviour. Neuroscience. 2001;104(1):71–9;
           and Weinstock M. The potential influence of maternal stress hormones on
           development and mental health of the offspring. Brain Behav Immun.
           2005 Jul;19(4):296–308 for scientific reviews of the mechanisms of gluco-
           corticoid programming of the fetal brain.

109   **Box 4.2: Turning On the Baby's Stress Gene** Meaney MJ, Szyf M, Seckl JR.
           Epigenetic mechanisms of perinatal programming of hypothalamic-pituitary-
           adrenal function and health. Trends Mol Med. 2007 Jul;13(7):269–77.

110   **"allostasis," which refers to the body's ability to maintain balance through
           change** Figures 4.1 & 4.2. Adapted from McEwen BS. Protective and damag-
           ing effects of stress mediators. N Engl J Med. 1998 Jan 15;338(3):171–9.

110   **Peter Nathanielsz, now at the University of Texas in San Antonio, uses**

an apt analogy of a thermostat Nathanielsz P. The prenatal prescription. New York: HarperCollins Publishers. 2001:91–92.

111 **This is when protection gives way to damage** McEwen BS. Stressed or stressed out: what is the difference? J Psychiatry Neurosci. 2005 Sep;30(5):3-15–8.

112 **Box 4.3: How Does Chronic Stress Cause Inflammation in Your Body?** Elenkov IJ, Chrousos GP. Stress hormones, proinflammatory and antiinflammatory cytokines, and autoimmunity. Ann N Y Acad Sci. 2002 Jun;966:2-90–303. Also see Chikanza IC, Grossman AB. Reciprocal interactions between the neuroendocrine and immune systems during inflammation. Rheum Dis Clin North Am. 2000 Nov;26(4):693–711.

114 *Merriam-Webster's Medical Dictionary* **defines resilience as** Merriam-Webster's Medical Dictionary, at Dictionary.com website: http://dictionary.reference.com/browse/resilience

115 **Furthermore, exercise appears to reduce your vulnerability to stress** Tsatsoulis A, Fountoulakis S. The protective role of exercise on stress system dysregulation and comorbidities. Ann N Y Acad Sci. 2006 Nov;1083:196–213.

115 **as demonstrated by improved insulin sensitivity and actions among individuals with diabetes who exercise regularly** Ostergard T, Jessen N, Schmitz O, Mandarino LJ. The effect of exercise, training, and inactivity on insulin sensitivity in diabetics and their relatives: what is new? Appl Physiol Nutr Metab. 2007 Jun;32(3):541–8.

116 **The National Institutes of Health and the 2005 Dietary Guidelines for Americans recommend that all adults set a long-term goal to exercise at least 30 minutes a day** National Institutes of Health. Physical Activity and Cardiovascular Health. NIH Consens Statement 1995 December 18–20;13(3):1–33. U.S. Department of Health and Human Services, U.S. Department of Agriculture (2005). Dietary Guidelines for Americans, 2005, 6th ed. Washington, DC: U.S. Government Printing Office. Also available online: http://www.healthierus.gov/dietaryguidelines/. Last accessed September 25, 2008.

116 **There are a number of websites** (e.g., the American Academy of Sleep Medicine, the Food and Drug Administration), Source: www.sleepeducation.com and www.sleepcenters.org, http://www.fda.gov/fdac/features/1998/498_sleep.html. Last accessed September 25, 2008.

118 **There is some evidence from animal studies that abdominal fat stores** Dallman MF, Pecoraro N, Akana SF, La Fleur SE, Gomez F, Houshyar H, et al. Chronic stress and obesity: a new view of "comfort food." Proc Natl Acad Sci U S A. 2003 Sep 30;100(20):11696–701.

119 **Here are some techniques that many of my patients have found helpful** You can learn these and other relaxation techniques at the Canadian Mental Health Association website: http://www.cmha.ca/english/coping_with_stress/physical_skills.htm. Last accessed September 25, 2008.

119 **In** *transcendental meditation* **(TM), the person sits with closed eyes**

You can get more information about TM from a number of useful websites including http://www.tm.org/maharishi/index.html. Last accessed September 25, 2008.

120   **A growing body of evidence suggests that TM may reduce risks for cardiovascular diseases** Walton KG, Schneider RH, Nidich S. Review of controlled research on the transcendental meditation program and cardiovascular disease. Risk factors, morbidity, and mortality. Cardiol Rev. 2004 Sep-Oct;12(5):262–6.

120   **There is even some preliminary evidence that TM may help remodel your brain** Lazar SW, Kerr CE, Wasserman RH, Gray JR, Greve DN, Treadway MT, et al. Meditation experience is associated with increased cortical thickness. Neuroreport. 2005 Nov 28;16(17):1893–7.

·120   **A special form of meditation is mindfulness meditation, popularized in the healthcare setting by Jon Kabat-Zinn** You can learn more about the mindfulness-based stress reduction (MBSR) program at http://www.umassmed.edu/content.aspx?id=41252. Last accessed September 25, 2008.

121   **Studies have shown the efficacy of mindfulness-based stress reduction (MBSR)** Carlson LE, Speca M, Patel KD, Goodey E. Mindfulness-based stress reduction in relation to quality of life, mood, symptoms of stress and levels of cortisol, dehydroepiandrosterone sulfate (DHEAS) and melatonin in breast and prostate cancer outpatients. Psychoneuroendocrinology. 2004 May;29(4):448–74.

128   **Peter Salovey at Yale and John Mayer at the University of New Hampshire were the first to use the term "emotional intelligence"** Salovey P, Mayer JD. "Emotional intelligence." Imagination, Cognition, and Personality, 1990;9:185–211.

128   **Daniel Goleman popularized the idea in his 1995 best-seller, *Emotional Intelligence*** Goleman D. Emotional Intelligence: why it can matter more than IQ. London: Bloomsbury. 1995.

128   **There are many self-help books and programs on how to improve your emotional intelligence** Bradberry T, Greaves J. The Emotional Intelligence Quick Book. New York: Fireside. 2005.

129   **There are a number of useful books and websites that can help you work on improving your communication skills** See Quilliam S. Relate: Stop arguing, start talking: The 10 point plan for couples in conflict. Vermilion (RAND). 2001. Also see the BBC's website on relationship at www.bbc.co.uk/relationships/. Last accessed September 25, 2008.

129   **I've long been a big fan of two books by these titles** Fisher R, Ury W, Getting to Yes: Negotiating Agreement Without Giving In. New York: Penguin Books, 1983; and Ury W. Getting Past No: Negotiating With Difficult People. New York: Bantam Books, 1991.

131   **Here are some recommendations from several noted psychologists** See Wallis C. The new science of happiness. TIME magazine. January 17, 2005. Also see Lyubomirsky S. Why are some people happier than others? The role of cognitive and motivational processes in well-being. American

Psychologist 2001;56:239–249 and Lyubomirsky S, Sheldon KM, Schkade D. Pursuing happiness: The architecture of sustainable change. Review of General Psychology 2005;9:111–131.

133   **You can learn more about how to develop positive mental health from Dr. Seligman's book** Seligman MEP. Learned Optimism: How to Change Your Mind and Your Life. New York: Vintage Books. 2006; or at his website on reflective happiness http://www.reflectivehappiness.com/Happiness/ . Last accessed September 25, 2008.

133   **I'd also recommend reading the Dalai Lama's book *The Art of Happiness.*** HH Dalai Lama, Cutler HC. The art of happiness: Handbook for living. New York: Riverhead Books. 1998.

136   **Social capital has been linked to maternal and infant health** Putnam RD, Leonardi R, Nanetti RY. Making Democracy Work: Civic Traditions in Modern Italy. Princeton, NJ: Princeton University Press. 1993; Also see Kawachi I, Kennedy BP, Lochner K, Prothrow-Stith D. Social capital, income inequality, and mortality. Am J Public Health 1997;87:1491–8.

136   **Spirituality has been found to be helpful in the prevention of physical and mental illness, and in coping with or recovery from illness** Anandarajah G, Hight E. Spirituality and medical practice: using the HOPE questions as a practical tool for spiritual assessment. Am Fam Physician. 2001 Jan 1;63(1):81–9; Also see American Family Physician patient education website: http://familydoctor.org/650.xml. Last accessed September 25, 2008.

137   **Some 4 to 8 percent of pregnant women are beaten up by their intimate partners *during* pregnancy** Gazmararian JA, Lazorick S, Spitz AM, et al. Prevalence of violence against pregnant women. JAMA 1996; 275(24): 1915–1920. See also: Lu MC, Lu JS. Domestic violence and sexual assault. In: DeCherney AH, Nathan L (eds). Current Obstetric and Gynecologic Diagnosis and Treatment. 9th ed. New York: Lange Medical Books/McGraw-Hill. 2003.

138   **If you answered yes to even one of these questions, call the National Domestic Violence Hotline** You can get more information from their website at http://www.ndvh.org/help/index.html. Last accessed September 25, 2008.

138   **Box 4.7: Diagnostic Criteria for Major Depression** Source: American Psychiatric Association 2000. *(DSM-IV-TR) Diagnostic and statistical manual of mental disorders*, 4th edition, text revision. Washington DC: American Psychiatric Press, Inc. 2000.

139   **Approximately one in eight pregnant women in the United States reported drinking alcohol during pregnancy, and nearly 3 percent reported binge drinking** Centers for Disease Control and Prevention. Alcohol use among women of childbearing age—United States, 1991–1999. MMWR Morb Mortal Wkly Rep. 2002;51:273–6.

140   **Stephen Covey, author of *First Things First*, talks about how we are so preoccupied in our daily** Covey SR, Merrill AR, Merrill RR. First Things First. New York: Simon & Schuster. 1994.

chapter 5: immune tune-up

141   **Infection is also a leading cause of preterm birth** Institute of Medicine.
        Preterm birth: Causes, consequences, and prevention. Washington DC:
        National Academies Press. 2007.

142   **Inflammation is the immune system's first line of defense against an in-
        fection** See Gorman C, Park A. The Fire Within. TIME Magazine cover
        story. February 23, 2004. for a review of the mechanisms of inflammation.
        http://www.time.com/time/magazine/article/0,9171,993419,00.html.

143   **Several studies have found that babies born to mothers who had chorio-
        amnionitis** Wu YW et al. Chorioamnionitis as a risk factor for cerebral
        palsy: A meta-analysis. JAMA. 2000;284:1417–24.

144   **One recent study showed that if you had the flu in the first half of preg-
        nancy** Brown AS. Prenatal infection as a risk factor for schizophrenia.
        Schizophr Bull. 2006 Apr;32(2):200–2.

144   **inflammation is thought to play a key role in the fetal origin of schizo-
        phrenia** Buka SL. Maternal cytokine levels during pregnancy and adult
        psychosis. Brain, Behavior, and Immunity. 2001;15:411–20.

144   **Box 5.1: Does Asthma Begin in the Womb?** Wjist M. Is the increase in
        allergic asthma associated with an inborn Th–1 maturation or with an
        environmental Th 1 trigger defect? *Allergy* 2004: 59: 148–50; Warner JA,
        Jones AC, Miles EA, Cowlell BM, Warner JO. Prenatal origins of asthma
        and allergy. Ciba Found Symp 1997: 206: 220–8; and Salvatore S, Keymo-
        len K, Hauser B, Vandenplas Y. Intervention during pregnancy and allergic
        disease in the offspring. Pediatr Allergy Immunol. 2005 Nov;16(7):558–66.

145   **children whose mothers smoked during pregnancy are more likely to
        develop allergies and asthma** Pattenden S, Antova T, Neuberger M, Niki-
        forov B, De Sario M, Grize L, Heinrich J, Hruba F, Janssen N, Luttmann-
        Gibson H, Privalova L, Rudnai P, Splichalova A, Zlotkowska R, Fletcher T.
        Parental smoking and children's respiratory health: independent effects of
        prenatal and postnatal exposure. Tob Control. 2006 Aug;15(4):294–301.

147   **Increasingly, periodontal disease is recognized as an important risk fac-
        tor in pregnancy** Xiong X, Buekens P, Fraser WD, Beck J, Offenbacher S.
        Periodontal disease and adverse pregnancy outcomes: a systematic review.
        BJOG. 2006 Feb;113(2):135–43.

148   **which has been shown to reduce the rates of preterm low birth weight
        births among pregnant women with periodontal disease** Xiong X, Buek-
        ens P, Fraser WD, Beck J, Offenbacher S. Periodontal disease and adverse
        pregnancy outcomes: a systematic review. BJOG. 2006 Feb;113(2):135–43.

149   **HIV, syphilis, and hepatitis B can be diagnosed with a blood test, and
        routine screening is recommended for all pregnant women at their first
        prenatal visit** American College of Obstetricians and Gynecologists and
        American Academy of Pediatrics. Guidelines for Perinatal Care. Fifth edi-
        tion. Washington DC: American College of Obstetricians and Gynecolo-
        gists. 2002.

151   routine screening of all pregnant women (with a simple urine test) for
        asymptomatic bacteriuria (bacteria in the urine) is recommended at
        their first prenatal visit American College of Obstetricians and Gyne-
        cologists and American Academy of Pediatrics. Guidelines for Perinatal
        Care. Fifth edition. Washington DC: American College of Obstetricians
        and Gynecologists. 2002.

152   You can get more information on toxoplasmosis from the CDC website
        on toxoplasmosis/ If You Are Pregnant or Getting Ready to Get Preg-
        nant and Own a Cat: http://www.cdc.gov/NCIDOD/dpd/parasites/toxo
        plasmosis/factsht_toxoplasmosis.htm and http://www.cdc.gov/healthypets/
        pregnant.htm. Last accessed September 25, 2008.

153   maternal rubella infection during pregnancy has also been implicated as a
        possible cause of schizophrenia in the offspring Brown AS. Prenatal infec-
        tion as a risk factor for schizophrenia. Schizophr Bull. 2006 Apr;32(2):200–2.

154   For more information on rubella, you can go to the CDC website http://
        www.cdc.gov/nip/diseases/rubella/default.htm. Last accessed September
        25, 2008.

155   You can get more information on CMV from the CDC website http://
        www.cdc.gov/cmv/. Last accessed September 25, 2008.

156   For more information on HSV, you can log on to the CDC website
        http://www.cdc.gov/std/Herpes/. Last accessed September 25, 2008.

156   You can get more information on syphilis from the CDC website http://
        www.cdc.gov/std/syphilis/STDFact-Syphilis.htm. Last accessed September
        25, 2008.

157   Box 5.3: Avoiding Foodborne Illnesses You can find more information
        on foodborne illnesses, including listeriosis, at the CDC websites: http://
        www.cdc.gov/ncidod/dbmd/diseaseinfo/foodborneinfections_g.htm
        #riskiestfoods and http://www.cdc.gov/nczved/dfbmd/disease_listing/liste-
        riosis_gi.html. Last accessed September 25, 2008.

160   You can also get information on food safety during pregnancy from the
        FDA website http://www.cfsan.fda.gov/~pregnant/safeats.html. Last ac-
        cessed September 25, 2008.

160   Several studies have shown elevated levels of inflammatory markers
        among current smokers Bazzano LA, He J, Muntner P, Vupputuri S,
        Whelton PK. Relationship between cigarette smoking and novel risk fac-
        tors for cardiovascular disease in the United States. Ann Intern Med.
        2003 Jun 3;138(11):891–7.

160   If you quit smoking, these inflammatory markers will gradually decline
        over time Bakhru A, Erlinger TP. Smoking cessation and cardiovascular
        disease risk factors: results from the Third National Health and Nutrition
        Examination Survey. PLoS Med. 2005 Jun;2(6):e160. Epub 2005 Jun 28.

160   Here are some tips from the American Medical Association http://jama
        .ama-assn.org/cgi/content/full/296/1/130. Last accessed September 25, 2008.

161   The National Institutes of Health also has a website: http://www.nlm.nih
        .gov/medlineplus/smokingcessation.html. Last accessed September 25, 2008.

162   Here are some recommendations from the American Academy of Allergy, Asthma, and Immunology (AAAAI) http://www.aaaai.org/patients/publicedmat/tips/indoorallergens.stm. Last accessed September 25, 2008.

163   or check out the EPA's website http://www.epa.gov/iaq/pubs/insidest.html #Look6. Last accessed September 25, 2008.

164   The new CDC guidelines recommend that all women receive a single dose of Tdap before they become pregnant http://www.cdc.gov/mmwr/preview/mmwrhtml/rr5517a1.htm. Last accessed September 25, 2008.

164   you should get a flu shot before you get pregnant http://www.cdc.gov/mmwr/preview/mmwrhtml/rr56e629a1.htm?s_cid=rr56e629a1_e. Last accessed September 25, 2008.

165   the vaccine is contraindicated during pregnancy See: http://www.cdc.gov/std/HPV/STDFact-HPV-vaccine.htm#hpvvac1. Last accessed September 25, 2008.

168   Exercise, in moderation, can boost your immune functions and reduce chronic inflammation Pederson BK. The anti-inflammatory effect of exercise: its role in diabetes and cardiovascular disease control. Essays Biochem. 2006;42:105–17.

168   regular exercise may also prevent several pregnancy complications, including gestational diabetes and preeclampsia, largely by reducing oxidative stress and chronic inflammation Weissgerber TL, Wolfe LA, Davies GA, Mottola MF. Exercise in the prevention and treatment of maternal-fetal disease: a review of the literature. Appl Physiol Nutr Metab. 2006 Dec;31(6):661–74.

168   Athletes engaged in high-intensity exercise are particularly susceptible to infections for up to 72 hours after exercise Nieman DC. Effects of exercise on the immune system: exercise effects on systemic immunity. Immunol Cell Biol. 2000 Oct;78(5):496–501.

chapter 6: healthy environment

171   this chemical can reduce the number of American children with far-above average intelligence (IQ above 130) by half Needleman HL, Leviton A, Bellinger D. Lead-associated intellectual deficit (letter), *N Engl J Med* 1982:**306**:367. Also see Grandjean P, Landrigan PJ. Developmental neurotoxicity of industrial chemicals. Lancet. 2006 Dec 16;368(9553):2167–78 for review of developmental neurotoxicity of lead and other industrial chemicals.

171–72 a mysterious outbreak of cerebral palsy, mental retardation, microcephaly (small head), and other neurological disorders in children born around the Minamata Bay in Japan. Cited in Schettler T, Solomon G, Valenti M, Huddle A. Generations at risk: Reproductive health and the environment. Cambridge MA: MIT Press. 2000:61.

172   fewer than half have ever been subjected to even token laboratory test-
       ing for toxicity to humans U.S. Environmental Protection Agency,
       *Chemical Hazard Data Availability Study: What Do We Really Know About
       the Safety of High Production Volume Chemicals?*, Office of Pollution Pre-
       vention and Toxics, Washington, DC (1998).

173   Philippe Grandjean at Harvard School of Public Health warns us about
       a silent pandemic Grandjean P, Landrigan PJ. Developmental neurotoxic-
       ity of industrial chemicals. Lancet. 2006 Dec 16;368(9553):2167–78.

174   Table 6.1. Chemicals that are known to be toxic to the human brain
       Source: Developmental neurotoxicity of industrial chemicals. Lancet. 2006
       Dec 16;368(9553):2167–78.

181   One survey found that 98 percent of households used pesticides at least
       once annually Davis JR, Brownson RC, Garcia R. Family pesticide use in
       the home, garden, orchard, and yard. Arch Environ Contam Toxicol. 1992
       Apr;22(3):260–6.

183   I will give you four major reasons why you should start to worry now
       and not later Schettler T, Solomon G, Valenti M, Huddle A. Generations
       at risk: Reproductive health and the environment. Cambridge MA: MIT
       Press. 2000.

184   Here are ten steps you can take to creating a healthy environment for
       your baby Schettler T, Solomon G, Valenti M, Huddle A. Generations at
       risk: Reproductive health and the environment. Cambridge MA: MIT
       Press. 2000 is heavily referenced in the development of the ten steps.

186   One consumer group found unacceptably high levels of lead in about 10
       percent of children's vinyl lunchboxes they tested See Center for Envi-
       ronmental Health website: http://www.cehca.org/lunchboxes.htm. Last ac-
       cessed September 25, 2008.

187   Box 6.1: Is Your Drinking Water Unleaded? Nakamura D. Water in D.C.
       exceeds U.S. EPA lead limit: random tests last summer found high levels in
       4,000 homes throughout city. Washington Post, January 31, 2004: A1.

187   another *Washington Post* story in October 2004 called attention to
       misrepresentation of water lead levels in cities across the United States
       Leonning CD, Becker J, Nakamura D. Lead Levels in Water Misrepre-
       sented Across U.S. Washington Post, 5 October 5, 2004: A1.

188   One 1998 study found that pregnant women in their first trimester
       Waller K, Swan SH, DeLorenze G, Hopkins B. Trihalomethanes in drink-
       ing water and spontaneous abortion. Epidemiology. 1998 Mar;9(2):134–40.

188   THMs have also been linked to cleft lip and palate, neural tube defects,
       cardiac defects, and other birth defects Bove F, Shim Y, Zeitz P. Drink-
       ing water contaminants and adverse pregnancy outcomes: a review. Envi-
       ron Health Perspect. 2002 Feb;110 Suppl 1:61–74.

189   simply log on to the EPA website at www.epa.gov to access local water
       information http://www.epa.gov/epahome/r2k.htm#waterquality. Last ac-
       cessed September 25, 2008.

189   **go to the non-profit National Sanitation Foundation (NSF) International website** http://www.nsf.org/consumer/newsroom/pdf/fact_water_dwtu.pdf. Last accessed September 25, 2008.

189   **The EPA website also provides some advice on tap water safety** http://www.epa.gov/safewater/wot/pdfs/book_waterontap_full.pdf. Last accessed September 25, 2008.

191   **The EPA recommends several steps you can take to protect your private water drinking supply** http://www.epa.gov/safewater/wot/pdfs/book_waterontap_full.pdf; Last accessed September 25, 2008. You can also get more information on well water safety at the NSF International website: http://www.nsf.org/consumer/drinking_water/dw_well.asp?program=WaterTre. Last accessed September 25, 2008.

191   **Box 6.2: How Safe Is Your Water Bottle?** McRandle PW. Plastic water bottles. National Geographic The Green Guide. http://www.thegreenguide.com/doc/101/plastic. Last accessed September 25, 2008.

191   **Recent evidence from rat studies suggests that fetal exposure to even low levels of BPA** Murray TJ, Maffini MV, Ucci AA, Sonnenschein C, Soto AM. Induction of mammary gland ductal hyperplasias and carcinoma in situ following fetal bisphenol A exposure. Reprod Toxicol. 2007 Apr-May;23(3):383–90

191   **Based on a review of over 500 studies, an expert panel convened by the National Institute of Health expressed "some concern"** See http://cerhr.niehs.nih.gov/chemicals/bisphenol/draftBPA_MtgSumm080807.pdf. Last accessed September 25, 2008.

193   **Smoking during pregnancy can cause miscarriage, fetal growth retardation, preterm birth, stillbirth, and placental separation** Cnattingius S. The epidemiology of smoking during pregnancy: smoking prevalence, maternal characteristics, and pregnancy outcomes. Nicotine Tob Res. 2004 Apr;6 Suppl 2:S125–40.

193   **Only about one in three pregnant women are able to quit smoking** Lumley J, Oliver SS, Chamberlain C, Oakley L. Interventions for promoting smoking cessation during pregnancy. Cochrane Database Syst Rev. 2004 Oct 18;(4):CD001055.

194   **Here are a few tips on how you can protect yourself and your future baby from these air pollutants** For more information on how to reduce indoor air pollutants from combustion products, you can access the EPA website at http://www.epa.gov/iaq/co.html. Last accessed September 25, 2008.

195   **Box 6.3: Dry-Cleaning and Your Reproductive Health** For more information on dry-cleaning, you can visit the EPA website: http://www.epa.gov/iaq/pubs/insidest.html#Look6. Last accessed September 25, 2008.

195   **The bedroom may have levels eight times as great** Schettler T, Solomon G, Valenti M, Huddle A. Generations at risk: Reproductive health and the environment. Cambridge MA: MIT Press. 2000:286.

196   **they are known to cross the placenta and can be absorbed by the fetus** Haque AK, Vrazel DM, Burau KD, Cooper SP, Downs T. Is there transpla-

cental transfer of asbestos? A study of 40 stillborn infants. Pediatr Pathol Lab Med. 1996 Nov-Dec;16(6):877–92.

198   **For more information on what you can do to safeguard indoor air quality in your home** visit the EPA (http://www.epa.gov/iaq/pubs/insidest. html#Look6) or NSF websites (http://www.nsf.org/consumer/indoor_air/ index.asp?program=IndoorAir) on indoor air quality. Sites last accessed September 25, 2008.

198   **Let's do a walkthrough, room by room, and start detoxifying your home before you start nesting** The article by Duncan DE. Chemicals within us. National Geographic. October 2006, and the website for the Green Guide were heavily referenced for this section. Accessed at http://www7 .nationalgeographic.com/ngm/0610/feature4/online_extra.html, and http:// www.thegreenguide.com/. Last accessed September 25, 2008.

198–99 **You can also compare the safety of common brands of personal care products at the Environmental Working Group's Skin Deep Cosmetics Safety Database website** at http://www.cosmeticsdatabase.com/splash.php ?URI= percent2Findex.php. Last accessed September 25, 2008.

199   **Bathroom cleaners** Go to the Green Guide website: http://www .thegreenguide.com/products/Housekeeping/Bathroom_Surface_Cleaners; also see McRandle PW DIY Household Cleaners for suggestions on non-toxic alternative cleaners http://www.thegreenguide.com/doc/120/diy, "Top Cleaning Product Ingredients to Avoid" and http://www.thegreenguide .com/doc/113/ingredients for a list of worst offenders. Last accessed on September 25, 2008.

199   **call the manufacturer and request the Material Safety Data Sheet (MSDS)** MSDS is also available online at http://www.msds.com/. If you need help understanding a MSDS, you can call the Teratogen Information Service in your state by clicking your state on the map at http://otispregnancy.org/otis_find_a_tis.asp. Last accessed September 25, 2008.

200   **For cleaning up grease, try a mixture of 1/2 teaspoon of washing soda, 2 tablespoons of distilled white vinegar, 1/4 teaspoon liquid soap, and 2 cups of hot water with a spray bottle**. For more suggestions, go to http:// www.thegreenguide.com/doc/120/diy and "Household Cleaning Supplies" at http://www.thegreenguide.com/reports/productprint.mhtml?id=15. Last accessed on September 25, 2008.

203   **Avoid Using Pesticides** You can find more information on alternatives to pesticides on the web at: http://www.pesticides.org/educmaterials.html. Last accessed September 25, 2008.

204   **Moth repellents contain paradichlorobenzene** See EPA website for more information on 1,4-Dichlorobenzene (para-Dichlorobenzene) http://www .epa.gov/ttn/atw/hlthef/dich-ben.html. Last accessed September 25, 2008.

205   **Start Nesting** Schettler T, Solomon G, Valenti M, Huddle A. Generations at risk: Reproductive health and the environment. Cambridge MA: MIT Press. 2000:286

206   **If you are going to install new carpets** For more information on selecting

carpet and rugs or care and cleaning, visit the Carpet and Rug Institute's website at http://www.carpet-rug.com/. Also see the Carpet and Rug Institute's installation guidelines http://www.carpet-rug.org/pdf_word_docs/105 .pdf. Last accessed September 25, 2008.

207 **Are you living next to one of the nation's worst toxic waste sites (a so-called Superfund site)?** Log on to the website for Environmental Defense Fund, a leading national nonprofit environmental advocacy group: http://www.scorecard.org/env-releases/land/, type in your zip code, and you will get the locations of the Superfund sites in your area, along with a list of top polluters and an environmental justice report for your County. Last accessed September 25, 2008.

208 **A 1995 study found New York City apartments** Leubuscher S. Dry Cleaning—Hidden Hazards. Amsterdam: Greenpeace International, 1992.

208 **In a study of the San Francisco Recreation and Parks Department between 1994 and 1995** Green Corps, Pesticide Watch Education Fund. An Evaluation of San Francisco's Recreation and Parks Department Pesticide Control Program. San Francisco: Pesticide Watch, January 1997.

209 **To find out more about air quality in your local area, visit the nonprofit Environmental Defense Fund's website** http://www.scorecard.org/envre leases/cap/ and type in your zip code. You will see how your county stacks up against other counties in the United States in terms of air pollution, how many days a year the air is healthy, and who are the top air polluters in your area. **You can also look up information about toxic chemicals released into your neighborhood at the EPA's Toxic Release Inventory (TRI) website** at http://www.epa.gov/tri/. **The EPA also maintains the Environfacts website** http://www.epa.gov/enviro/html/tris/tris_query.html, which allows users to identify the facilities (with street addresses) monitored by the EPA in their area and the amount of air emissions released by the facilities into the neighborhood. Last accessed September 25, 2008.

210 **A growing body of evidence now suggests that noise pollution from airports and other sources may reduce birth weight** Schell LM, Gallo MV, Denham M, Ravenscroft J. Effects of pollution on human growth and development: an introduction. J Physiol Anthropol. 2006 Jan;25(1):103–12.

210 **You may also want to check out Noise Free America's website** http://www.noisefree.org/ Last accessed September 25, 2008.

211 **You can find examples of healthy cities and healthy communities all over the United States on the Healthy Cities/Healthy Communities website** http://www.well.com/user/bbear/hc_articles.html#how Last accessed September 25, 2008.

211 **If you are like most Americans, you spend on average 24 minutes commuting to work each day** http://www.census.gov/Press-Release/www/releases/archives/american_community_survey_acs/004489.html. Last accessed September 25, 2008.

211 **Increased exposure to carbon monoxide and ozone in the second month of pregnancy** Ritz B, Yu F, Fruin S, Chapa G, Shaw GM, Harris JA. Ambi-

ent air pollution and risk of birth defects in Southern California. Am J Epidemiol. 2002 Jan 1;155(1):17–25. Also see Wilhelm M, Ritz B. Local variations in CO and particulate air pollution and adverse birth outcomes in Los Angeles County, California, USA. Environ Health Perspect. 2005 Sep;113(9):1212–21.

213 **Do your part to reduce air pollution** For more information on ways to reduce air pollution, check out http://www.epa.gov/oar/epa450.txt Last accessed September 25, 2008.

213 **There are now more than 84,000 chemical compounds in the workplace** Lawson CC, Grajewski B, Daston GP, Frazier LM, Lynch D, McDiarmid M et al. Workgroup report: Implementing a national occupational reproductive research agenda—decade one and beyond. Environ Health Perspect. 2006 Mar;114(3):435–41.

214 **Log onto the Organization of Teratology Information Services (OTIS) website** at http://www.otispregnancy.org/ You can also access an updated list of chemicals known to cause cancer and reproductive toxicity at California's Proposition 65 website: http://www.oehha.ca.gov/prop65/prop65_list/files/P65single081106.pdf. Last accessed September 25, 2008.

215 **You can learn more about the 1970 OSHA Act by logging onto the OSHA website:** http://www.osha.gov/ Last accessed September 25, 2008.

chapter 7: preconception care

218 **preconception care is a set of prepregnancy interventions that aim to identify and modify biomedical, behavioral, and social risks** Johnson K, Posner SF, Biermann J, Cordero JF, Atrash HK, Parker CS, Boulet S, Curtis MG; CDC/ATSDR Preconception Care Work Group; Select Panel on Preconception Care. Recommendations to improve preconception health and health care—United States. A report of the CDC/ATSDR Preconception Care Work Group and the Select Panel on Preconception Care. MMWR Recomm Rep. 2006 Apr 21;55(RR–6):1–23; or access on line at http://www.cdc.gov/mmwr/preview/mmwrhtml/rr5506a1.htm See also March of Dimes' website on preconception care: http://www.marchofdimes.com/pnhec/173.asp. Last accessed September 25, 2008.

221 **A reproductive life plan is a set of personal goals about having (or not having) children** See: http://www.cdc.gov/ncbddd/preconception/QandA.htm#5. Last accessed September 25, 2008.

221 **Box 7.1: How Fast Is Your Biological Clock Ticking?** Source: http://www.asrm.org/Patients/patientbooklets/agefertility.pdf. Last accessed September 25, 2008.

226 **Box 7.2: If you've had a preterm baby** Source: Lu MC, Kotelchuck M, Culhane J, Hobel CJ, Klerman LV, Thorp J. Preconception care between pregnancies: The content of internatal care. Matern Child Health J. 2006;10(S7):107–122.

229   **Box 7.3: If you have chronic hypertension (high blood pressure)** Source:
        Chobanian AV, Bakris GL, Black HR, Cushman WC, Green LA, Izzo JL Jr,
        Jones DW, Materson BJ, Oparil S, Wright JT Jr, Roccella EJ. Seventh report
        of the Joint National Committee on Prevention, Detection, Evaluation,
        and Treatment of High Blood Pressure. Hypertension 2003;42:1206–52.

230   **A healthy eating plan** Log on to the National Institutes of Health website
        for Dietary Approaches to Stop Hypertension (DASH) eating plan http://
        www.nhlbi.nih.gov/health/public/heart/hbp/dash/. Last accessed Septem-
        ber 25, 2008.

231   **Box 7.4: If you have diabetes (high blood sugar)** American Diabetes As-
        sociation. Preconception care of women with diabetes. Diabetes Care
        2004;27(Suppl 1):S76–8.

236   **You should talk to your doctor about your family history and genetic
        risks** Shapira SK, Dolan S. Genetic risks to the mother and the infant:
        assessment, counseling, and management. Matern Child Health J. 2006
        Sep;10(5 Suppl):S143–6.

238   **although the American College of Obstetricians and Gynecologists now
        recommends that *all* couples who are pregnant or contemplating preg-
        nancy be offered cystic fibrosis screening** American College of Obstetri-
        cians and Gynecologists. ACOG Committee Opinion. Number 325,
        December 2005. Update on carrier screening for cystic fibrosis. Obstet
        Gynecol. 2005 Dec;106(6):1465–8.

240   **For example, if you have phenylketonuria (PKU)** For more information
        on PKU, you can log on to the March of Dimes website at: http://www
        .marchofdimes.com/professionals/14332_1219.asp. Last accessed September
        25, 2008.

239–40 **Tell your doctor, or call the National Domestic Violence Hotline at
        1–800–799-SAFE (7233)** For more information, log on to http://www
        .ndvh.org/. Last accessed September 25, 2008.

243   **Box 7.5: Diagnostic Criteria for Eating Disorders** Source: Adapted
        from American Psychiatric Association. Eating Disorders. In: Diagnostic
        and Statistical Manual of Mental Disorders, (DSM-IVTR), fourth edition,
        Washington, DC: American Psychiatric Association, 2000, p.583–97.

245   **Box 7.6: Diagnostic Criteria for Anxiety Disorders** Source: Adapted
        from American Psychiatric Association. Eating Disorders. In: Diagnostic
        and Statistical Manual of Mental Disorders, (DSM-IVTR), fourth edition,
        Washington, DC: American Psychiatric Association, 2000, p.583–97.

246   **Box 7.7: Recommended Preventive and Primary Health Services for
        Women of Childbearing Age** Source: U.S. Preventive Services Task
        Force; access on line at http://www.ahrq.gov/clinic/uspstfix.htm. Last ac-
        cessed September 25, 2008.

247   **Box 7.8: All Women Should Have an Annual Pelvic Exam But Not All
        Women Need Annual Pap Tests** Source: ACOG Practice Bulletin: clini-
        cal management guidelines for obstetrician-gynecologists. Number 45,
        August 2003. Cervical cytology screening. Obstet Gynecol. 2003;102:417–27.

248   The first eight tests on my list are routine prenatal labs, typically ob-
        tained during your first prenatal visit American College of Obstetri-
        cians and Gynecologists and American Academy of Pediatrics. Guidelines
        for Perinatal Care. Fifth edition. Washington DC: American College of
        Obstetricians and Gynecologists. 2002.

249   If left untreated, up to 40 percent of pregnant women with asymptom-
        atic bacteriuria will develop a kidney infection Smaill F, Vazquez JC.
        Antibiotics for asymptomatic bacteriuria in pregnancy. Cochrane Data-
        base Syst Rev. 2007 Apr 18;(2):CD000490.

252   One recent study tested the IQ of children born to women who were
        mildly deficient in thyroid hormones in early pregnancy Pop VJ et al.
        Maternal hypothyroxinaemia during early pregnancy and subsequent
        child development: A 3-year follow-up study. Clin Endocrinol
        2003;59:282–8.

252   Genetic screen for cystic fibrosis you can talk to your doctor or go to
        ACOG's website http://www.acog.org/from_home/wellness/cf001.htm.
        Last accessed September 25, 2008.

chapter 8: from here to paternity

256   The DNA carried in your sperm can get damaged in a lot of different
        ways Aitken RJ, Koopman P, Lewis SE. Seeds of concern. Nature. 2004
        Nov 4;432(7013):48–52. Also see: Hampton T. Researchers discover a
        range of factors undermine sperm quality, male fertility. JAMA. 2005 Dec
        14;294(22):2829–31; and Zini A, Libman J. Sperm DNA damage: clinical
        significance in the era of assisted reproduction. CMAJ. 2006 Aug
        29;175(5):495–500; and Alvarez JG. Nurture vs nature: how can we opti-
        mize sperm quality? J Androl. 2003 Sep-Oct;24(5):640–8.

257   Kids growing up in families with high levels of father involvement have
        better cognitive and socioemotional development Lamb ME. The role of
        the father in child development. New York: Wiley. 1997.

258   the life cycle of sperm lasts about 42 to 76 days Misell LM, Holochwost
        D, Boban D, Santi N, Shefi S, Hellerstein MK, Turek PJ. A stable isotope-
        mass spectrometric method for measuring human spermatogenesis kinet-
        ics in vivo. J Urol. 2006 Jan;175(1):242–6.

261   Box 8.1: Do men have a biological clock, too? Source: Biological clock
        ticks for men, too: genetic defects linked to sperm of older fathers. JAMA.
        2004 Apr 14;291(14):1683–5.

263   Certain medical conditions, such as diabetes, varicoceles, or sexually
        transmitted infections, can cause damage to your sperm DNA Agbaje
        IM, Rogers DA, McVicar CM, McClure N, Atkinson AB, Mallidis C,
        Lewis SE. Insulin dependant diabetes mellitus: implications for male re-
        productive function. Hum Reprod. 2007 Jul;22(7):1871–7. Also see: Ber-
        tolla RP, Cedenho AP, Hassun Filho PA, Lima SB, Ortiz V, Srougi M.

Sperm nuclear DNA fragmentation in adolescents with varicocele. Fertil Steril. 2006 Mar;85(3):625–8.

265 **Men who are overweight have reduced fertility** Sallmen M, Sandler DP, Hoppin JA, Blair A, Baird DD. Reduced fertility among overweight and obese men. Epidemiology. 2006 Sep;17(5):520–3.

266 **On average, chronic smokers show a 75 percent decline in fertilizing capacity when compared to non-smokers** See study cited in Science Daily: Men Who Smoke Heavily May Impair Sperm, Fertility: http://www.sciencedaily.com/releases/2005/10/051018080741.htm. Last accessed September 25, 2008.

267 **Some studies have shown that moderate drinking may be protective** Marinelli D, Gaspari L, Pedotti P, Taioli E. Mini-review of studies on the effect of smoking and drinking habits on semen parameters. Int J Hyg Environ Health. 2004 Jul;207(3):185–92.

267 **In a study of alcoholics in an addiction treatment center** Muthusami KR, Chinnaswamy P. Effect of chronic alcoholism on male fertility hormones and semen quality. Fertil Steril. 2005 Oct;84(4):919–24.

268 **You can get help by . . . or going to the U.S. Substance Abuse and Mental Health Services Administration** at http://www.findtreatment.samhsa.gov/ to find an alcohol treatment program near you. Last accessed September 25, 2008.

268 **In a small study of 15 men who were using anabolic steroids** Cited in Hampton T. Researchers discover a range of factors undermine sperm quality, male fertility. JAMA. 2005 Dec 14;294(22):2829–31.

268 **One Brazilian study found that men who drank more than six cups of coffee per day had _higher_ sperm motility** Sobreiro BP, Lucon AM, Pasqualotto FF, Hallak J, Athayde KS, Arap S. Semen analysis in fertile patients undergoing vasectomy: reference values and variations according to age, length of sexual abstinence, seasonality, smoking habits and caffeine intake. Sao Paulo Med J. 2005;123:161–6.

269 **What does your stress level now have to do with your baby in the future?** Giblin PT, Poland ML, Moghissi KS, et al. Effects of stress and characteristic adaptability on semen quality in healthy men. Fertil Steril. 1988;49:127–132; their finding of a link between stress and poorer sperm quality was not supported by the study by Hjollund NH, Bonde JP, Henriksen TB, Giwercman A, Olsen J; The Danish First Pregnancy Planner Study Team. Reproductive effects of male psychologic stress. Epidemiology. 2004 Jan;15(1):21–7.

270 **Nutritional deficiencies in several micronutrients, especially zinc and folate, have been shown to lower sperm production and impair male fertility** Wong WY, Thomas CM, Merkus JM, Zielhuis GA, Steegers-Theunissen RP. Male factor subfertility: possible causes and the impact of nutritional factors. Fertil Steril. 2000 Mar;73(3):435–42.

270 **Several randomized, placebo-controlled trials have found daily supplementation with 5 mg of folic acid and 66 mg of zinc sulfate** Ebisch IM, Thomas CM, Peters WH, Braat DD, Steegers-Theunissen RP. The impor-

tance of folate, zinc and antioxidants in the pathogenesis and prevention of subfertility. Hum Reprod Update. 2007 Mar-Apr;13(2):163–74.

270   **In one study, the combination of vitamin C and E at high doses resulted in sperm DNA damage** Donnelly ET, McClure N, Lewis SE. The effect of ascorbate and alpha-tocopherol supplementation in vitro on DNA integrity and hydrogen peroxide-induced DNA damage in human spermatozoa. Mutagenesis. 1999 Sep;14(5):505–12.

271   **Exposures to a number of xenobiotics have been shown to reduce male fertility and sperm quality** See Aitken RJ, Koopman P, Lewis SE. Seeds of concern. Nature. 2004 Nov 4;432(7013):48–52 for a review of xenobiotics and male reproductive health.

272   **Polychlorinated biphenyls (PCBs)** You can get more information on PCBs at the CDC website: http://www.atsdr.cdc.gov/tfacts17.html#bookmark04. Last accessed September 25, 2008.

273   **Infections and inflammation have been shown to cause oxidative stress and sperm DNA damage** Erenpreiss J, Hlevicka S, Zalkalns J, et al. Effect of leukocytospermia on sperm DNA integrity: a negative effect in abnormal semen samples. J Androl 2002; 23: 717–23.

274   **High temperature inside the scrotum (the sac that contains the testes) has been shown to cause sperm DNA damage and lower male fertility** Evenson DP, Jost LK, Corzett M, et al. Characteristics of human sperm chromatin structure following an episode of influenza and high fever: a case study. J Androl 2000;21:739–46. Also reviewed in: Zini A, Libman J. Sperm DNA damage: clinical significance in the era of assisted reproduction. CMAJ. 2006 Aug 29;175(5):495–500.

275   **There is no conclusive evidence that exposure to computers is harmful to sperm** Sun YL, Zhou WJ, Wu JQ, Gao ES. Does exposure to computers affect the routine parameters of semen quality? Asian J Androl. 2005 Sep;7(3):263–6.

275   **There are conflicting reports regarding the effects of electromagnetic fields on sperm quality** Irgens A, Kruger K, Ulstein M. The effect of male occupational exposure in infertile couples in Norway. J Occup Environ Med 1999; 41:1116–20; and Akdag MZ, Dasdag S, Aksen F, Isik B, Yilmaz F. Effect of ELF magnetic fields on lipid peroxidation, sperm count, p53, and trace elements. Med Sci Monit. 2006 Nov;12(11):BR366–71.

275   **Exposure to mobile phone radiation also remains controversial** Aitken RJ, Bennetts LE, Sawyer D, Wiklendt AM, King BV. Impact of radio frequency electromagnetic radiation on DNA integrity in the male germline. Int J Androl. 2005 Jun;28(3):171–9.

275   **One recent study found that men who used mobile phones for four hours or more a day** Agarwal A, Deepinder F, Sharma RK, Ranga G, Li J. Effect of cell phone usage on semen analysis in men attending infertility clinic: an observational study. Fertil Steril. 2008;89:124–8.

275   **"Mindfulness means paying attention in a particular way"** See Kabat-Zinn J. Wherever you go there you are. New York: Hyperion. 2005.

277   **The website breaks down financial planning for a baby into seven steps**
       See March of Dimes website: http://www.marchofdimes.com/pnhec/
       173 _14007.asp. Last accessed September 3, 2007.

280   **a national survey found that about a third of women return to work less
       than six weeks after giving birth** Cantor D, Waldfogel J, Kerwin J, McKinley-
       Wright M, Levin K, Rauch J et al. Balancing the needs of families and em-
       ployers: Family and medical leave surveys. Rockville, MD: Westat. 2001.

282   **Learn to perceive and respond to each other's needs and expectations**
       See Rodriguez, R. What's your pregnant man thinking? A book for ex-
       pectant mothers about expectant dads. Lulu Press. 2004.

epilogue

285   **pregnancy may reveal a woman's risk for chronic disease in later life**
       See Kaaja RJ, Greer IA. Manifestations of chronic disease during preg-
       nancy. JAMA. 2005; 294(21):2751–7, and Kim C, Newton K, Knopp R.
       Gestational diabetes and the incidence of type 2 diabetes: a systematic
       review. *Diabetes Care.* 2002;25:1862–1868.

285   **If you had gestational diabetes, you have a 40 percent chance of develop-
       ing type 2 diabetes** Lauenborg J, Hansen T, Moller D, et al. Increasing inci-
       dence of diabetes after gestational diabetes. *Diabetes Care.* 2004;27:1194–1199,
       and Kim C, Newton K, Knopp R. Gestational diabetes and the incidence of
       type 2 diabetes: a systematic review. *Diabetes Care.* 2002;25:1862–1868.

285   **If you had preeclampsia, you have a greater risk of suffering a heart at-
       tack** Smith GC, Pell JP, Walsh D. Pregnancy complications and maternal
       risk for ischaemic heart disease: a retrospective cohort study of 129 290
       births. *Lancet.* 2001;357:2002–2006, and Bellamy L, Casas JP, Hingorani
       AD, Williams DJ. Pre-eclampsia and risk of cardiovascular disease and
       cancer in later life: systematic review and meta-analysis. BMJ. 2007 Nov
       10;335(7627):974.

286   **It is perhaps not surprising that prenatal care has not been more effec-
       tive in preventing low birth weight and preterm births** See Lu MC,
       Tache V, Alexander G, Kotelchuck M, Halfon N. Preventing LBW: is pre-
       natal care the answer? J Matern Fetal Neonat Med 2003;13;362–80.

289   **That was what happened to Ikea** Case study presented by Mathur SK,
       Hacker CS, Aday LA. Sustainable development. In: Aday LA. Reinvent-
       ing Public Health: Policies and Practices for a Healthy Nation. San Fran-
       cisco: Jossey-Bass. 2005:93–98.

289   **One such study is the National Children's Study** For more information,
       go to the website for the National Children's Study: http://www.national
       childrensstudy.gov/. Last accessed September 25, 2008. For full disclosure
       of potential conflict of interest, I am a lead investigator for the National
       Children's Study in Los Angeles, and I receive funding from the Na-
       tional Institute of Child Health and Development for my research.

INDEX

abdominal fat, 32, 118
abortion, 195, 224
açaí, 67, 76
Accutane, 232
ACE inhibitors, 230, 232
achondroplasia, 239, 262
acrylamides, 256–57, 273
action steps, 6–7
  for fathers. *See* fatherhood action
    plan
  for healthy environment. *See*
    environmental action plan
  for immune system. *See* immune
    system action plan
  for nutritional preparedness. *See*
    nutritional preparedness plan
  for preconception care. *See*
    preconception visit
  for smart and healthy baby, 20–24
  for stress. *See* stress resilience
addictions (addictive behaviors),
    242–44
  of fathers-to-be, 265–68
ADHD (attention deficit hyperactivity
    disorder)
  maternal stress and anxiety and, 17,
    23, 24, 107–9, 245
  smoking and, 193
adrenalin, 26, 110, 111, 115–16
aerobic exercise, 115–16, 168
African ancestry, and genetic disorders,
    237–38

age, 221–23
  genetic risks and maternal, 238–39
  genetic risks and paternal, 261–62
agricultural operations, 208
air-conditioning, 162, 206
air fresheners, 199
airports, noise pollution from, 210
air quality, 193–98, 209–10, 212
Alaskan wild salmon, 53–54, 62,
    84–85
alcohol, and eating right, 40, 118
alcohol abuse, 139–40, 242, 267–68
alfalfa sprouts, 75, 98, 157
alkylphenols, 182–83, 199
allergies
  environmental triggers for, 162–63
  peanuts and, 82
  smoking and, 145
allostasis (allostatic overload), 25–27,
    285, 286–87
  chronic inflammation and, 184
  nutritional stress and, 30–31
  psychological stress and, 26–27,
    110–11, 113, 116
almonds, 62, 80–81
alpha-linolenic acid (LnA), 52, 53, 64
alpha-tocopherol. *See* vitamin E
American Academy of Allergy,
    Asthma, and Immunology
    (AAAAI), 162, 163
American Cancer Society, 161
American Lung Association, 161

ammonia, 199, 200
amniocentisis, 239
anemia, 71, 72
    blood test for, 248–49
anencephaly, 24, 40, 68
angiotensin-converting enzyme (ACE)
    inhibitors, 230, 232
animal proteins, 58–62
Annual Water Quality Report, 189
anorexia nervosa, 243
anthocyanins, 66, 92, 94
antibacterial soaps, 198
antibody screen tests, 249–50
antioxidants
    in beans, 77
    in fruits and vegetables, 39, 65–68,
        92, 94
    for male sperm, 270–71
    in nuts and seeds, 81
    in olive oil, 83
    oxidative stress and, 39, 81, 166–67, 270
antivirals, for genital herpes, 155–56
anxiety disorders, 244–45
apples, 67
arginine, 81
arsenic, 180–81
artificial sweeteners, 100–101, 240
Art of Happiness (Dalai Lama), 133
asbestos, 196–98
Ashkenazi Jewish ancestry, and genetic
    disorders, 237–38
Asian ancestry, and genetic disorders,
    237–38
asparagus, 64, 68, 167
aspartame, 101, 240
aspirin, 232
astaxanthin, 84–85
asthma, 144–45, 193, 289
atherosclerosis, 168
attention deficit hyperactivity disorder.
    See ADHD
attic detoxification, 202
autism, 289
    maternal infections and, 18, 24,
        144, 145
    paternal age and, 262
automobiles. See cars
autonomy (self-governance), 130
auto repair shops, 208

bacterial vaginosis (BV), 86, 142,
    149–50, 169
bacteriuria, 151, 249
balanced diet, 38–42. See also
    nutrition; nutritional
    preparedness plan
Barker, David (Barker hypothesis), 16
barley, 87, 90
basement detoxification, 202–3
bathroom cleaners, 199
bathroom detoxification, 162, 198–200
beans, 39, 61–64, 77–78
bedding, 162–63, 201
bedrooms
    detoxifying, 201–2
    sleeping tips, 117
bedtime rituals, 117
beef (red meat), 40, 57, 59, 61, 62,
    97–98, 157
behavioral problems, and maternal
    stress, 23, 24, 107–9
behavioral risk factors, 242–44
    of fathers-to-be, 265–68
belly (abdominal) fat, 32, 118
Benson, Herbert, 120
benzene, 175, 181, 199
beta-blockers, 230
beta-carotene, 64, 66, 71, 92, 94
binge drinking, 139–40
binge eating disorder, 243–44
bioaccumulation, 183
biological clock, 221–23
    for men, 261–62
biotin (vitamin B7), 70, 79, 103
birth defects
    alcohol and substance use, 139
    infections and, 141–42, 145,
        148–49, 156
    medications and, 232
    multivitamins and, 40, 68
    overweight and, 34
    saccharin and, 101
    soy consumption and, 78
    sperm DNA and, 5, 22
    vitamins and minerals and, 65, 69,
        71, 99
birth spacing, 31, 223–24
bisphenol-A (BPA), 24, 191, 200
blessings, counting your, 132, 140

blood pressure
    checking your, 246, 265
    high. *See* hypertension
    medications for, 230, 232
blood sugar (glucose), 30–31, 46–50
    high. *See* diabetes
    stress and, 30, 111–12
blood tests, 248–50
blood type tests, 249–50
Bloom syndrome, 238
blueberries, 67, 92–93
blue fruits and vegetables, 67, 92–93
body image, 38
Body Mass Index (BMI), 34, 35
boiling water, 189
books, about prepregnancy, 6
bottled water, 190–92
BPA (bisphenol-A), 24, 191, 200
Bradberry, Travis, 128
brain, fetal. *See* fetal brain
brain foods, 72–95
    Alaskan wild salmon, 84–85
    dark green vegetables, 91–92
    dark purple fruits, 92–93
    eggs, 78–80
    legumes, 77–78
    nuts and seeds, 80–82
    olive oil, 82–84
    orange/red fruit and vegetables, 93–95
    whole grains, 87–91
    yogurt and kefir, 85–87
brainstorming solutions, 126–27
breakfast, 41, 49, 89
breast cancer, 83, 182, 191, 246
breast examination, 246
breathing clean air, 193–98
breathing exercises, 119, 140
broccoli, 66, 67, 91–92
brushing teeth, 147–48
building blocks, 22–23. *See also*
    nutritional preparedness plan;
    sperm
bulimia nervosa, 243
butter, 40, 57, 58
BV (bacterial vaginosis), 86, 142,
    149–50, 169

cadmium, 180, 213, 273
caffeine, 117, 268

CAGE questions, 139–40, 267–68
Cajun ancestry, and genetic disorders,
    237–38
calcium, 64, 72
    recommended daily intake, 70
    sources of, 40, 45, 54, 81, 87
caloric intake, 42–44, 48–49
    weight gain and, 37
    weight loss and, 35–36
calories, 42–44
Campbell, Joseph, 14, 20
Canavan disease, 237–38
cancer. *See also specific types of cancer*
    genetic risks for, 19
    pesticides and, 182, 184
    positive mental health for, 131
    smoking and, 272
    sperm DNA and, 22, 181, 184, 257
cancer prevention
    diet and, 39, 45, 94
    olive oil and, 83
canola oil, 39, 51, 52
    for frying, 57, 84
Capoten, 230, 232
carbohydrates, 46–50
    glycemic index of, 46–50
    low-carb diets, 44–46
    recommendations for choosing,
        48–50
carbon monoxide, 184, 194, 195,
    209, 211
carbon monoxide detectors, 195
cardiovascular exercise, 116
career goals, 122
carotenoids, 94, 167, 270
carpets (carpeting), 162, 201–2,
    206–7, 213
cars
    air pollution, 209–10, 212
    commuting tips, 211–13
    maintenance of, 212–13
Carver, Charles, 133
category A medications, 233, 234
category B medications, 233, 234
category C medications, 233, 234
category D medications, 233, 234
category X medications, 233, 234
cats, 152–53
cause(s) of problems, 126

CDC (Centers for Disease Control and Prevention), 40, 68, 152, 154–57, 159, 160, 217, 260
celery, 44, 67
central air handling systems, 194
cereals, 38, 45, 49, 50
cerebral palsy, 11, 144, 145, 171
cervical cancer, 165, 251
cheating husbands, 280–83
cheeses, 62, 96–97, 159–60
chemical toxins. See environmental toxins
cherries, 66, 67
chicken, 39–40, 52–53, 57, 59, 62
chickenpox (varicella) vaccine, 165, 166, 223, 246
childhood obesity, fetal origins of, 17
chilling foods, 158
chlamydia, 142, 148–49, 250
chlorine bleach, 199, 200
cholesterol
    alternative medications for, 230
    eggs and, 54, 79
    LDL, 55, 83, 99
choline (vitamin B4), 69, 70
chores, 278–79
chorioamnionitis, 143–44
chorionic villus sampling (CVS), 239
chromium, 54, 79, 94, 181
chronic medical conditions, 228–32
    of fathers-to-be, 263
cigarette smoking. See smoking
cinnamon, 104
circadian rhythms, 117
clean air, 193–98, 209–10, 212
cleaning foods, 67, 98, 158
CMV (cytomegalovirus), 154–55
cobalamine. See vitamin B12
cockroaches, 163, 205
coconut oil, 51, 55, 57, 63
cod liver oil, 51, 52
coffee, 72, 117, 268
colds, 131, 142, 168
coldwater fish, 52, 53–54, 62
collard greens, 64, 91
colors, of fruits and vegetables, 65–67, 91–95
comfort foods, 32, 44, 118

communication skills, 128–29, 270, 277
community
    connecting with your, 136
    environmental survey, 207–11
community health, 210–11
community service, 133, 137
commuting (commutes), 211–13
conception, 224, 235–36
conflict resolution, 127–29, 270
connectedness with others, 134–37
Consolidated Omnibus Budget Reconciliation Act (COBRA), 125
consumer products, lead in, 186
cooking foods, 94, 157
    eggs, 80, 157
    oils for, 55, 57, 84
    whole-wheat pasta, 49–50
cooking stoves, 194
cookware, 200
copper, 65, 70, 103
core conditioning, 116
core values, 131
corn syrup, 100–101
corticotropinreleasing hormone (CRH), 41, 106, 108
cortisol, 107–12, 169
    ADHD and, 17
    eating right, 118
    exercise and, 168
    HPA and, 26
    placenta and, 22
    sleep and, 116
cosmetics, 198–99
countertop cleaners, 200
Covey, Stephen, 140
cranberries, 66
CRH (corticotropinreleasing hormone), 41, 106, 108
cross-contaminating foods, 157–58
Cryptosporidium, 190
cryptoxanthin, 66, 92, 94
current medical conditions. See medical conditions
CVS (chorionic villus sampling), 239
cystic fibrosis, 237–38
    genetic screen for, 252–53
cytomegalovirus (CMV), 154–55

dads-to-be, 255–83. *See also* fatherhood
    action plan
  what women want, 256–58
daily acts of kindness, 133, 134
dairy (dairy products), 40, 45, 57, 61.
    See also cheeses; milk
Dalai Lama, 133
dark leafy greens, 51, 52, 66–67,
    91–92
dark purple fruits, 67, 92–93
deep breathing, 119
deep-fried foods, 56, 58
dehumidifiers, 162, 206
deli meats, 97, 159
dental care, 147–48
dentists, 147–48, 265
depression, 138–39, 244–45
DES (diethylstilbestrol), 4, 182, 247
detoxifying your environment.
        See environmental action
        plan
DHA (docosahexaenoic acid), 51–54,
    84, 272
DHA eggs, 53, 54, 62, 79, 80
diabetes, 24–25, 231–32, 289
    cod liver oil for, 52
    exercise for, 168
    screen for, 252
    weight loss for, 34
diaries, food, 36
1,2-dibromo-3-chloropropane, 271
diet. *See* nutrition; nutritional
        preparedness plan
Dietary Guidelines for Americans, 40,
    90–91, 116
diethanolamine, 199, 200
dieticians, 37, 42, 63
diet sodas, 100–101, 240
dining room detoxification, 200–201
dioxins, 4–5, 182–83, 272. *See also*
        environmental action plan;
        environmental toxins
docosahexaenoic acid. *See* DHA
doctor visit. *See* preconception visit
domestic violence, 137–38, 240–41
douching, 149–50
Down syndrome, 221–23, 238–39
drain cleaners, 200–201

drinking water, 188–92
    ensuring safety and quality of,
        188–91
    lead testing of, 186–88
    vs. sodas, 100–101
Drinking Water Hotline, 187
drug abuse, 139–40, 242, 268
dry-cleaning (dry-cleaners), 24,
    195–96, 208
dryers, 202
dumb fats, 55–58, 99–100, 118
    recommendations for reducing, 56–58
dust mites, 162–63

eating disorders, 242–44
eating right. *See also* nutritional
        preparedness plan
    for fathers-to-be, 270–71
    for immune fitness, 166–67
    for stress resilience, 118
eating safely, 96–99, 157–60
E. coli, 75, 98
eggs, 39–40, 78–80
    DHA-fortified, 53, 54, 62, 79, 80
    safety tips for, 79–80
eicosapentaenoic acid (EPA), 51–54, 84
ellagic acid, 81
emotional intelligence, 127–28, 270, 277
Emotional Intelligence (Goleman), 128
Emotional Intelligence Quick Book
        (Bradberry and Greaves), 128
emotional support, 275–77
empathy, 128, 129, 276
empty calories, 42, 43, 100
endocrine disruptors, 4–5, 59, 182–83
endorphins, and exercise, 115
energy conservation, 211–13
environmental action plan, 4–5,
        184–216
    avoiding harmful exposures at work,
        213–15
    avoiding pesticides, 203–5
    breathing clean air, 193–98
    choosing cleaner commute, 211–13
    detoxifying your home, 198–203
    drinking clean water, 188–92
    for immune fitness, 161–63
    knowing your rights at work, 215–16

environmental action plan (*continued*)
  making your home lead-free zone,
    185–88
  remodeling your home, 205–7
  surveying your neighborhood, 207–11
Environmental Defense Fund, 54,
  207, 209
environmental toxins, 171–84
  action plan for. *See* environmental
    action plan
  known neurotoxic chemicals, 174–83
  reasons to worry about, 183–84
Environmental Working Group (EWG),
  67, 199–200
EPA (Environmental Protection
  Agency)
  Drinking Water Hotline, 187
  Fish Advisory, 60
  pesticide residues in food, 182
  Toxic Release Inventory (TRI), 209
EPA (eicosapentaenoic acid), 51–54, 84
epigenetics, 18–20, 109
epilepsy, 144, 145, 232
EQ (emotional quotient), 128
Equal, 101, 240
essential oils, 104
ethanol, 181
ethnic background (ethnicity), and
  genetic risks, 236–38, 264
exercise
  before bedtime, 117
  for immune fitness, 168
  for stress reduction, 115–16
  for weight loss, 36
exhalation breathing, 119
exhaust fans, 194
extra-virgin olive oil, 83–84

fabric softeners, 202
fad diets, 36
faith, 136–37
familial dysautonomia, 237–38
family history and genetic risks,
  236–40, 264
family therapy, 129, 241
family violence, 137–38, 240–41
farm-raised fish, 60–61, 62, 85
fast-foods, 44, 56, 95
father-absent families, 257–58

fatherhood action plan, 259–83
  eating right, 270–71
  giving up biggest vices, 265–68
  instrumental support, 277–79
  learning to give emotional support,
    257, 275–77
  making a reproductive life plan,
    260–62
  managing stress, 269–70
  protecting your sperm DNA,
    271–75
  reprioritizing, 279–80
  staying faithful, 280–83
  visiting your doctor, 262–65
fathers-to-be, 255–83
  action plan for. *See* fatherhood
    action plan
  what women want, 256–58
fats, 51–58, 118. *See also* saturated fats;
  trans fats
  dumb, 55–58, 99–100
  glycemic index and, 48
  smart, 51–54, 63–64
FDA (Food and Drug Administration),
  68, 98
  drug categories, 233–34
  egg safety, 80
  Fish Advisory, 60, 85
  food safety during pregnancy, 160
fetal brain
  cortisol and, 17, 22
  dioxins and, 4, 59, 99, 171–73, 185
  inflammation and, 18, 143–44
  minerals and, 69
  omega-3 fatty acids and, 51, 52
fetal goiter, 78
fetal programming, 15–18, 27
  epigenetic basis of, 18–20
  of immune system, 144–46
  maternal stress and, 107–9
  placental role in, 21–22
fiber
  in beans, 77
  in carbs, 45, 50
  in dark purple fruits, 93
  glycemic index of, 48
  in whole grains, 89, 103
fight-or-flight response, 26, 108–12
financial planning, 122, 277–78

fireplaces, 194
First Things First (Covey), 140
fish and seafood, 39–40, 52–54, 59–62
  Alaskan wild salmon, 53–54, 62,
    84–85
  to avoid, 60, 62, 96, 160
Fisher, Roger, 129
fish oil, 51–52, 54
flavanones, 94
flavonals, 77
flavonoids, 66, 77, 94
flaxseed oil, 39, 52, 81
flaxseeds, 52, 53, 64, 81, 82
flexibility training, 116
flossing teeth, 147–48
flu (influenza), 18, 24, 144
  shots, 164, 246
fluoride, 181
folate. *See* vitamin B9
folic acid, 65–71
  in beans, 77
  carbs as source of, 45
  for fathers-to-be, 270
  in fruits and vegetables, 66, 67, 68
  methylation and, 19
  multivitamin with, 40, 68–69, 71
  in nuts and seeds, 81
  for preventing neural tube defects,
    24, 33, 65, 69
  in whole grains, 89, 103
food. *See* nutrition; nutritional
    preparedness plan
Food and Drug Administration. *See* FDA
foodborne illnesses, 96–99, 157–60
food diaries, 36
food labels, and "whole grain," 90, 102–4
food substitutions, 43
forgiveness, 132
formaldehyde, 181, 205, 213, 289
  in furniture, 201, 206
  in personal care products, 198
free thyroxine (free T4) tests, 251–52
French Canadian ancestry, and genetic
    disorders, 237–38
friendships, 130, 133, 134–37
fruits, 39, 50, 65–68. *See also specific fruits*
  by color, 65–67, 92–95
  folic acid in, 66, 67, 68
  preparation tips, 157–58

fruit juices, 50, 98–99
fruit rolls, 50
furniture, 201, 206

garage detoxification, 202–3
garbanzo beans, 64, 77
gasoline, 181
  lead additives in, 171, 173
gas stations, 208, 212
gas stoves, 194
Gatorade, 50
Gaucher disease, 237–38
genes, 15–16
  epigenetics, 18–20, 109
genetic risks and disorders, 236–40
  age and, 221–23, 238–39
  ethnic background and, 236–38
  family history and, 236, 264
genistein, 78
genital herpes, 155–56
German measles, 153–54
Getting past NO (Ury), 129
Getting to YES (Fisher and Ury), 129
Giardia, 190
ginger, 104
gingivitis, 147–48
glass cleaners, 200
glucose. *See* blood sugar
glucosinolates, 67
glutathione, 167, 270
glycemic index (GI), 46–50, 88, 100
glycemic load (GL), 46–50, 77
glycol ethers, 198, 199, 200, 213
glycoprotein, 45
goals. *See also* reproductive life
    plans
  for exercise, 116, 168
  in life, 131
  for weight gain, 37
  for weight loss, 34–35
  at work, 122, 125
Goleman, Daniel, 128
golf courses, pesticide use on, 208–9
gonorrhea, 142, 148–49, 250
Grandjean, Philippe, 173, 174
grapes, 66, 67
gratitude journals, 132, 140
gratitude letters, 132
Greaves, Jean, 128

green fruits and vegetables, 66–67, 91–92
grocery lists, 41

half-life, 235
  of dioxins, 5, 32
hand washing, 97, 98, 152, 153,
  154–55
happiness, 132–33
  exercising for, 115–16
harm's way, keeping out of, 24. See also
  environmental action plan
hazardous waste sites, 207
health behaviors. See lifestyle behaviors
health insurance, 122, 125, 241, 278
Health Insurance Portability and
  Accountability Act (HIPPA), 125
Healthy Cities/ Healthy Communities,
  210–11
Healthy Eating Pyramid, 40
healthy environment, action plan for.
  See environmental action plan
healthy weight, 34–38
heart defects, 153, 184, 240, 250
heart disease, 16, 29, 147
heaters, 194
heavy metals, 174–75, 180–81, 273
hematocrit tests, 248–49
hemoglobin tests, 248–49
hepatitis B, 149
  screening, 250–51
  vaccines, 164, 246
herbal preparations, 104, 236
herpes simplex viruses, 155–56
hesperedin, 94
high blood pressure. See
  hypertension
high blood sugar. See diabetes
high-fructose corn syrup, 100–101
high-intensity exercise, 168
high temperature, and sperm DNA, 274
hippocampus, 107, 109
Hippocrates, 75
Hispanic ancestry, and genetic
  disorders, 237–38
HIV (human immunodeficiency virus),
  149, 247
  screening, 251
hobbies, 202–3, 264
home detoxification, 198–203

homeostasis, 110–11
home remodeling, 122, 205–7
homocysteine, 94
hot dogs, 97, 159
household chores, 278–79
household toxins. See environmental
  toxins
HPA (hypothalamic-pituitary-adrenal),
  26, 108–13, 118
human genome, 15–16
human papilloma virus (HPV) vaccine,
  165–66, 223, 246
humidity, 162, 163, 205, 206
hummus, 78
husbands. See fathers-to-be
hydrops, 156
hypercholesterolemia, 18
hypertension, 229–30, 286
  stress and, 111, 121
hypoglycemia, 231
hypothyroidism, 252

Ikea, 201, 289
immune system action plan, 146–70
  avoiding environmental triggers,
    161–63
  check-ups for STIs, RTIs, and UTIs,
    148–51
  dental care, 147–48
  eating right, 166–67
  eating safely, 157–60
  exercising, 168
  immunizations, 163–66
  quitting smoking, 160–61
  reducing stress, 169–70
  TORCH infections, 151–56
immunity, 141–70
  action steps for. See immune system
    action plan
  fetal programming and, 144–46
  infections and inflammation,
    141–44
  stress and, 106–7, 112–13
immunizations, 163–66, 246, 265
implantation, 2–3, 22, 25, 28, 81
indigo fruits and vegetables, 67, 92–93
indoles, 67
infant mortality, 106, 141–42, 257,
  286–87

infections, 141–46
  autism and schizophrenia and, 18, 24,
    144, 145
  sperm DNA and, 273–75
infertility, 148–49, 221–23
  male, 265, 268, 270–71
inflammation, 141–46
  chronic stress and, 112–13
  fetal brain programming and, 143–44
  omega-3 fatty acids and, 51–54
  sperm DNA and, 273–75
influenza, 18, 24, 144
  vaccines, 164, 246
inorganic compounds, 174–75, 180–81
instrumental support, from
    fathers-to-be, 277–79
insulin, 30–31, 46–48
Integrated Pest Management (IPM), 209
interpersonal conflicts, 127–29, 270
interpersonal relationships, 130, 133,
    134–37
iodine, 64–65, 70, 78
IQ (intelligence quotient), 171, 173,
    181, 252
iron, 64, 72
  blood test for deficiency, 248–49
  recommended daily intake, 70
  sources of, 64, 91, 93, 167

job. See work
John Q (movie), 14–15
junk foods, 31–32, 44, 56

Kabat-Zinn, Jon, 120, 275–76
kale, 66, 91–92
kefir, 85–87
kidney beans, 64, 77, 78
king mackerel, 60, 62, 96
kitchen detoxification, 200–201

laboratory tests, 247–53
  for fathers-to-be, 265
Lactobacillus, 85–86
laundry detergents, 202
LDL cholesterol, 55, 83, 99
lead (lead compounds), 173, 174, 273
  in drinking water, 186–88
  in gasoline, 171, 172, 173
  in paint, 185–88, 273

lead-free home zone, 185–88
Learned Optimism (Seligman), 133
learning disabilities, 107–9, 173
leflunomide, 263–64
legumes, 39, 64, 77–78
lentils, 39, 64, 77–78
leptin, 47–48
lettuce, 67, 98, 158
life, personal satisfaction with, 130–31,
    132
life insurance, 278
lifestyle behaviors, 242–44
  of fathers-to-be, 265–68
listening skills, 128–29, 276
listeriosis, 96–97, 158–60
litter boxes, 152
liver, 99
living room detoxification, 201–2
Lotensin, 230, 232
low birth weight, 16, 31, 106
low-carb diets, 44–46
luncheon meats, 97, 159
lutein, 66, 67, 92
lycopene, 66, 94
lysine, 63
Lyubomirsky, Sonja, 132

McEwen, Bruce, 26–27, 113
magnesium, 70, 81
mammography, 246
managing stress. See stress
    resilience
manganese
  recommended daily intake, 70
  sources of, 94, 103
manganese compounds, 180–81
Marfan syndrome, 239, 262
margarine, 52, 56, 58
marital infidelity, 280–83
marriage counseling, 129, 241
mass transit, 213
Material Safety Data Sheet
    (MSDS), 199, 214, 215, 241,
    264, 273
maternal nutrition. See nutrition
maternal stress. See stress
Matthews, Kathy, 72
mattresses, 162–63, 201
meaning, sense of, 130, 131

meaningful work, 124–25
meat spreads, 97, 159, 160
medical conditions, 228–32
  of fathers-to-be, 263
medical records, 225
medications, 232–36
  benefits vs. risks, 235
  dosages, 235
  of fathers-to-be, 263–64
  FDA categories, 233–34
  safer alternatives to, 233, 235
meditation, 119–21
Mediterranean ancestry, and genetic
    disorders, 237–38
men. *See* fatherhood action plan
mental health. *See* positive mental
    health
mentors, seeking out at work, 135–36
menu planners, 41, 43
mercury, 172
  in fish and shellfish, 39, 52, 59–60, 96
metals, 174–75, 180–81, 273
methyl (methylation), 19, 109
methylmercury, 32
  in fish and seafood, 39, 52, 59–60, 96,
    183
  in fish oil, 54
microalgae DHA supplement, 54, 64
microwaving plastic, 200
milk, 40, 51, 58–59, 61, 63
  low-fat or skim, 5, 40, 57, 62
  unpasteurized, 96–97
Minamata Bay, Japan, 171–72
mindfulness, 120–21, 275–76
mindfulness-based stress reduction
    (MBSR), 120–21
minerals. *See also specific minerals*
  recommended daily intake, 70
miscarriages, 221–22, 224, 239
  BPA and, 191
  environmental toxins and,
    180–82
  formaldehyde exposure and, 201
  infections and, 145, 159
  medications and, 232
  stress and, 106
  tap water and, 188
mission statements, 131, 135
MMR vaccine, 164–65, 166, 223, 246

molds and mildew, 162
molybdenum, 70, 94
monoethanolamine, 199
monounsaturated fat, in olive oil, 82–83
moth repellents, 204–5
Motrin, 232
MSDS (Material Safety Data Sheet),
    199, 214, 215, 241, 264, 273
multivitamins, 40, 68–72
mumps-measles-rubella (MMR)
    vaccine, 164–65, 166, 223, 246
mushrooms, 64, 167
MyPyramid Menu Planner, 41, 43

naps (napping), 117
Nathanielsz, Peter, 110–11
National Children's Study, 289–90
National Domestic Violence Hotline,
    138, 241
National Drug and Alcohol Treatment
    Referral Routing Service,
    139–40, 268
National Heart, Lung, and Blood
    Institute, 34, 36
National Institute for Occupational
    Safety and Health (NIOSH),
    203, 215
National Institutes of Health (NIH), 191
  body mass index, 34–35
  exercise guidelines, 116, 168
  smoking cessation, 161
National Sanitation Foundation (NSF),
    189–91
National Weight Control Registry, 36
negotiation skills, 129
neighborhood environmental survey,
    207–11
neighbors, connecting with your, 136
neural tube defects, 24–25, 32–33, 65,
    68, 94, 188
niacin (vitamin B3), 70, 103
nickel, 181
Niemann-Pick disease, 238
NIH. *See* National Institutes of Health
nitric oxide, 81
nitrogen dioxide, 194, 209, 216
noise pollution, 210
nonsteroidal anti-inflammatory drugs
    (NSAIDs), 232

non-stick pans, 200
nonylphenois, 271
"no," saying, 123
Nutrasweet, 101
nutrition, 29–104
    action plan for. *See* nutritional
        preparedness plan
    fetal programming and childhood
        obesity, 17
    before pregnancy, 30–33
nutritional preparedness plan, 33–74
    achieving healthy weight, 34–38
    dumping dumb fats, 55–58
    eating balanced diet everyday, 38–42
    eating high-quality proteins,
        58–65
    eating less toxic foods. *See* toxic foods
    eating more brain foods. *See* brain
        foods
    eating rainbow of fruits and
        vegetables, 65–68
    eating safely, 96–99, 157–60
    for fathers-to-be, 270–71
    going low on glycemic load, 44–50
    for immune fitness, 166–67
    loading up on smart fats, 51–54
    making every calorie count, 42–44
    taking daily multivitamin containing
        folic acid, 68–72
nutritional supplements, 104, 236
    for weight gain, 37–38
nuts and seeds, 39, 52, 80–82
    benefits of, 80–81
    safety tips, 81–82

oatmeal, 38, 88, 89
obesity, weight-loss steps for, 34–37
Occupation Safety and Health Act
    (OSHA), 215–16
oleic acid, 83
olive oil, 39, 57, 82–84
    benefits of, 82–83
    recommendations for, 83–84
omega-3 fatty acids, 51–54, 77, 79,
    81, 166
omega-6 fatty acids, 52, 53
optimism, 131, 133, 134
orange fruits and vegetables, 66, 93–95
oranges, 50, 64, 66, 93–95

organic foods, 67–67, 94–95
organic solvents, 175–76, 181
oven cleaners, 200
overcooking water, 189
overweight, weight-loss steps for, 34–37
oxalic acid, 91
oxidative stress, 55–56, 166–67
    antioxidants and, 39, 81, 166–67, 270
    dioxins and, 272
    exercise and, 168
    fats and, 55–56, 83
    sperm damage and, 270, 273
Oxygen Radical Absorbance Capacity
    (ORAC), 92

packaged vegetables, 98
palm oil, 51, 55, 57, 63
pancreas, 16, 29, 47–48
Papanicolau smears (Pap tests),
    246, 247, 251
paradichlorobenzene, 204–5
parks, pesticide use in, 208–9
partially hydrogenated oils, 56, 58, 95,
    99–100
particleboard, 206, 213
partner. *See also* fathers-to-be
    connecting with your, 134–35
    domestic violence, 137–38, 240–41
passion for your work, 124–25
passive smoking, 193–94
past pregnancy history, 224–28
pâtés, 97, 160
paying attention, by fathers-to-be,
    275–76
PCBs (polychlorinated biphenyls),
    183, 272
peaches, 66, 67
peanuts (peanut butter), 62, 81, 82
peas, 39, 64, 67, 77–78
pelvic exams, 246, 247
perchloroethylene (PCE), 24, 195–96,
    208
periodontal disease, 147–48
periodontitis, 148
Perricone Promise (Perricone), 72–73
personal care products, 198–99
personal relationships, 130, 133, 134–37
personal satisfaction with life,
    130–31, 132

personal strengths, 131–32
pertusis (whooping cough), 164
pest control, 203–4
pesticides, 181–82
    list of known, 177–80
    steps for reducing exposure, 203–5,
        208–9
phenols, 181, 206
phenylketonuria (PKU), 101, 240
phosphorus, 65, 70, 87, 103
phthalates, 182–83, 198–202, 256,
    272–73
physical exams, 246, 265
physician visit. See preconception visit
phytic acid, 81
phytoesterols, 81
PKU (phenylketonuria), 101, 240
placenta, 21–22
    inflammation and, 143–44
    maternal stress and, 107–9
    preeclampsia and, 21, 25
plant oils, 39. See also specific plant oils
plant proteins, 63–65
plaque build-up, 148
playgrounds, pesticide use in, 208–9
plywood paneling, 205, 206
polybrominated diphenyl ethers
    (PBDEs), 201
polycarbonate, 191, 192, 200
polychlorinated biphenyls (PCBs),
    183, 272
polycyclic aromatic hydrocarbons
    (PAHs), 272
polyethylene, 192
polyphenols, 81, 83, 94
polyunsaturated vegetable oils,
    52, 55, 57
pomegranates, 66, 76, 81
pork, 59, 98, 159
portion sizes, 43
positive mental health, 23–24, 129–33
    characteristics of, 130–31
    pathways to, 131–33
positive psychology, 130
postpartum cardiomyopathy, 225
potatoes, 50, 67
poultry, 39–40, 52–53, 57, 59, 62
Power of Myth (Campbell), 14, 20
Pratt, Steven, 72

preconception care, 217–53
    five Ws of, 217–20
    topics to discuss with your doctor.
        See preconception visit
preconception visit, 220–53
    chronic medical conditions, 228–32
    depression and anxiety, 244–45
    family history and genetic risks,
        236–40
    for fathers-to-be, 262–65
    health behaviors, 242–44
    laboratory tests, 247–53
    medications you are taking, 232–36
    past pregnancy history, 224–28
    preventive and primary care, 245–47
    reproductive life plan, 221–24
    social history, 240–41
preeclampsia
    Angie's story, 1–3, 220
    heart attacks and, 285
    hypertension and, 229
    overweight and, 34
    oxidative stress and, 166, 168
    Paula's story, 11–14, 25
    placental development and, 21, 25
    stress and, 106
Pregnancy Readiness Quotient (PRQ),
    27–28, 291–98
prenatal care, 24–25, 28, 217, 286–87
preparation
    to avoid stress, 121–22
    getting ready for pregnancy, 21
    importance of, 3–4
prescription drugs. See medications
pressed wood products, 205–6
preterm birth
    fish oil and, 51–52
    infections and, 141–42, 145, 148–49,
        151
    multivitamins and, 69
    past pregnancy history and, 224–28
    placental development and, 21, 25
    skipping meals and, 41
    stress and, 106–7
    underweight and, 34
preventive care, 245–47
primary care, 245–47
prioritizing your life, 125, 279–80
probiotics, 85–86

problem-solving, 125–27
processed foods, 43, 52, 56, 101
product labels, 199–200, 206
professional help, 137–40
progesterone, 228
progressive relaxation, 119
proteins, 58–65
    animal, 58–62
    in low-carb diets, 46
    plant, 63–65
    sources of, 77–81, 84, 86
proteoglycan, 45
prunes, 67, 92–93
psoriasis drugs, 232
pumpkin seeds, 52, 62, 81
purple fruits and vegetables, 67, 92–93
purpose in life, 130, 131
pyridoxine. See vitamin B6

quick fixes, 286–87

radiation, 22, 213, 256, 274–75
radon, 196–97
raisins, 67, 92–93
Rank, Otto, 20
raw foods, 97–99, 157–60
reactive oxygen species (ROS), 270–71
red bell peppers, 67, 93–95
red fruits and vegetables, 66, 93–95
red meat, 40, 57, 59, 61, 62, 97–98, 157
reducing stress. See stress resilience
refined carbohydrates, 40, 44, 118
refined flour, 48, 87, 89, 102–4
refined grains, 87–89
relational resilience, 134–37
relaxation, 118–21
    ritual before bedtime, 117
    techniques for, 119–21
relaxation response, 120
religious faith, 136–37
remodeling your home, 122, 205–7
reprioritizing your life, 279–80
reproductive history, 224–28
    of fathers-to-be, 263
reproductive life plans, 221–24
    of fathers-to-be, 260–62
reproductive tract infections (RTIs),
    142, 149–50
resilience. See stress resilience

resolving conflicts, 127–29, 270
respect, 128–29, 276–77
Rhogam, 249–50
riboflavin. See vitamin B2
right cues, 23–24. See also stress; stress
    resilience
risk factors. See also behavioral
    risk factors; genetic risks and
    disorders
    for pregnancy complications,
    225–27
rubella, 153–54, 250

saccharin, 101
Safe Drinking Water Act, 187, 188
safe eating, 96–99, 157–60
sage, 104
salmon, Alaskan wild, 53–54, 62,
    84–85
salmonella, 75, 79–80, 98
Salovey, Peter, 127–28
Santayana, George, 224
satisfaction with life, 130–31, 132
saturated fats, 55–58, 59, 99–100, 118
savings account, nutritional, 31
saying "no," 123
scaling and root planing, 148
Scheier, Michael, 133
schizophrenia, 18, 24
    maternal flu and, 24, 164
    maternal infections and, 144, 145
    paternal age and, 239, 262
    rubella and, 153, 250
scrambled eggs, 80
seafood. See fish and seafood
sea vegetables, 64–65
secondhand smoke, 193–94
seeds. See nuts and seeds
selenium, 69, 71, 167
    recommended daily intake, 70
    sources of, 65, 81, 103
self-acceptance, 130, 134
self-awareness, 128, 129
self-esteem, 130, 134
self-governance (autonomy), 130
self-regulation, 110, 128
Seligman, Martin, 132, 133
separating foods, 157–58
setting limits, 123

sexual infidelity, 280–83
sexually transmitted infections (STIs), 142, 148–49, 156, 274
shampoo, 198–99
shark, 60, 62, 96
shifting your perspective, 133
shopping lists, 41
sickle cell, 237–38, 239–40
SIDS (sudden infant death syndrome), 193
silica, 200
single-parent families, 257–58
Six Million Dollar Man (TV series), 15
skin examination, 246, 265
skipping meals, 41
sleep, 116–17
smart fats, 51–54, 63–64, 118
    recommendations for increasing, 53–54
smoked seafood, 97, 160
smoke-free zones, 193–94
smoking
    by fathers-to-be, 266–67
    quitting, 160–61, 242, 266–67
    for stress, 107
snacks (snacking), 41, 43–44, 50
social capital, 136
social history, 240–41
sodas, 50, 100–101, 240
sodium hydroxide, 199, 200
sodium hypochlorite, 199, 200
sodium lauryl sulfate, 199
sofas, 201
soft cheeses, 96–97, 159–60
soft drinks, 50, 100–101, 240
solutions to problems, 126–27
solvents, 175–76, 181
solving problems, 125–27
sore throats, 142, 168
Soriatane, 232
soybeans, 62, 63–65, 77, 78
soy milk, 61, 85
space heaters, 194
sperm, 5, 22, 256–59
    making good sperm in 90 days, 258–59
sperm DNA, 256–59, 261–62
    protecting your, 271–75
spices, 75–76

spina bifida, 24, 40, 68
spinach, 67, 91–92
spirituality, 136–37
Splenda, 101
spouse. *See also* fathers-to-be
    connecting with your, 134–35
    domestic violence, 137–38, 240–41
stain removal, 202
starch, 48, 50
statin medications, 230
STIs. *See* sexually transmitted infections
storage, of pesticides, 204
storage areas, 202
stoves, 194
stovetop cleaners, 200
strawberries, 66, 67
strength training, 116
stress, 23–24, 105–40
    abnormal response, 111, 112
    action plan for. *See* stress resilience
    ADHD link to, 17, 24
    allostasis and, 26–27, 30
    fetal programming and, 107–9
    inflammation and, 112–13
    normal response, 110, 111
    pregnancy complications due to, 106–7
    "stressed" vs. "stressed out," 109–14
stress avoidance, 122
stress genes, 23, 108–9
stress prevention, 121–25
stress resilience, 23–24, 114–40
    connections with others, 134–37
    defined, 114
stress resilience (*continued*)
    eating right, 118
    exercising, 115–16
    for fathers-to-be, 269–70
    good night's sleep, 116–17
    for immune fitness, 169–70
    learning to prevent stress, 121–25
    learning to relax, 118–21
    positive mental health, 129–33
    problem-solving, 125–27
    resolving conflicts, 127–29
    seeking professional help, 137–40
substance abuse, 139–40, 242, 267–68
sucralose, 101

sudden infant death syndrome (SIDS), 193

sugars, added, 100–101

superfoods, 72–76. *See also* brain foods

Superfoods Rx (Pratt and Matthews), 72

Superfund sites, 207

supplements, 104, 236
    for weight gain, 37–38

support groups, for smokers, 161

Sweet'N Low, 101

swordfish, 60, 62, 96

sympathetic response, 26, 111

syphilis, 148–49, 156

syphilis screen, 250

taking back our nation, 288–90

tap water. *See* drinking water

tartar, 148

Tay-Sachs disease, 237–38

tea, 72

teeth care, 147–48

Tegison, 232

Teratology Information Services (TIS), 214

testicular cancer, 265

testicular hyperthermia, 22, 256, 259

tests. *See* laboratory tests; Pregnancy Readiness Quotient; *and specific tests*

Tetanus-diphtheria-pertussis (Tdap) vaccine, 164, 246

thiamin. *See* vitamin B1

thimerosol-free flu shots, 164

thrifty genes, 17

thyroid-stimulating hormone (TSH) tests, 251–52

tilefish, 60, 62, 96

timing, 3, 224
    developmental toxicity and, 184
    nutrition and, 32–33

tofu, 40, 61, 64

toluene, 176, 181

tomatoes, 66, 94

TORCH infections, 141–42, 151–56

touch (touching), 277

toxic foods, 73–74, 95–104
    added sugars, 100–101
    herbal preparations, 104

hot dogs, luncheon meats, deli meats, raw or smoked seafood, 97

liver, 99

raw or undercooked meat, 97–98

refined flour, 102–4

saturated fats, trans fats, and partially hydrogenated oils, 99–100

soft cheeses and unpasteurized milk, 96–97

swordfish, shark, king mackerel, and tilefish, 96

unwashed vegetables, raw vegetable sprouts, and unpasteurized juices, 98–99

Toxic Substance Control Act (TSCA), 206

toxins. *See* environmental toxins

Toxoplasma, 97–98, 151–52

toxoplasmosis, 97–98, 151–53, 157

tracking your weight and nutrition, 36

transcendental meditation (TM), 120

trans fats, 51, 52, 53, 55–58, 99–100

trichomoniasis, 150

triclocarban, 198

triclosan, 198

trihalomethanes (THMs), 24, 188

TSH (thyroid-stimulating hormone) tests, 251–52

underweight, steps for weight gain, 37–38

unpasteurized juices, 98–99

unpasteurized milk, 96–97

urea-formaldehyde, 201, 206

urinary tract infections (UTIs), 142, 151

urine testing, 249

vaccinations, 163–66, 246, 265

vacuuming, 162

vapor-lock gas pumps, 212

varicoceles, 22, 256, 263

Vasotec, 230, 232

vegans, 63–65, 69

vegetable oil spreads, 58

vegetables, 39, 65–69. *See also specific vegetables*
    by color, 65–67, 91–95
    preparation tips, 157–58
    unwashed or packaged, 98–99

vegetable sprouts, 75, 98–99, 157

vegetarians, 63

vices. *See* behavioral risk factors

vinaigrette dressing, 50

violet fruits and vegetables, 67, 92–93

vitamins. *See also specific vitamins*
  multivitamins, 40, 68–72
  recommended daily intake, 70

vitamin A, 71
  birth defects and, 71, 99, 233
  liver and, 99
  recommended daily intake, 70, 99
  sources of, 64, 79, 91, 94

vitamin B1 (thiamin)
  recommended daily intake, 70
  sources of, 66, 93, 94, 103

vitamin B2 (riboflavin), 71
  recommended daily intake, 70
  sources of, 64, 67, 79, 87, 91, 103

vitamin B3 (niacin), 70, 103

vitamin B4 (choline), 69, 70

vitamin B5 (panththenic acid), 70

vitamin B6 (pyridoxine), 71, 79
  recommended daily intake, 70
  sources of, 54, 91, 94

vitamin B7 (biotin), 70, 79, 103

vitamin B9 (folate)
  deficiency, 65
  recommended daily intake, 70, 81
  sources of, 66, 67, 79

vitamin B12 (cobalamine), 64
  deficiency, 65, 71, 249
  recommended daily intake, 70

vitamin C, 72, 167
  recommended daily intake, 70
  sources of, 66, 93–94

vitamin D, 64, 71
  recommended daily intake, 70
  sources of, 65, 79

vitamin E (alpha-tocopherol), 167
  recommended daily intake, 70
  sources of, 81, 103

vitamin K, 67, 70, 91, 94

volunteer work, 133, 137

wallpapers, 201, 272

walnuts, 51, 52, 64, 81

washing foods, 67, 98, 158

washing hands, 97, 98, 152, 153, 154–55

washing machines (washers), 202

water, drinking. *See* drinking water

water bottles, 190, 191–92

water filters, 187, 189, 192

Water Quality Report, 189

weight, 34–38
  Body Mass Index and, 34, 35
  of fathers-to-be, 265

weight gain, steps for, 37–38

weight loss, steps for, 34–37

weight-loss programs, 36–37

Weight Watchers, 36

Weil, Andrew, 102

well water, 190–91

whole grains, 38–39, 87–91
  benefits of, 88–89
  best, 87
  for breakfast, 49
  on food labels, 90, 102–4
  nutritional content of, 103
  recommendations for increasing,
    38–39, 89–90

whole-wheat pasta, 49–50

wild Alaskan salmon, 53–54, 62, 84–85

Willett, Walter, 40

William, Ury, 129

wills, 278

window blinds, 201

window cleaners, 200

woodstoves, 194

work
  commuting tips, 211–13
  harmful exposures at, 213–15, 241
  healthy snacks for, 43–44
  managing stress at, 124–25
  mentors at, 135–36
  your rights at, 215–16

work overload, 125

work relationships, 125

xenobiotics, 271–73

yeast infections, 150

yellow fruits and vegetables, 66

yogurt, 57, 61, 85–87

zeaxanthin, 66, 92

zinc, 103, 167
  deficiency, 64, 65, 270
  recommended daily intake, 70

ABOUT THE AUTHOR

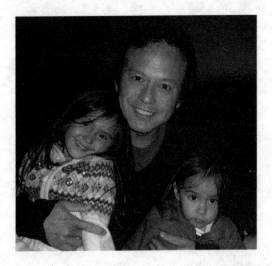

Michael C. Lu, MD, MPH, is an associate professor of obstetrics and gynecology and public health at UCLA. Dr. Lu received his bachelor's degrees from Stanford University, master's degrees from UC Berkeley, medical degree from UC San Francisco, and residency training in obstetrics and gynecology from UC Irvine. Dr. Lu is widely recognized for his research, teaching, and clinical care. He received the 2004 American Public Health Association Young Professional Award in Maternal and Child Health for his research on pregnancy outcomes. He recently served on the National Academy of Sciences Institute of Medicine Committee on Understanding Prematurity and the Centers for Disease Control and Prevention (CDC) Select Panel on Preconception Care. Dr. Lu teaches obstetrics and gynecology at the David Geffen School of Medicine at UCLA, and maternal and child health at the UCLA School of Public Health. He has received numerous awards for his teaching, including Excellence in Teaching Awards from the Association of Professors of Gynecology and Obstetrics. Dr. Lu is the CoDirector of the UCLA Preconception Care Clinic, and has been voted one of the Best Doctors in America since 2005.